Henry E. Sigerist

Correspondences with
Welch, Cushing, Garrison,
and Ackerknecht

T0200097

Marcel H. Bickel (ed.)

Henry E. Sigerist

Correspondences with
Welch, Cushing, Garrison,
and Ackerknecht

Peter Lang

Bern · Berlin · Bruxelles · Frankfurt am Main · New York · Oxford · Wien

Bibliographic information published by Die Deutsche Nationalbibliothek
Die Deutsche Nationalbibliothek lists this publication in the Deutsche
Nationalbibliografie; detailed bibliographic data is available on the Internet at
‹http://dnb.d-nb.de›.

British Library and Library of Congress Cataloguing-in-Publication Data:
A catalogue record for this book is available from *The British Library,*
Great Britain.

Library of Congress Cataloging-in-Publication Data

Sigerist, Henry E. (Henry Ernest), 1891-1957.
Henry E. Sigerist : correspondences with Welch, Cushing, Garrison, and Ackerknecht /
Marcel H. Bickel (ed.).
p. ; cm.
Includes bibliographical references and index.
ISBN 978-3-0343-0320-0 (alk. paper)
1. Sigerist, Henry E. (Henry Ernest), 1891-1957–Correspondence. 2. Medical historians–
Switzerland–Zurich–Correspondence. 3. Welch, William Henry, 1850-1934–
Correspondence. 4. Cushing, Harvey, 1869-1939–Correspondence. 5. Garrison,
Fielding H. (Fielding Hudson), 1870-1935–Correspondence. 6. Ackerknecht, Erwin Heinz,
1906-1988–Correspondence. I. Bickel, Marcel H. II. Title.
[DNLM: 1. Sigerist, Henry E. (Henry Ernest), 1891-1957. 2. History of Medicine–
Collected Correspondence. 3. Physicians–Collected Correspondence. WZ 100 S576 2010]
R566.S53A3 2010
610.92'2–dc22

2010003561

Cover design: Eva Rolli, Peter Lang AG

ISBN 978-3-0343-0320-0

© Peter Lang AG, International Academic Publishers, Bern 2010
Hochfeldstrasse 32, CH-3012 Bern, Switzerland
info@peterlang.com, www.peterlang.com, www.peterlang.net

Printed in Germany

Table of Contents

4. *Correspondence Henry E. Sigerist – Erwin H. Ackerknecht*
   1931–1957

Preface

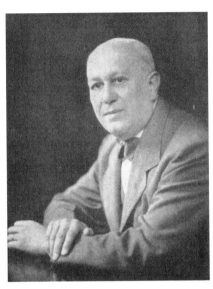

Henry E. Sigerist (1891–1957) is recognized as the foremost historian of medicine of his time. He was, in addition, an activist in the fight for a reform of the American health system and, last but not least, a scholar with an exceptional breadth of interests and with engaging human qualities.

Sigerist was born in 1891 in Paris, the son of Swiss parents. After schooling in Paris and Zurich he started out with studies of Oriental languages in Zurich and London, then studied medicine in Zurich and Munich. After obtaining his MD in 1917 he entered the field of the history of medicine as an independent scholar in Zurich and became so productive and successful that in 1925 he was called to fill the first chair of medical history in Leipzig as the successor of the famous Karl Sudhoff. After successful years at his new department he was offered the Chair of the first American institute of the History of Medicine at Johns Hopkins University. Glad to leave Germany before a Nazi takeover he moved to Baltimore in 1932. His Institute soon became the center of medico-historical activities in America, and the history of medicine became professionalized. Sigerist became the outstanding scholar in the field, creating a wealth of publications; he also proved a successful organizer as well as an engaged propagator of new forms of health care systems, based on his conviction that health care was a right rather than a privilege. After 15 fruitful years of having left marks on American medicine he eventually resigned his post at Hopkins in 1947 in order to find the time to write his multi-volume *History of Medicine*. As Professor in absentia of Yale University Sigerist was able to retire to the

Swiss village of Pura for the final decade of his life where he wrote parts of his opus magnum and many more publications. He died in Pura in 1957.

An undefatigable writer, Sigerist produced many books and hundreds of papers (Miller 1966), (Sigerist Beeson 1966) which, together with his rhetorical talent and his charisma stimulated many authors to deal with Sigerist during his time. This secondary literature has even increased in the half century since his death (Berg-Schorn 1978), (Fee/Brown 1997).

In addition to his scientific work Sigerist also wrote an enormous amount of letters. They were his link to hundreds of correspondents all over the world, among them physicians, medical historians as well as representatives of a large spectrum of cultural life. We know that in the early 1950s he wrote some 1000 letters per year (Bickel 1997), a fact which his friend John F. Fulton commented:

> Sigerist was as greatly interested in men as he was in books – men of all lands, persuasions, and occupations – and so conscientious was he in maintaining lines of communication with his ever-widening circle of friends that, toward the end of his life, his correspondence became so vast that it interfered with his more serious writing. (Fulton 1960)

Most of Sigerist's correspondence is a hidden treasure; only the incomplete correspondences with George Rosen (Viseltear 1978) and with George Urdang (Sonnedecker 1983) have been published. More recently an edition of the Sigerist correspondence with four Swiss historians of medicine (Arnold C. Klebs, Bernhard Milt, Hans Fischer, Erich Hintzsche) has also been published (Bickel 2008).

There are several reasons that make an edition of more of Sigerist's correspondences worth-while:

1) Most of the correspondences are stored in only two archives in a well-organized and accessible form.
2) Stored are not only the letters conscientiously collected by Sigerist, but also the carbon-copies of his own letters since about 1923.
3) These correspondences are almost complete with very few letters missing.

These three facts are rarely combined and are therefore an invaluable advantage for an edition of complete correspondences. To this must be added the interest in both Sigerist and selected representatives of his correspondents.

For the technicalities I have tried to adopt modern criteria for the edition of correspondences (Steinke 2004). The three reasons given above allowed for an edition of the letters to and from Sigerist (in a chronological sequence) and using all (existing) letters, i.e., without a selection, which in any case would have been questionable. An unselected edition was also feasible because even the large correspondences are not overwhelming in size and contain very few trivialities. Thus, all the letters were transcribed in their totality. Future editors would then only have to alter the annotations. This edition is therefore likely to allow a true insight into a part of the lives and mentalities of the correspondents, including their private lives and scientific work as well as relationships with persons, books, and topics. Hence the correspondences are sources for the correspondents' biographies and for many topics and features of the 20th century.

Problems of transcription are dealt with in the introductions to the four individual correspondences. The annotations are given in small print following each transcribed letter. They are meant to help understanding the contents of the letters rather than to interpret them and are therefore kept at a minimum. They also serve as links to former letters and annotations so that persons or things can be explained once only. Persons explained in the text may not appear in the annotations if sufficiently characterized; persons not explained and mentioned only once or twice in a correspondence may be marked as not identified. However, all persons mentioned in the letters are listed in the name index of each individual correspondence. A bibliography of all literature mentioned in the letters and annotations is also given for each correspondence.

The bulk of the letters to and from Sigerist is stored in the following archives:

1) Manuscripts and Archives
   Yale University Library
   P.O. Box 208240
   New Haven, CT 06520-8240

2) The Alan Mason Chesney Medical Archives
   The Johns Hopkins Medical Institutions
   5801 Smith Avenue, Suite 235
   Baltimore, MD 21209

1) contains Sigerist's correspondences of his time in Zurich (prior to 1925 and incomplete) and of the years in Pura (1947–1957, almost complete). 2) contains the correspondences of his years at Johns Hopkins (1932–1947, almost complete). Both archives have lists of the correspondences under the heading "Sigerist Papers" or "Sigerist Collection", respectively. Letters of Sigerist's Leipzig years are at the Universitätsarchiv Leipzig

9

(1925–1932, incomplete). The archive of the Department of the History of Medicine at the University of Zurich has a large collection of Sigristiana, however, next to no letters belonging to the four correspondences in question.

The value of correspondences as historical sources is obvious, particularly in former centuries. Compared with today's technical means of communication the Sigerist correspondences of the first half of the 20th century may in a way still belong to that era. They clearly do not yet belong to our age of mobility and of an excessive use of the telephone and of quickly deleted, unprinted e-mail.

After a first edition of complete Sigerist correspondences with four medical historians in Switzerland (Bickel 2008), I have selected in the present edition the correspondences with a number of famous Americans in medicine and medical history. This selection of the correspondents aimed at the inclusion of important colleagues and friends of Sigerist who played a major role in academic life in the United States and whose epistolar opus was not of an excessive size. This volume contains Sigerist's relatively short correspondences with William H. Welch, Harvey Cushing, and Fielding H. Garrison, as well as the extended correspondence with Erwin H. Ackerknecht.

W. H. Welch was the architect and organizer not only of the Johns Hopkins Medical School but also of American Medicine in the critical half century around 1900 when Medicine in America was transformed from provinvial to world-leading. The few years of the correspondence are Welch's last active ones, yet for Sigerist the critical time of his turning from Europe to America.

Cushing, during his final years as a world famous neurosurgeon in Boston and his switching to medical history at Yale, also was in personal contact and in correspondence with Sigerist who was 22 years younger. This correspondence covers Sigerist's final years in Europe and the first ones in the US.

Garrison, also a distinguished medical historian, corresponded during the final decade of his life with the 21 years younger Sigerist. The two eventually became colleagues at Johns Hopkins. Garrisons letters, revealing and full of thoughts, were praised by other authors.

The more voluminous correspondence with Erwin Ackerknecht, 15 years younger than Sigerist, lasted for a quarter century until Sigerist's death. It is a touching document of a pupil-teacher relationship that becomes a relationship among close colleagues and eventually a friendship. In addition, it reveals Ackerknecht as an astute observer as well as a victim of the the political convulsions of the 20th century. This correspondence comes close to a double biography of the two correspondents.

All four correspondences discuss problems of medicine and its history, they tell of the correspondents' work and experiences, their plans and achievements, books read and people met. The reader becomes acquainted with the personalities of the five correspondents and watches as the first half of the 20th century unfolds in many of its aspects. All four correspondents are introduced with a biographical sketch and a general comment on their correspondence; there is a list of the literature mentioned and a name index for each individual correspondences.

There are plans for further editions of Sigerist correspondences with American and international medical historians, in particular the extensive correspondence with his colleague and friend of about the same age, John F. Fulton.

The editor ows gratitude to many who have helped him in various ways. The archives of Yale, Johns Hopkins and the University of Leipzig mentioned above were kind enough to let me publish the correspondences. Their personnel's competence, cooperation, and friendly advice is highly appreciated. I extend my thanks to my colleagues of the Departments of the History of Medicine in Bern and Zurich for stimulation and help with the transcription and annotations: Urs Boschung, Pia Burkhalter, Gertraud Gamper, François Ledermann, Iris Ritzmann, Hubert Steinke. Help was kindly offered by Nora Sigerist Beeson, Sylvia Bonner, Theodor M. Brown of The University of Rochester Press, and last but not least my wife Leni and our daughter Susanne. Martina Fierz of Peter Lang Publishers once more proved her competent and cooperative ways. Thanks are also due to the Swiss National Science Foundation for carrying the cost of publication of this book.

Marcel H. Bickel
Bern 2009

Berg-Schorn, Elisabeth: *Henry E. Sigerist (1891–1957)*. Köln 1978.
Bickel, Marcel H.: *Henry E. Sigerist's Annual "Plans of Work" (1932–1955)*. Bull. Hist. Med. 71, 489–498, 1997.

Bickel, Marcel H., ed.: *Henry E. Sigerist. Vier ausgewählte Briefwechsel mit Medizinhistori-kern der Schweiz.* Peter Lang Publishing Group, Bern 2008.

Fee, Elizabeth / Brown, Theodore M.: *Making Medical History. The Life and Times of Henry E. Sigerist.* Baltimore / London, 1997.

Fulton, John F.: *Foreword.* In: F. Marti-Ibañez, ed.: "Henry E. Sigerist on the History of Medicine". New York 1960, ix–xi.

Miller, Genevieve: *A Bibliography of the Writings of Henry E. Sigerist.* Montreal 1966.

Sigerist Beeson, Nora: *Henry E. Sigerist: Autobiographical Writings.* Montreal 1966.

Sonnedecker, Glenn, ed.: *The American Correspondence Between George Urdang and Henry E. Sigerist 1941–1948.* Graz, 1983 (21 pages).

Steinke, Hubert: *Why, What and How? Editing Early Modern Scientific Letters in the 21st Century.* Gesnerus (Swiss J. Hist. Med. Sci.) 61, 282–295, 2004.

Viseltear, Arthur J., ed.: *The George Rosen – Henry E. Sigerist Correspondence.* J. Hist. Med. Allied Sci. 33, 281–313, 1978.

1. Correspondence
Henry E. Sigerist – William H. Welch
1927–1933

1.1. Introduction

1.1.1. William H. Welch (1850–1934)

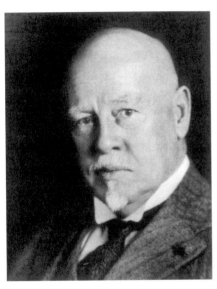

William Henry Welch was born in Norfolk, CT, on 8 April 1850, the son of a physician. He studied at Yale University in New Haven, CT, and at the College of Physicians and Surgeons in New York, obtaining his M.D. degree in 1875. During an internship at the Bellevue Hospital he developed a keen interest in pathology. After one year he started for a training tour in Europe, as did many colleagues interested in scientific medicine. For two years he studied research methods in Strasburg, Leipzig, Breslau, and Vienna under medical leaders like Waldeyer, von Recklinghausen, Hoppe-Seyler, Ludwig, Weigert, Cohnheim and others. He returned with a scientific, laboratory-based training in pathology. Back in New York Welch inaugurated the first teaching laboratory in pathology in the U.S., however, with restricted possibilities to do research. The way out of frustration was his being offered the professorship in pathology at the newly founded Johns Hopkins University in 1884. Before moving to Baltimore Welch spent another year in Germany, concentrating on the rapidly emerging fields of bacteriology and public health and studying with Robert Koch in Berlin and Max von Pettenkofer in Munich.

In 1885 Welch started work at the Johns Hopkins University where, in collaboration with President Gilman, John S. Billings, and H. Newell Martin he succeeded to recruit the best possible men for the new Hopkins Hospital and Medical School: Osler, Halsted, Kelly, Mall, Abel, Howell,

15

Hurd, and others. Welch became the first dean of a unique medical school, based on the German system of laboratory and clinical teaching, of students in residency and teachers as researchers. Thus, he created a new kind of scientifically based medicine in America. He now also had able assistants and pupils like Simon Flexner as well as adequate laboratory facilities, allowing for his successful research in pathology and bacteriology. Though he made excellent summations of current scientific work, his future was not in pathological research. Rather, he became one of the most influential organizers and spokesmen for American medicine. He was the leader in creating the Rockefeller Institute in New York, heading its Board of Scientific Directors and serving as trustee. He also was on the Board of the Carnegie Institution in Washington and of the Milbank Memorial Fund. He was president of the American Medical Association, the American Association for the Advancement of Science, and of the National Academy of Sciences. He was editor of the Journal of Experimental Medicine. He was rightfully considered the mastermind of modern American medicine.

His interest in bacteriology, tuberculosis and tropical medicine as well as his serving on the Maryland State Department of Health let him give up his chair at the Medical School in 1916 to become dean of the School of Hygiene and Public Health, another unique Hopkins medical institution, financed by the Rockefeller Foundation. He continued as dean until 1925, when the foundation's General Education Board under its secretary, Abraham Flexner, persuaded him to accept the newly established chair of the history of medicine the following year. Welch agreed to do this as an interim until a trained medical historian would be found and also if an institute would be created in conjuction with a central medical library. Once more he spent months in Europe, this time to study how medical history was institutionalized and taught there, and to buy books for the new library. Thus, Welch met Sigerist in Leipzig. In 1929, when Welch was almost 80, the Johns Hopkins Institute of the History of Medicine was inaugurated, together with the "Welch Medical Library". In 1931 he resigned as chairman of this institute, and his final success was to find his successor: Henry E. Sigerist of the Institute of the History of Medicine in Leipzig. He took over the Hopkins Institute in 1932. Welch's health then soon deteriorated; he spent most of 1933 at the Hopkins Hospital as a patient and died on 30 April 1934, at the age of 84.

For biographical literature on Welch see (Flexner/Flexner 1941), (Shryock 1950), (Fleming 1954), (Brieger 1976).

1.1.2. The Correspondence

This is a small and obviously incomplete correspondence. There is a total of only 11 letters of Sigerist to Welch and 15 letters of Welch to Sigerist. Clearly, all of Welch's letters of 1927 to 1930 are missing, and so are presumably some of Sigerists letters of 1929 to 1933.

Sigerist's first letters, written in Leipzig, are in German, all of the remaining correspondence is in English. The German letters have been translated by the editor.

In most of the letters the dates are given, but not the places the letter have been written. Sigerist's letters are typed, while Welch's are in longhand. The sign [ ] was used for Sigerist's signature which was missing on the carbon copies used. Literary works are given as, e.g., (d'Irsay 1928) and listed in chapter 3 (Literature).

The annotations in small print following each letter are meant to help understanding the contents of the letters rather than to interpret them and are therefore kept at a minimum. They also serve as links to former letters and annotations so that persons or things can be explained once only. A few persons sufficiently characterized and explained in the letter may not appear in the annotations. A few persons, most of them mentioned only once, could not be identified and are marked as such in the annotation. However, all persons mentioned in the letters are listed in the name index (chapter 4). A bibliography of all literature mentioned in the letters and annotations is also given in chapter 3.

This correspondence consists of relatively few letters not only because of missing ones but also because it spans the short period of 1927 to 1933. However, these were seven decisive years in the biographies of both correspondents, times when there was mutual dependence; when the mutual respect and gratitude is outspoken, often touching.

The correspondence starts in 1927 and is likely to be the first contact between Sigerist and Welch. Sigerist, the 36 year old professor of the history of medicine in Leipzig, in the early phase of his brilliant career; Welch, 77, architect of modern American medicine, at the end of his overwhelmingly rich career, yet at the beginning of its final chapter of creating the first American institute of the history of medicine in conjunction with a medical library.

It is Welch in 1931 who organizes Sigerists lecture and study tour in the U.S. It is Sigerist who then is offered and accepts Welch's chair at Johns Hopkins University. There is mutual relief and a warm welcome when Sigerist arrives in Baltimore in 1932. The following year is the beginning of Sigerist's successful career in America as well as of Welch's illness leading to death in 1934.

1.2. The Letters

SIGERIST to WELCH, Leipzig, 18 January 1927
(Original in German)

Dear Doctor Welch,

Dr. Garrison tells me you wish to become a member of our Society. The Society is happy to welcome you as a new member and so am I. The by-laws and your member-card will be sent to you. You will regularly receive our journal.

I am very glad that a chair of the history of medicine has been created in the United States, and I am sure that this will decisively further our studies. My congratulations for your appointment.

Faithfully yours,

[Henry E. Sigerist]

S.'s address: Talstrasse 38, Leipzig; A.'s address: 807 Paul Street, Baltimore. "Dear Dr. Welch" may be the adequate translation of "Hochgeehrter Herr Kollege". Fielding H. Garrison (1870–1935) medical historian, at that time librarian at the Surgeon Generals's Library (now National Library of Medicine) in Washington. S. was treasurer of the German Society of the History of Medicine and Sciences (DGGMN); its journal was *Mitteilungen zur Geschichte der Medizin und der Naturwissenschaften*. W. had been elected Professor of the History of Medicine at Johns Hopkins University in 1926 at age 76.

SIGERIST to WELCH, Leipzig (?), 24 May 1927
(Original in German)

Dear Dr. Welch,

Thank you very much for your good letter of April 30th and for your interesting news. I am particularly glad to see you this year in Leipzig. Dr. Klebs, who was here at the end of March, had already

19

informed me of your visit. It will be a pleasure to show you my Institute.

> With kindest regards, I am,
> Faithfully yours,
> [Henry E. Sigerist]

W.'s letter is missing. Arnold C. Klebs (1870–1943) Swiss-American physician and historian of medicine, son of Edwin Klebs, friend of W. and S.

SIGERIST to WELCH, Leipzig (?), 21 November 1927 (Original in German)

Dear Dr. Welch,

I have recently written a memorandum on my institute for the Saxonian Department of Education. In it I have tried to describe the institute's develoment during the past two years, and particularly I wanted to delineate the needs for the future development. Maybe you are interested to see this memorandum which I enclose as a copy. Perhaps you may make use of it for your own plans.

> Hoping you are fine, I am,
> With my best regards,
> Sincerely yours,
> [Henry E. Sigerist]

W.'s London address is Brown, Shipley and Co. (a private bank), 123 Pall Mall. W. had visited S.'s Institute in order to learn what could be done for the planned Baltimore Institute which was to be inaugurated in 1929. It was his first visit of the Leipzig Institute for the History of Medicine, founded in 1905. W. spent the year 1927/28 in Europe, buying books for his future Institute.

SIGERIST to WELCH, Leipzig (?), 9 January 1928 (Original in German)

Dear Dr. Welch,

Very many thanks for your kind letter of December 3rd I was very glad to receive. It is a pleasure to enclose another copy of my memorandum which, of course, you may show to Abraham Flexner or use however you please. I do hope you will succeed in obtaining the funds for your Institute for I am increasingly of opinion that institutes of this kind will play an ever greater role in medical education. This winter again we have a large number of students, and there is much activity. In a few weeks I hope to be able to send you the first volume of our year-book which provides an overview of the past year's work. I also enclose proofs of an article published in the year-book on "The History of Medicine in Academic Teaching". In it you find how this teaching is organized in several countries, as well as a list of the teaching personnel with their addresses. Possibly it will provide the material you need for your lecture in London. Excuse the printing errors still in the text.

Dr. d'Irsay and I have become good friends. He is well settled here and is working assidiously through whole nights. Half of his "History of Physiology" is written and is likely to become a most remarkable book. In it he shows how our views have developed, and I am sure that the book will be a great success among physiologists. He has also dealt with several more limited topics such as the early Middle Ages, using paleography. In addition, he intends to edit a Greek manuscript text. You will find a short philosophical study in our year-book. And last but not least he wants to write a short book on Haller as long as he is in Leipzig. I am sure that for your new Institute you will have an excellent coworker in Dr. d'Irsay for he belongs to the few young historians who are able to work in the whole field of medical history and have an excellent knowledge of its methods and literature. Personally I regret that he will leave in spring; I would have liked to keep him in Leipzig.

I am glad that you will stay some more time in Europe, and I hope that you will visit Leipzig once more.

With best regards and wishes for the New Year, I am,

Faithfully yours,

[Henry E. Sigerist]

W.'s London address see S. to W. of 21 November 1927. W. spent a year in Europe in preparation for his future Institute. W.'s letter is missing. S.'s memorandum see S. to W. of 21 November 1927. Abraham Flexner (1866–1959) (medical) educator, at that time at the Rockefeller Foundation which made the endowments for the new Welch Medical Library and the Institute of the History of Medicine. Year-book: Kyklos: The Year-book of the Leipzig Institute. *Geschichte der Medizin im akademischen Unterricht* (Sigerist 1928). Stephen d'Irsay (1894–1934) medical historian, see (Sigerist 1935), at that time in Leipzig in preparation for his collaboration with W. Apparently d'Irsay's planned book *History of Physiologie* has not been published. "philosophical study" (d'Irsay 1928), book on Haller (d'Irsay 1930).

Sigerist to Welch, Leipzig (?), 23 March 1923 (sic) correct 1928 (Original in German)

Dear Dr. Welch,

Many thanks for your long letter I was delighted to receive. This is just a line to tell you that I will travel to Italy with my wife and that presumably we shall be in Florence from April 1 to 21. Our address will be: Pensione Ravasso, Via Curtatone 5. Dr. d'Irsay will also be in Florence from April 1 to about 10. Should you happen to be near-by, we would be very pleased to see you.

Our year-book has recently appeared, and I take pleasure in sending you a copy by separate mail.

With kind regards, I am,
    Sincerely yours,
      [Henry E. Sigerist]

W.'s London address see S. to W. of 21 November 1927. W.'s letter is missing. d'Irsay and year-book see S. to W. of 9 January 1928. W. was also in Italy during his European year 1927/28.

Sigerist to Welch, Leipzig ?, 19 November 1928 (Original in German)

Dear Dr. Welch,

It would be a great honor and a pleasure if you would agree that the second volume of our "Kyklos" were dedicated to you, and I would like to ask if you were ready to accept such a dedication. The volume will appear in March, and I hope that it will be possible to hand it over to you at the inauguration of your new Institute. I would very much like to add a photo of you to the volume and would be delighted if you sent me one.

I hope you are fine. Here the activities of the term are in full swing; there are many students attending the courses and seminars, and a total of 20 % of the medical students are using the Institute.

With kind regards I am, dear Dr. Welch,

Sincerely yours,

[Henry E. Sigerist]

This is S.'s last letter to W. written in German. The second volume of the "Kyklos" yearbook contains a photograph of W., a dedication to W. and his Institute, and a foreword (Sigerist 1929) in the form of an open letter to W.

For 1929 and 1930 there are no letters at the Archives used.

SIGERIST to WELCH, Leipzig ?, 5 May 1931

Dear Dr. Welch,

I received a very kind invitation from President Ames asking me to be Visiting Lecturer in the History of Medicine at the Johns Hopkins University during the next academic year.

I know that the invitation was sent to me on your proposal; so allow me to thank you very much for it. It has long been my wish to visit the United States and most especially your Institute, so it was with the greatest pleasure that I accepted the invitation.

I will sail at the end of September and so be in Baltimore for the opening of the Medical School in October.

I hope to see you soon in Leipzig and we might then perhaps discuss the subject of my lectures.

Believe me, dear Dr. Welch,

sincerely yours

[Henry E. Sigerist]

This is S.'s first letter in English of this correspondence. Joseph S. Ames (1864–1943) physicist, president of Johns Hopkins University. Teaching at W.'s Institute started in 1930 with guest lecturers and Garrison (see S. to W. of 18 January 1927) as a new member of staff.

SIGERIST to WELCH, Leipzig ?, 30 May 1931

Dear Dr. Welch,

I send you enclosed the list of my lectures etc. If you think that any change would be advisable, I should be grateful for any suggestion you might have.

I have not yet discovered the address of the Shelton Hotel but in any case you will be able to reach me through the American Express Co. in New York.

Would you kindly give d'Irsay the enclosed letter when you meet him in Cologne. I don't know his address.

It was a great pleasure for us all to have you in Leipzig.

With kindest regards in which Mrs. Sigerist joins

I am sincerely yours

[Henry E. Sigerist]

Letter addressed to W. at Hotel Adlon, Berlin. Shelton Hotel, S.'s first lodging in New York in fall 1931. d'Irsay see S. to W. of 9 January 1928. Once more W. spent the summer of 1931 in Europe. S.'s wife Emmy Escher from Zurich.

WELCH to SIGERIST, Berlin, 31 May 1931

Dear Sigerist.

Nothing could be more satisfactory than the material which you have sent and which I received to-day – the documents contain precisely the information desired. I shall send one of the copies to Dr. Alan Chesney, the dean of our Medical School, and ask him to make copies and prepare announcements for distribution, and I shall communicate with Dr. Duggan and others.

I am delighted with your choice of subjects for the six lectures and six seminary or conference exercises in Baltimore, as well as with the topics available for lectures elsewhere.

There should be no difficulty in arranging for lectures, with suitable honorarium, in various places which you will care to visit.

I am confident that you will do more to arouse interest in medical history than any previous similar event has ever done. It is a great thing for us in Baltimore that you are coming.

I enjoyed immensely my visit in Leipzig – It was a great pleasure to see you and Sudhoff, and the two midday meals with you and Mrs. Sigerist in your charming home was a sheer delight.

I am comfortably settled here at the Adlon where I shall probably remain until Friday. There came to-day a telegram from d'Irsay asking if I could meet him on the 8th – I shall wire that the 7th is the latest date for our conference, as the 8th I must be in London. I shall hand him your letter.

I am already deep in engagements here for the next few days. To-morrow I shall hope to see Diepgen in his Institute. I have not yet communicated with him. Several of my friends were away on vacation when I arrived but they are now returning.

Please give my cordial regards to Geheimrath Sudhoff – especially remember me most kindly to Mrs. Sigerist and your young daughters.

Thanking you very much for your kindness and hospitality during my stay in Leipzig, I am, with all good wishes,

Ever faithfully yours,
William H. Welch

Allen M. Chesney (1888–1964). Duggan not identified. Karl Sudhoff (1853–1938) medical historian in Leipzig, S.'s teacher and predecessor. Emmy Sigerist see S. to W. of 30 May 1931. Adlon: Hotel in Berlin. d'Irsay see S. to W. of 9 January 1928. Paul Diepgen (1878–1966) director of the newly founded Institute of the History of Medicine in Berlin. S.'s daughters Erica (1918–2002) and Nora (born 1922).

SIGERIST to WELCH, Leipzig ?, 1 September 1931

Dear Dr. Welch,

My address in New York will be: Shelton Hotel, Lexington Ave. and 49th Str. I will wait there for you. Please let me know when you will arrive and on what steamer.

I enclose a few photos. With kindest regards from Mrs. Sigerist and myself

Yours very sincerely
[Henry E. Sigerist]

Dear Sigerist –

I am sorry to miss you. I am returning to Baltimore to-day, having delayed my arrival there much longer than I intended.

You have probably received from Dean Chesney the announcement, giving the dates of your lectures and of the Seminar Course: the first lecture coming on October 15th at 5 p.m. and the others following at weekly intervals. The Seminar Conference is on the day following each lecture, also at 5 p.m.

I understood you to say that you were coming to Baltimore on the 10th. If there should be any reason why you may prefer a later date before the 15th, please let me know.

It would be well to drop a line to the Baltimore Club, corner of Madison and Charles Streets, giving the time of your arrival, so that the room will be ready.

If you will let me know the train, I shall try to meet you; at any rate I shall see you soon after you arrive.

There are two railways from New York to Baltimore – the most travelled and in some ways the most convenient is the Pennsylvania R.R. – the other, which I generally prefer, is the Baltimore and Ohio, which runs motor coaches (without extra charge) carrying passengers and hand baggage from the B and O Station on 42nd Street opposite the Commodore Hotel. By the latter you cross by ferry to Jersey City, whence the train starts. I enclose a time-table of the B&O, which I am about to take.

We shall have a meeting of our Medical-Historical Club while you are in Baltimore. If you have anything to give us at the meeting, it will of course be most welcome.

I hope that you are enjoying your stay, and getting all the lecture engagements you desire. With best regards, I am, very sincerely yours

William H. Welch

Chesney see W. to S. of 31 May 1931. The Johns Hopkins Medical-Historical Club had been founded in 1889 by William Osler with W. as its first president.

Dear Sigerist –

I am glad to get your letter of September 1st, received this morning while I am spending a few days at Klebs's.

I am sailing from Cherbourg on September 19th on SS. Volendam of the Holland America Line, which should land me in New York about September 26th. I shall try to get into touch with you at the Hotel Shelton soon after landing. I expect to go first to my nephew's Senator F. C. Walcott, Norfolk, Connecticut, before returning to Baltimore, where I shall probably arrive about October 5th or 6th.

I think your first lecture might come about a week or so after that. Perhaps the Dean of the Medical School, Dr. Chesney, has arranged the dates after communicating with you.

I imagine that you will have as many lecture engagements as you can manage. The Paris office of the Rockefeller Foundation called me on the telephone while I was in Paris to say that the International Education Bureau (I am not sure of official title), which had learned of your desiring engagements to lecture, wished to know about what honorarium you would expect. I suggested that for engagements in the East perhaps $75 would be suitable, but this in no way commits you.

I am delighted with the photographs, and thank you very much for sending them. Arnold Klebs and Harvey Cushing, who is here after the Berne Congress, consider them excellent.

I leave to morrow [sic] for Paris, where my address until Sept. 19 will be the Grand Hotel, Boulevard des Capucines. Best greetings to Mrs. S., yourself and Sudhoff –

very sincerely yours,
William H. Welch

P. S. I shall arrange for a room for you in Baltimore at the Baltimore Club and shall have a visitor's card sent to your N. Y. address for the University Club. W. H. W.

Nyon, a town on Lake Geneva in Switzerland, since WWI home of Arnold C. Klebs, see S. to W. of 24 May 1927. Cherbourg: Port in Normandy. Frederic C. Walcott: Republican senator of Connecticut. Chesney and Sudhoff see W. to S. of 31 May 1931. Harvey Cushing (1869–1939) neurosurgeon and historian of medicine. "Berne Congress", international, of Neurology.

WELCH to SIGERIST, Baltimore ?, 15 November 1931

Dear Sigerist –
    I will call for you about ten minutes after one o'clock with a taxi to go
out to Adolf Meyer's
    Sincerely yours
        William H. Welch

Adolf Meyer (1866–1950) Swiss psychiatrist, professor of psychiatry at Hopkins and
first director of the Phipps Clinic. W. had resigned his chair on 1 July 1931; Garrison
(see S. to W. of 18 January 1927) was head of the Institute ad interim.
    S.'s success during his lecture tour in the U.S. made Cushing renounce the offer to
to succeed W., even though he previously had hoped for the position for the time after
his career as a neurosurgeon. The Advisory Board of the Hopkins Medical School
voted unanimously on 18 December 1931 to offer W.'s chair to S. At a convention in
Minneapolis at the end of December S. received the news of a call to Hopkins.

WELCH to SIGERIST, Minneapolis, 31 December 1931

Dear Sigerist –
    I called your room and found you out. I am sorry not to say good-by
[sic] personally. It has been a delight to see you here and to find you so
happy and cheerful. I congratulate you upon the great success you are
having everywhere with your lectures and personal impressions.
    Above all I am happy over the prospect that we may have you with us
permanently in Baltimore. I have written Chesney that I feel encouraged,
but explaining that your decision must await your return to Germany.
    I am particularly pleased with the idea that Mrs. Sigerist may join you
in Baltimore. Good luck, Happy New Year, pleasant continuance of your
travels.
    Rowntree is here with his car.
        Sincerely yours,
            William H. Welch

Chesney see W. to S. of 31 May 1931. S.'s "decision" to accept the call to Johns
Hopkins University. At the end of S.'s U. S. tour he was joined by his wife Emmy. "Your
travels": After Minneapolis and other Midwestern cities S. proceeded to California
and Hawaii. Leonard G. Rowntree (1883–1959) physician and pharmacologist.

Sigerist to Welch, San Francisco ?, 22 January 1932

My dear Dr. Welch,

Just a line to tell you that I had a cable from Mrs. Sigerist saying that she will join me in New York on the 5th of March. I am very happy indeed that she could make it possible to come. It is a very good sign because it proves that she too is interested in the matter and I am so glad to know that she will be able to see Baltimore and to meet my friends there.

I expect to be in New York one day before Mrs. Sigerist arrives and we will be in Baltimore about the 7th of March.

I had a very delightful time in San Francisco, although the weather was rather bad in the beginning.

I gave eight lectures at Stanford University as well as the University of California. It was a great pleasure to meet the very brilliant group of young scholars doing excellent work in Medical History here.

I feel rather tired now and am looking forward to having a holiday in the Hawaiian Islands. I am sailing tomorrow morning and I expect to be back in San Francisco on Feb. 16th.

With kindest regards I am,
Very sincerely yours,
[Henry E. Sigerist]

"The matter": S.'s call to Johns Hopkins. "Brilliant group", led by Chauncey D. Leake (see correspondence Sigerist-Leake).

Welch to Sigerist, Baltimore, 5 March 1932 (Telegram)

CORDIAL GREETINGS TO YOU AND MRS SIGERIST ON HER ARRIVAL EAGERLY EXPECTING YOU MONDAY GLAD TO MEET YOU ON ARRIVAL IF YOU WILL INFORM ME OF TRAIN HAVE ACCEPTED MR HUBERS INVITATION TO HIS BOX FOR SYMPHONY CONCERT WEDNESDAY NIGHT THE NINTH FOR YOU MRS SIGERIST AND MYSELF AND MRS HEMSLEY JOHNSONS INVITATION TO LITTLE SUPPER AT HER RESIDENCE AFTER CONCERT ROOMS ENGAGED FOR YOU AT THE STAFFORD
W H WELCH

Mr. Huber, Mrs. Hemsley Johnson not identified.

Welch to Sigerist, Baltimore, 30 April 1932 (Telegram)

AM REJOICED AND JACOBS GARRISON AND OTHERS JOIN IN OUR DELIGHT
GREETINGS MRS SIGERIST AND SUDHOFF
    WELCH

A congratulation to S. in Leipzig on his acceptance of the call to Baltimore. Sigerist after his U.S. tour had returned to Leipzig and there made the decision to have his future in Baltimore. Henry Barton Jacobs (early 20th ct.) physician and medical historian; donated his collection to Johns Hopkins University. Garrison and Sudhoff see S. to W. of 18 January 1927 and W. to S. of 31 May 1931, respectively.

Welch to Sigerist, Atlantic City, NJ, 6 May 1932

Dear Sigerist –

Nothing could have given me greater joy and satisfaction than the receipt of your cablegram last Saturday, April 30th – and everybody, both at Johns Hopkins and elsewhere, feel likewise.

I can hardly tell you the sense of relief which your decision has given me. As you know, I have been greatly concerned about the future of the Institute of Medical History at the Hopkins. I felt a unique opportunity for the development of such an Institute in America existed provided the right man could be found for the position. Now we are assured of the best man in the world for the place, the future is assured, and I feel "O Lord! Let thy Servant depart in peace".

I came down to Atlantic City on May 1st before the reporters could reach me, so that the account of your acceptance in the Baltimore 'Sun', which I sent you does not contain my comments.

I came to attend the meetings of various medical Societies which have been held here this week, including a session and dinner meeting of the Association of the History of Medicine on Monday. This latter was well attended and some of the papers quite good. All the amateur historians were delighted when I told them of your decision.

I am returning to Baltimore to-day in time to attend the first of three lectures by Charles Singer (perhaps one will be by Dorothea) who will spend a week with us.

I shall move my things out of the big rooms at the Institute this summer into one of the small rooms, which will serve me as a pied à terre, so that all will be in readiness for you to move in.

I imagine Sudhoff will never forgive us for stealing you away. Give him my cordial regards, and also my heartiest greetings to Mrs. Sigerist –

Yours ever

William H. Welch

S.'s telegram is missing. The Baltimore Sun, newspaper. Charles Singer (1876–1960) English historian of medicine in Oxford and London; his wife Dorothea. Sudhoff see W. to S. of 31 May 1931.

WELCH to SIGERIST, New York ?, 19 September 1932

Dear Sigerist –

I was not certain of your arrival on this side until I picked up the Baltimore 'Sun' this morning and read the interview with you. Garrison had told me that you were to be on the 'Deutschland' and he thought that you would stop at the Shelton for a day or so before going to Baltimore. I made an ineffectual effort to meet you at the dock on Friday. The Deutschland was advertised to arrive at one o'clock, and I was so informed over the telephone from the office of the Hamburg-American line. So I went to the dock and waited an hour, but having an engagement soon after two o'clock I was obliged to leave before the ship arrived. I left a letter for you at the Shelton and called the hotel later, but was told you had not arrived there. I assume that you went on directly to Baltimore, which was sensible.

I am sorry not to have been in Baltimore to welcome you to your new home. I have made a mental vow not to leave here until I have finished some writing for which the printers are waiting, but I am incorrigibly lazy and have been much interrupted.

I told Garrison to tell you to clean out my disordered leavings from the two rooms which I have occupied at the Library and to take possession. Anyone of the small rooms will serve me as a pied à terre, if it can be spared.

I have seen your programme of lectures and courses – a perfectly delightful one. The Advisory Board – of which you will be a member –

should arrange to have your courses counted as optional subjects for the degree and made examinable. Furthermore the Academic Council or the University should provide that work with you should be eligible for either a major or minor for the PhD degree. I have no doubt this will be arranged.

You and Mrs. Sigerist are doubtless home-hunting. My love to you both and your daughters and all my best wishes until I see you, which I hope will be in a week or so.

Very sincerely yours,
William H. Welch

Garrison see S. to W. of 18 January 1927. Shelton Hotel in New York. Pied à terre: Base. Advisory Board (of the Medical School): The faculty. S.'s daughters see W. to S. of 31 May 1931.

WELCH to SIGERIST, Baltimore ?, 11 October 1932 (?)

Dear Sigerist –

I dropped in, thinking that you may have arrived – but it seems not. I shall try to see you in the morning, but if Garrison or Oliver are to take you to the Library I shall see you there about noon. I have an appointment which will occupy me part of the morning.

Welcome –

Yours sincerely
William H. Welch

Garrison see S. to W. of 18 January 1927. John Rathbone Oliver (1872–1943) MD, PhD, psychiatrist and associate professor at the Institute of the History of Medicine in Baltimore, also novelist and priest.

SIGERIST to WELCH, Baltimore ?, 16 November 1932

Dear Dr. Welch:

We would very much like to commemorate the anniversary of Leeuwenhoek and we all thought that the best way to do it would be to ask you to give a lecture on Leeuwenhoek and bacteriology for the medical students and the members of the faculty. Having just had the Rabelais celebration, we would not care to repeat the proceedings and therefore thought it would be nicer to limit the audience to the medical school. The lecture could be given on an afternoon and I think the beginning of December would be the best time. We would appreciate your acceptance very much.

John Fulton will address the Medical History Club on November 28th. I asked him to have dinner with us before the lecture, at six o'clock, at our house, and Mrs. Sigerist and myself would be very delighted if you could join us.

With kind regards, I am
Very sincerely
Henry E. Sigerist

Antony van Leeuwenhoek (1632–1723) Dutch scientific biologist, discoverer of micro-organisms. François Rabelais (1494–1553) French writer. John F. Fulton (1899–1960) physiologist and medical historian at Yale University.

WELCH to SIGERIST, Baltimore ?, 17 November 1932

Dear Sigerist,

I shall be delighted if you can dine with me at seven o'clock on Friday, November 25th, at the University Club to meet Mr. John Kingsbury, Secretary of the Milbank Memorial Fund, who is to give a field-night talk at nine o'clock on his and Sir Arthur Newsholme's studies of the public health system in Russia last summer.

I am very glad that I am to meet you and Mrs. Sigerist next Tuesday night at the Harry Black's. They have a charming home, and Mrs. Black, who is from England, is most interesting.

Hoping that you can come on the 25th, I am,
Sincerely yours,
William H. Welch

The Milbank Memorial Fund is an endowed national foundation that supports analysis, study, and research on issues in health policy. Arthur Newsholme (1857–1943) British public health physician, developed models of socialized medicine. Harry Black not identified.

Dear Sigerist –

There is a Mr. Beveridge here at the University Club – a Scotsman, who studied at Edinburgh – who has a collection – perhaps 20 or 40 volumes – of illustrated works especially on Egyptology. The few he has shown me are official publications of governments and exploration funds, handsomely illustrated – e.g. one on zoology by Naville of Geneva – others by Flinders Petrie etc.

Beveridge, who was a teacher at the Tome Institute in this state, is out of a job and hard up – and wishes to sell his archeological books, and proposes to offer them to David Robinson.

It occurs to me that you and Garrison might be interested and would like to see the books, so I told Beveridge that I would write you. He will be glad to show his collection to you, and I really think it may be worth while for you to see them with the view of possible purchase, or at least some for our library. If so, you can doubtless by telephone or by letter make an appointment with James Beveridge – he resides near the Club, and is at the Club much of the time, and would be very glad to show you the books.

I thought our Leeuwenhoek celebration went off very well, thanks to you and Cohen and the film.

With best wishes and greetings of the season for you and Mrs. Sigerist
 I am, very sincerely yours,
  William H. Welch

Henri E. Naville (1844–1926) Swiss egyptologist. Flinders Petrie (1853–1942) British egyptologist. Tome Institute (School) at Port Deposit, MD. David Robinson not identified. Garrison see S. to W. of 18 January 1927, since 1930 head of the Welch Medical Library and S.'s staff member. Leeuwenhoek see S. to W. of 16 November 1932. Cohen, probably I. Bernard Cohen (1914–2003) historian of science.

WELCH to SIGERIST, Baltimore, summer 1933 ?

Bon voyage and safe return to America.
  Affectionately
    William H. Welch

Probably for the Sigerists' first summer vacation in Europe 1933, written at the Johns Hopkins Hospital.

WELCH to SIGERIST, Baltimore, 2 November 1933

Dear Sigerist –
  I have never been in the habit of keeping letters, but now that we have a collection of autographed letters at the Institute, it occurs to me that you may like to add the three which I enclose to the collection.
  Morgan's letter is in reply to my congratulations on the award of the Nobel Prize in Medicine – Otto Warburgs steamer letter I have acknowledged – John C. Finley is one of the editors of the N. Y. Times. His verse is also in reply to my congratulations on his 70th birthday. He and Morgan are Johns Hopkins graduates.
  Yours sincerely
    William H. Welch

The letter-head reads "The Johns Hopkins Hospital", where W. was since February 1933 and until his death in April 1934. Thomas H. Morgan (1866–1945) geneticist and embryologist. Otto Warburg (1883–1970) German biochemist and Nobel Prize laureate.

WELCH to SIGERIST, Baltimore, late 1933 ?

Thank you so much for 'The Great Doctors' a delightful book.
  W. H. W.

Great Doctors (Sigerist 1933).

1.3. Literature

Brieger, Gert H.: *Welch, William Henry*. In "C.C. Gillispie, ed.: Dictionary of Scientific Biography", vol. XIV, New York 1976.

d'Irsay, Stephen: *Time-implied Function: An Historical Aperçu*. Kyklos 1, 52–59, 1928.

d'Irsay, Stephen: *Albrecht von Haller: Eine Studie zur Geistesgeschichte der Aufklärung*. Leipzig 1930.

Fleming, Donald: *William Henry Welch and the Rise of Modern Medicine*. Boston 1954.

Flexner, Simon / Flexner, James T.: *William Henry Welch and the Heroic Age of American Medicine*. New York 1941.

Shryock, Richard H.: *Dr. Welch and Medical History*. Bull. Hist. Med. 24, 325–332, 1950.

Sigerist, Henry E.: *Die Geschichte der Medizin im akademischen Unterricht. Ergebnisse einer Rundfrage des Instituts*. Kyklos 1, 147–156, 1928.

Sigerist, Henry E.: *Foreword* (Open letter to William H. Welch). Kyklos 2, 5–7, 1929.

Sigerist, Henry E.: *Great Doctors. A Biographical History of Medicine*. (Translation of "Grosse Aerzte"). New York 1933.

Sigerist, Henry E.: *Stephen d'Irsay, 1894–1935*. Bull. Hist. Med. 3, 431–442, 1935.

1.4. Name Index

2. Correspondence
Henry E. Sigerist – Harvey Cushing
1926–1939

2.1. Introduction

2.1.1. Harvey Cushing (1869–1939)

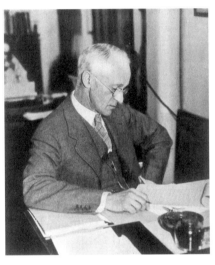

Born in Cleveland in 1869, the son of a physician, Harvey Cushing was raised in a family with a long tradition of medicine. He obtained his B.A. at Yale in 1891 and an M.D. at Harvard in 1895. From 1896 to 1912 Cushing worked at the Johns Hopkins Medical School under the famous surgeon and teacher William Halsted, doing research on the structure and physiology of the nervous system. The years 1900–1901 provided further training in England, France, Switzerland, and Germany. Back in Baltimore he became associate professor, further specializing in neurosurgery and the pituitary gland. During all these years at Hopkins he also felt the influence of Osler, Kelly, and Welch who also awakened an interest in the history of medicine in Cushing.

In 1912 Cushing continued his career at Harvard. At Peter Bent Brigham Hospital he became the world leader in the new speciality of neurosurgery. He introduced technical innovations, operated with impeccable technique and careful handling of tissues, showing concern for the welfare of his patients. He also directed laboratories for experimental surgery and created a classification of brain tumors. During WWI he was head of the Harvard Base Hospital in France. When he retired in 1932 at age 63 he had operated 2000 brain tumors, written over 300 scientific papers and had dramatically improved the field of neurosurgery.

In 1931 Cushing declined Welch's chair of the History of Medicine at Hopkins in favor of Sigerist, but he accepted a professorship of neurology at Yale which he held until 1937. For his two final years he was director of studies in medical history. As a medical historian he had written the famous biography of William Osler (Cushing 1925), a biobibliography of Vesalius (Cushing 1943) in addition to many essays. In more general terms he enhanced the position of the humanities in the study of medicine. A bibliophile, he inherited and collected books and convinced A. C. Klebs and J. F. Fulton to combine their libraries with his own 8000 volumes, which after WWII resulted in the Yale Medical School Historical Library with 25,000 books.

Cushing belongs to the most distinguished physicians in the history of American medicine. The 23 honorary degrees bestowed upon him are a sign of acknowledgment of his achievements. No wonder is there a large literature on Cushing. Suffice it therefore to indicate but a few biographical titles: (Baumgartner 1940), (Fulton 1946), (Sigerist 1954), (Davey 1969), (Bliss 2005).

2.1.2. The Correspondence

Sigerist and Cushing corresponded from 1926 to Cushing's death in 1939. They had known each other before, mainly through their common friend, Arnold C. Klebs. When they first met in October 1931 Cushing, 62 years old, was at the end of his career as the world-famous neurosurgeon in Boston, while Sigerist, 40, professor in Leipzig, was on a study tour in the United States. Most of the correspondence then is between Cushing as elderly professor at Yale University in New Haven and Sigerist during his first years as professor at Johns Hopkins in Baltimore. Both were obviously impressed by each other and remained in respect and empathy. The salutation in Cushing's letters goes from "Dear Professor Sigerist" to "Dear Sigerist" to "Dear Henry" while for Sigerist it is always "Dear Dr. Cushing".

The correspondents discuss books and problems in the history of medicine, tell of their work and travels, of past and future invitations, they also exchange invitations for lectures. 25 books and articles are mentioned as well as 54 names, foremost among the latter are their common friends Fulton, Klebs, and Welch. Occasionally Cushing mentions his increasing health problems in general terms.

There are 40 letters by Sigerist and 36 by Cushing with little evidence of missing letters. Thus, the frequency of exchanged letters is moderate, but then there were likely telephone calls and quite a few personal encounters in New Haven, New York, and Baltimore. The first three letters of Sigerist from Leipzig are written in German. They have been fully translated by the editor. All letters are typed. They are written in very good style and choice of words, concise, and often with a grain of humor. The letters of 1926–1929 are at the University Archive Leipzig, the letters of 1931–1932 at the Yale University Library, all the following ones at the Alan Mason Chesney Medical Archives of The Johns Hopkins Medical Institutions.

2.2. The Letters

SIGERIST to CUSHING, Leipzig, 10 June 1926
(Original in German)

Dear Dr. Cushing,
Many thanks for your check of 21 Mark as your annual dues for 1926. We have acknowledged your change of address.
Yours faithfully
[Henry E. Sigerist]

Letter addressed to H. Cushing, Peter Bent Brigham Hospital, Boston, Mass. S. was treasurer of the German Society of the History of Medicine and Sciences (DGGMN) collecting the annual dues.

CUSHING to SIGERIST, Boston, 10 January 1927

Dear Dr. Sigerist:
I wish to acknowledge with pleasure the receipt of your New Year's greeting. I was speaking of you only last evening with our mutual friend, Arnold C. Klebs, who is in Boston paying a visit.
With assurances of my regard, I am
Sincerely yours,
Harvey Cushing

Arnold C. Klebs (1870–1943), son of Edwin Klebs, physician and medical historian in the U.S. and Switzerland, friend and major correspondent of both S. and C., an expert on incunables (early prints before 1500).

SIGERIST to CUSHING, Leipzig, 20 October 1927
(Original in German)

Dear Dr. Cushing,
    Many thanks for your check of 21 Mark as your annual dues for 1926.
        Yours faithfully,
            [Henry E. Sigerist]

CUSHING to SIGERIST, Boston, 16 January 1928

Dear Professor Sigerist:
    What a delightful New Year's remembrance from your Institute for the
History of Medicine! I had never seen a copy of this 1564 Paracelsus and
shall treasure this facsimile with much appreciation.
    With sincere regards, I am
        Most truly yours,
            Harvey Cushing

Paracelsus facsimile (Sigerist 1928).

CUSHING to SIGERIST, Boston, 17 January 1929

Dear Professor Sigerist:
    I am greatly pleased to have your New Year's greeting in the form of
this most delightful reproduction of a portrait of Karl Sudhoff.
    I am hoping to see Sudhoff here in America next October, for Profes-
sor Welch tells me that he is coming over to give an address at the opening
of the Welch Library.
    With assurances of my regard, I am
        Very sincerely yours,
            Harvey Cushing

Karl Sudhoff (1853–1938) German medical historian, director of the Leipzig Institute
of the History of Medicine from 1905 to 1925, S.'s teacher. William H. Welch (1850–

45

1934) pathologist, hygienist, medical historian at Johns Hopkins University. He would
be the first director of the newly created Hopkins Institute for the History of Medicine.
In October 1929 Sudhoff was invited to the U.S. for the inauguration of the Institute of
the History of Medicine and the Welch Medical Library in Baltimore.

CUSHING to SIGERIST, Boston, 6 August 1929

Dear Dr. Sigerist:

I am delighted to see your second volume of KYKLOS and am so
pleased that it has been issued in honour of my revered master and friend,
William H. Welch. I hope you will ask the publishers to put my name
down as one of the subscribers to KYKLOS and hope that they will send
me the first volume as well as the present one.

Very sincerely yours,

Harvey Cushing

KYKLOS: Year-book of the Institute for the History of Medicine of the University of
Leipzig. Welch see C. to S. of 17. January 1929.

SIGERIST to CUSHING, Leipzig, 21 August 1929
(Original in German)

Dear Dr. Cushing,

Thank you for your letter of 8 August. I am glad that you liked our
volume of 'Kyklos' in which we duly honored Welch. I have just asked our
publisher to send you the two volumes of 'Kyklos'. Learning of your coming to Europe, I would be happy if time allowed you to visit our institute.
I shall be in Leipzig from 18 September on.

With kind regards I am,

Yours faithfully

[Henry E. Sigerist]

Kyklos see C. to S. of 6 August 1929. Welch see C. to S. of 17. January 1929. Volume
2 of Kyklos was dedicated to Welch and his Institute of the History of Medicine in
Baltimore (Sigerist 1929). In the weeks before 18 September S. and his associates
were on a tour in Vienna, Prague, and Budapest.

Cushing to Sigerist, Boston, 21 October 1929

Dear Prof. Sigerist:

Thanks for your kind letter of August 21st. I am so glad to be a subscriber to the KYKLOS which promises to be a most important and delightful journal.

I am just back from the ceremonies at Baltimore which were highly interesting. Dr. Welch was in good form and full of enthusiasm – Sudhoff no less so.

With warm regards, I am
Sincerely yours,
Harvey Cushing

KYKLOS see C. to S. of 6 August 1929. "Ceremonies at Baltimore", Welch, and Sudhoff see C. to S. of 17 January 1929.

Sigerist to Cushing, Baltimore ?, 17 October 1931

My dear Dr. Cushing:

It is very kind of you to want me to stay with you while I am in Boston. I do not know yet when I shall be in Boston, as I am waiting for a letter from Dr. Edsall. As I told you in New York, any time between the 23rd of November and the 1st of December would be convenient. On December 2, I intend to go to Rochester, New York, on my way to Chicago.

It was a very great pleasure to have met you in New York and I am looking forward to seeing you in Boston next month.

Yours very sincerely,
[Henry E. Sigerist]

S. knew of C.'s medico-historical interests years before, see correspondence between S. and A. C. Klebs. S. is on his study tour in the U.S. of 1931/1932 which would result in the call to the Johns Hopkins University, i. e., he was on leave from the University of Leipzig. C. was at Peter Bent Brigham Hospital in Boston at the end of his spectacular career as a neurosurgeon. Edsall, probably David L. (1869–1945) at Massachussets General Hospital in Boston.

CUSHING to SIGERIST, Boston, 9 November 1931

Dear Professor Sigerist:

We are looking forward eagerly to your coming here the end of the month. I hope at least that you will spend the week-end with me, and I am planning to get some of the Mediaevalists in Cambridge to meet you at a small dinner on Saturday evening.

I trust that you have been having a pleasant time in Baltimore. I hear from all sides most complimentary things about your lectures. I am still hoping that I may be able to come down sometime before you leave.

Please give my greetings to Dr. Welch and Garrison, and believe me
 Most cordially yours,
  Harvey Cushing

Welch see C. to S. of 17 January 1929. Fielding H. Garrison (1870–1935) medical historian, at that time librarian of the Welch Medical Library at Johns Hopkins.

SIGERIST to CUSHING, Baltimore ?, 13 November 1931

My dear Dr. Cushing:

Thank you so much for your kind letter of November 9. I shall be delighted to spend the week-end with you. I expect to arrive in Boston on Saturday morning, November 28, at 10:45 A.M., coming from Rochester where I shall spend all of Friday with Dr. Corner.

I am looking forward with much pleasure to seeing you soon. With kindest regards, I am
 Very sincerely yours,
  [Henry E. Sigerist]

George Washington Corner (1889–1982) anatomist and medical historian in Rochester, NY.

CUSHING to SIGERIST, Boston, 18 November 1931

Dear Professor Sigerist:

I have your note of November 13th saying you will be here Saturday morning, November the 28th. You will be coming directly from Rochester so that I will expect you to get off at the Huntington Avenue station rather than at the terminus, and Dr. Corner will explain this to you. Indeed, I will write him about this myself.

The local Historical Society was planning to have a meeting for you on Friday afternoon and it will be a great disappointment to them not to have you here. I have asked a few people to meet you for dinner Saturday and will make plans for you to see something of the libraries during the all-too-few days you are to be here. I suppose you have changed your plans somewhat, for I believe you told me you were expecting to leave here Tuesday night so that you could be in Rochester on December 2nd, but Corner has evidently persuaded you to change the date to Friday, the 27th. I trust this means you may be able to prolong your visit here.

It is the greatest disappointment that I cannot join my friend, Fulton, from New Haven and come down for your last lecture, but I find myself more involved with work than I had expected. Please give my affectionate regards to Drs. Welch, Garrison and Oliver.

Most cordially yours,
Harvey Cushing

Corner see S. to C. of 13 November 1931. John F. Fulton (1899–1960) physiologist and medical historian at Yale University in New Haven, CT. Welch, Garrison see C. to S. of 9 November 1931. John Rathbone Oliver (1872–1943) MD, PhD, psychiatrist.

SIGERIST to CUSHING, Baltimore ?, 23 November 1931

My dear Dr. Cushing:

I have your note of November 18 and expect to arrive in Boston, Saturday morning, November 28. I shall leave Boston on Wednesday afternoon, December 2, as I intend to spend December 3 at

Cleveland. I am very sorry that I will not be able to stay longer in Boston.

Looking forward with great pleasure to seeing you, I am
Very sincerely yours,
[Henry E. Sigerist]

On his study tour S. spent several weeks in October and November at the Johns Hopkins Institute of the History of Medicine in Baltimore before lecturing in Boston, Cleveland, Michigan, and Madison. At the end of November C. sent Welch the following telegram:

"Sigerist has captivated everyone here by his modesty, learning, lively interest in everything, and personal charm. I cannot imagine a more suitable person for the post or one more certain to develop it in the way you would desire. He is certain to have a great following. America fascinates him and I believe he would find an offer difficult to refuse" (Fulton 1946, 613). This made C. to renounce the succession of Welch offered to him, even though he previously had hoped for the position for the time after his career as a neurosurgeon. At a convention in Minneapolis at the end of December S. received the news of a call to Hopkins as a result of the unanimous decision by the faculty.

CUSHING to SIGERIST, Boston, 31 December 1931

Dear Sigerist:

I was so happy to have a glimpse of you again at Atlantic City and enjoyed your brilliant talk about the Smith Papyrus more than I can possibly say.

I meant to speak to you at the time about my friend and one-time pupil, Dr. S. C. Harvey, who is Professor of Surgery at Yale. He is going abroad for a sabbatical year and has taken on the task of writing a surgical book for Charles Thomas along the lines of Fulton's Studies in Physiology and Long's Studies in Pathology. No one could possibly do it better than Harvey for, though untrained like myself, he has strong historical leanings.

He plans to go to Zurich as a convenient place where he can put his children to school, and I have urged him to come down and have a talk with you about his programme, for I am sure you could help him greatly. So if you hear from him, do give him a welcome and such hints

50

and suggestions as to where he could find material in Zurich or elsewhere.

Always with warm regards and compliments to your wife, I am
Sincerely yours,
Harvey Cushing

During S.'s visit in Boston of the final days of November he also was a highly impressed spectator of one of C.s brain operations. Atlantic City, NJ, a place where many scientific and medical meetings take place. Papyrus Smith, one of the medical papyri from Ancient Egypt. Harvey, probably Samuel C., has written about the history of surgery. Charles Thomas, publisher. Fulton see C. to S. of 18 November 1931. Esmond R. Long (1890–1979) pathologist and medical historian. Both Fulton and Long have written on the history of their disciplines.

Cushing to Sigerist, Boston, 4 January 1932

Dear Sigerist:

I am enclosing for your information a note from Captain F. L. Pleadwell, who was formerly a medical officer in the navy – a very good fellow, with historical interests. He is just the man to take you in charge in Honolulu and to show you the country.

I have been getting news of you from roundabout sources – particularly from Fulton, who was recently with you in Minneapolis. I wish I might have been there too. I gather that the J. H. U. people have made ouvertures to you in regard to taking Welch's position. I am highly jelous of you, but you are so obviously the right man for them that I gladly withdraw in your favor and sincerely trust that you will see your way clear to accept this blue-ribbon position in American medicine.

We look back upon your visit here with joy.
Always yours,
H. C.

Fulton see C. to S. of 18 November 1931. See also comment to S. to C. of 23 November 1931.

SIGERIST to CUSHING, on tour in Northern states, 5 January 1932

Dear Dr. Cushing:

It was delightful to see you again and I only regret that you could not stay longer in Atlantic City. Your paper interested me extremely. What splendid material you have! I do hope that you will publish this paper with all the illustrations. It would be of great service to all of us.

I remember very well having met Dr. S.C. Harvey in New Haven and I know the book he wrote on the history of transfusion. I am very pleased to hear that he is preparing a book on the history of surgery and I am sure that he is the best man for it.

Zürich is quite a good place for such a work. The library in which I worked for so many years has a good collection of old medical and surgical books and I am sure that he will find there all he needs. The University of Basel has a good medical library too and is just an hour's ride from Zürich.

I would be delighted to see Dr. Harvey and he can be assured of a warm welcome.

　　　　With kind regards, I am
　　　　　　Very sincerely yours,
　　　　　　　[Henry E. Sigerist]

Atlantic City, NJ, see C. to S. of 31 December 1931. Harvey's two book titles not identified.

SIGERIST to CUSHING, San Francisco ?, 22 January 1932

My dear Cushing:

Thank you so much for your kind letter of December 22nd which I received in San Francisco.

You have been in Baltimore by now and you will have heard that the Chair of Dr. Welch has been offered to me. It is a great honor and the offer is very tempting because I am sure that it gives great opportunity for excellent work to be done there. You know, however, that I would never accept the Chair if I thought that you would like to have it. You know my views on the subject and you know how much I would have liked to see you in Baltimore.

I asked Mrs. Sigerist to join me in America and I just had a cable saying that she would be in New York the beginning of March. I am very glad that she will be able to see Baltimore and I would very much like for her to meet Mrs. Cushing and yourself.

I had a very delightful and very busy time in San Francisco and am sailing tomorrow morning for the Hawaiian Islands, but I expect to be back at the St. Francis on February 16th.

Please remember me to Mrs. Cushing and with kind regards, I am

Very sincerely your,

[Henry E. Sigerist]

Cushing's letter of 22 December 1931 is missing. See also comment on S. by C. of 23 November 1931. St. Francis: Hotel in San Francisco.

Cushing to Sigerist, Boston, 2 February 1932

Dear Sigerist:

Thanks for your letter from the St. Francis. By the time you get this, you will probably be back there again and I hope will have had a delightful time in the Islands, though they seem to be in a sort of turmoil at present. The whole Orient seems to have gone mad just now, and the Hawaiian Islands are near enough to it to feel the general uneasiness.

I had a delightful time in Baltimore and tried to make a speech, but I am afraid they may have thought I was somewhat frivolous [sic], which I didn't mean to be. I was only poking a little fun at my old housemate H. B. Jacobs.

I rejoice to know that Mrs. Sigerist is coming over for a visit and I sincerely hope that both Mrs. Cushing and I will have an opportunity to meet her either here or in Baltimore. Your old room will be ready for you should you ever find your way here again either alone or in company with your wife.

Sincerely yours,

Harvey Cushing

Turmoil in the Orient: Probably the Japanese occupation of Manchuria. Henry Barton Jacobs 1858–1939) physician, medical historian, collector. There are no letters during S.'s final half year in Leipzig from March to September 1932.

SIGERIST to CUSHING, Baltimore ?, 20 February 1933

Dear Dr. Cushing:

We have just discovered buried among other books the enclosed edition of Vesalius. The title-page and the last pages are missing and I am not quite sure what it is. It looks to me as if it were the Cologne edition 1600, which has 48 leaves and 40 plates. However, I am not sure and would very much appreciate if you could help us in identifying this copy.

Very sincerely yours,

[Henry E. Sigerist]

Beginning in fall 1932 S. was William H. Welch Professor of the History of Medicine and head of the Hopkins Institute for the History of Medicine in Baltimore. Andreas Vesalius (1514–1564) anatomist. C. was an expert on Vesalius.

SIGERIST to CUSHING, Baltimore ?, 27 February 1933

Dear Dr. Cushing:

Thank you very much for your kind letter of February 24th. I am awfully glad to have the book and the other plate identified. I shall complete the book by having photostats of the missing pages made.

I showed the book to the students in our seminar and asked them how they would identify such a book. They suggested looking up all kinds of reference books, but finally I told them that where-ever Vesalius was concerned there was a much more reliable method, namely to consult Harvey Cushing. The result has shown that I was right.

With kind regards from us all,

Very sincerely yours,

[Henry E. Sigerist]

C.'s letter of 24 February 1933 is missing. Vesalius see S. to C. of 20 February 1933.

Dear Sigerist:

You will see by the above my change of address. I was only here for a week toward the end of October when I went abroad for a month in order to give a lecture in London and to go to Paris for a degree. But much more than that, it was to try and get a little change of scene before taking up my new work here, whatever it may prove to be.

I only returned yesterday and the first thing I saw on my desk was your new book which I am sure will be a most important one, and I am most eagerly looking forward to reading it. How you have managed to grasp all this information about the history of American Medicine in so short a time is astonishing. But still, I could see during that first delightful visit you made to us in Brookline how interested you were already coming to be in the history of Medicine in this new and still in many respects highly uncouth country.

But more of this another time. Fulton just dropped in on me a few minutes ago and told me that you were coming Friday, and I said of course that you were to stay with us, and your wife also if she comes with you. John told me that he had already bespoken you, but I protested and said I had a prior claim of friendship. So either he or I will meet you at the train (and you will of course let us know just when you are going to arrive) and we will deposit you quietly here. John has arranged for a tea for you, and I believe there is a dinner before the meeting which I am looking forward to with the greatest interest.

Do drop in on Dr. Welch before you leave and give him my love and tell him I hope to come down soon to see him, to give him an account of my brief sojourn abroad. People everywhere asked eagerly for him. I was asked by the Faculty to go with them to the public funeral which was held at Notre Dame for Roux. It was a marvellous experience, an account of which I would like to give him at first hand.

Always affectionately yours,
Harvey Cushing

This is C.'s first letter after he had moved from the Peter Bent Brigham Hospital in Boston to Yale University in New Haven, CT. New book (Sigerist 1934a); S. must have sent C. the German original of 1933. Brookline, MA. Fulton see C. to S. of 18 November 1931. S. was to attend a meeting of the Yale Beaumont Club. Welch see C. to S. of 17 January 1929. C. attended the funeral with the Paris Medical Faculty. Pierre P. E. Roux (1853–1933) French microbiologist.

SIGERIST to CUSHING, Baltimore ?, 21 November 1933

Dear Dr. Cushing:

I wish to thank you for your extremely kind letter, but first of all let me congratulate you most highly upon the honorary degree coferred upon you by the Sorbonne. It was great news.

I, of course, am looking forward with greatest pleasure to seeing you soon, and will be delighted to stay with you. I intend to arrive in New Haven on Friday morning at 10:15.

I hope to see Dr. Welch tomorrow morning and will bring him your love, and shall tell him about your experience.

So à bientôt and kindest regards from
    Yours ever
      [Henry E. Sigerist]

Sorbonne, University of Paris. Welch see C. to S. of 17 January1929.

SIGERIST to CUSHING, Baltimore ?, 28 November 1933

Dear Dr. Cushing:

I forgot to make a note of your home address and so I have to write you through the Medical School.

I want to thank you and Mrs. Cushing most heartily for the perfectly delightful days I spent with you. I was glad to find that you are well settled in New Haven and that you feel happy there. I went to see Dr. Welch yesterday and told him all about you and your new home. I found him very cheerful, and he is looking forward to seeing you here some day.

I found a letter from Dr. Klebs in my mail yesterday, saying that he expects to arrive in this country by the middle of December. It would be nice if we could arrange a meeting of our History Club on incunables some time in January, and I hope that you will be able to join us.

The two days I had in New Haven were very refreshing. It is always good to see that there are other medical schools besides your own, and I was extremely interested in what Winternitz is doing and planning.

With kind regards to Mrs. Cushing and yourself, I am,
    Very sincerely yours,
      [Henry E. Sigerist]

Welch see C. to S. of 17 January 1929. In a letter of 25 November 1933 Cushing tells Welch what a delightful guest S. was and what an excellent lecture he had delivered. Klebs see C. to S. of 10 January 1927. Milton C. Winternitz (1885–1959) Dean of Yale Medical School 1920–1935.

SIGERIST to CUSHING, Baltimore ?, 29 November 1933

Dear Dr. Cushing:

I just had a letter from Dr. Harvey, telling me that you have to spend several weeks in the hospital. I felt extremely sorry about the news, but, of course, felt that this was the wisest thing to do. I do hope you will recover soon.

Dr. Harvey wants me to deliver an address on the occasion of the 150th anniversary of the New Haven County Medical Association. All of you gave me such a delightful reception in New Haven last week that I have accepted this new invitation, although I have a good many engagements in January already. I am sure your address would have been far better.

With best wishes, I am,

Very sincerely yours,

[Henry E. Sigerist]

Dr. Harvey see S. to C. of 31 December 1931. C. was treated in hospital for his circulatory problems in legs and feet.

CUSHING to SIGERIST, New Haven, 2 December 1933

Dear Henry:

I am perfectly delighted that you are coming on to give this address in January as my substitute. You could do it so much better anyway that I would have backed out if I had known how to do so. I don't know how you will want to attack it. I myself had a sort of idea of giving some hints about the general gregarious character of the profession and how in this new country they came together in small groups and made societies, which were first county societies, this one happening to be one of the early ones. The early figures here were perhaps not so interesting as were the early figures in Boston, let us say, or Charleston or Philadelphia. Nevertheless they were very worthy people.

I suppose they have told you that there will be two papers in the afternoon dealing specifically with the local history, and they rather wanted a general paper in the evening where you will have a large audience, I am sure. And if I can come there, whether in a wheel chair or not, you can depend upon my being in the front row.

One suggestion I would make would be to send out to Morris Fishbein for a dossier of papers relating to the early county medical societies throughout the country. He once sent me a large batch of these things, but I was much too busy to look at them then and sent them back, expecting to get them again.

I am beastly sorry to be laid up just at this time, and you were perhaps conscious of the fact that I was hobbling around and sidestepping activity of any kind when you were here. Nevertheless I enjoyed your address hugely. It was, as Osler would have said, simply A++.

Always sincerely yours,
Harvey Cushing

Morris Fishbein (1889–1976) editor, of the Journal of the American Medical Association. William Osler (1849–1919) professor of medicine at McGill University, Johns Hopkins, and Oxford, England.

SIGERIST to CUSHING, Baltimore ?, 4 December 1933

Dear Dr. Cushing:
Although you are hardly recognizable on the picture, I thought you would like to have this article, which I found in Le Siècle Médicale.

I was delighted to hear that you are comfortable at the hospital, and I hope that you will recover soon.

With best wishes, I am,
Very sincerely yours,
[Henry E. Sigerist]

Dear Dr. Cushing:

Thanks ever so much for your very charming letter of December 2nd. I thought of calling my address MEDICAL SOCIETIES PAST AND PRESENT. I intended to trace briefly the general development of medical societies abroad, then to give the eighteenth century European background, to proceed by describing the first organizations in this country without going into details as to the New Haven County Medical Association, which will be discussed by other speakers, then I would end by making some general remarks on the functions of medical societies. I have a few ideas on the subject, which may interest the audience.

Dr. Blumer very kindly sent me a whole batch of reprints on medical history in Connecticut, which will save me a great deal of trouble. However, I will certainly write to Morris Fishbein, and I am sure that this will be a great help also.

I am so glad that you liked my Beaumont lecture, and I hope that I will not disappoint the New Haven audience on January 5th.

With best wishes, I am,

Very sincerely yours

[Henry E. Sigerist]

S.'s address given in New Haven was published (Sigerist 1934b). George Blumer, Professor of Medicine at Yale and Dean 1910–1920, predecessor of Winternitz. Fishbein see C. to S. of 2 December 1933. S.'s lecture at the Beaumont Club (of the History of Medicine) see C. to S. 19 November 1933.

Cushing to Sigerist, New Haven, 15 March 1934

Dear Henry:

Thanks so much for your letter. I am glad to say that I am home again, and though I haven't ventured to start in work at the Hospital I am now at least sojourning at home and am picking up rapidly after my long incarceration.

It is nice of you to have thought of asking me to give the Noguchi Lectures next autumn and equally considerate of you to let me off so graciously. I do not think that I ought to think of undertaking anything so responsible as this until I am really once more in the swim.

I am glad to know that you are going to resume the publication of the Bulletin, for I have always looked forward to it eagerly. W. G. MacCallum gave me the pleasure of a visit two or three days ago and we talked much about you and the fine work that is being done in the Institute under your wise and active direction. I am glad that Klebs' talk pleased you, but I rather gathered from what he said that he feared he had not quite pulled it off successfully.

Always with warm regards, I am
 Most sincerely yours,
  Harvey Cushing

S.'s mentioned letter seems to be missing. "I am home again" after a prolonged stay in the hospital as a patient, see S. to C. of 29 November 1933. Noguchi Lecture Series at S.'s Institute in Baltimore. "Bulletin" of the Institute of the History of Medicine, founded by S. in 1933 as a supplement of the Johns Hopkins Hospital Bulletin; it became an independent journal in 1935 and was renamed Bulletin of the History of Medicine in 1939; it is still a leading journal of the history of medicine. William George MacCallum (1874–1944) pathologist and medical historian at Hopkins. Klebs see C. to S. of 10 January 1927.

SIGERIST to CUSHING, Baltimore ?, 19 March 1934

Dear Dr. Cushing:

I was so glad to hear that you are at home again and that you feel better. I saw MacCallum and he told me of the delightful time he had with you in New Haven.

I just spent a few days in New York, attending a very interesting meeting of the Milbank Memorial Fund, and had an extremely pleasant evening with the Klebs family just before they sailed. I also met Mr. Ivins of the Metropolitan Museum, whom you probably know. He has an extremely interesting and rather revolutionary theory about Vesalius and Kalkar, and believes that most of the credit should be given to Kalkar. We spent almost the whole night discussing this point.

Do not forget that we are expecting you next winter and that your lectures will be welcome at any time you choose to give them.

With kind regards, I am,
 Very sincerely yours,
  [Henry E. Sigerist]

MacCullum see C. to S. of 15 March 1934. Milbank Memorial Fund: A national foundation supporting studies in health policy. Klebs see S. to C. of 10 January 1927. William M. Ivins, curator of the Metropolitan Museum in New York. Vesalius see S. to C. 20 February 1933. Jan Stephan Kalkar (ca. 1499 – ca. 1546) anatomist, Vesalius' illustrator.

CUSHING to SIGERIST, New Haven, 23 April 1934

Dear Henry:

I have been looking over the last number of the <u>Bulletin of the Institute</u> which makes up half of the <u>Hospital Bulletin</u> – all very excellent. I see that copies of your admirable Syllabus are available. I hope it won't be hoggish of me to ask for a hundred of them so that I can scatter them about. Enclosed please find ten dollars for the same.

Much power to your elbow.

 Always yours,
  Harvey Cushing

"Bulletin of the Institute" of the History of Medicine, see C. to S. of 15 March 1934. Syllabus (Sigerist 1934c).

SIGERIST to CUSHING, Baltimore ?, 25 April 1934

Dear Dr. Cushing:

I will be glad to let you have a hundred reprints of my Syllabus. We have not gotten the reprints yet, but they may come at any time. Our Bulletin is developing very nicely and I intend to print about 800 pp. this year. It will be high time for us to separate from the Hospital Bulletin at the end of the year.

I am glad to say that our financial situation has improved somewhat. Some of the money that we lost last year has come back so that I am rather optimistic about the future.

We are sailing from Baltimore on May 30. I am not anxious at all to go to Europe and would prefer to spend my vacation somewhere in the mountains of New Mexico, but I want to complete my mediaeval work as soon as possible before the next European war breaks out. I intend to spend some time in France, Belgium and Holland, and to finish my work at the Vatican library. We have rented a little house near Lucerne right on the Lake, and make this our headquarters for the summer.

With kind regards, I am,
    Very sincerely yours,
        [Henry E. Sigerist]

Syllabus (Sigerist 1934c). "Bulletin" of the History of Medicine. "Sailing from Baltimore": From 1933 to 1939 S. and his family spent the summer months in Europe. "Not anxious to go to Europe": because of the political situation created by Nazi-Germany. House near Lucerne: Utohorn in Kastanienbaum.

CUSHING to SIGERIST, New Haven, 23 May 1934

Dear Sigerist:

Thanks so much for your letter. I doubt very much whether we will be able to pull off the symposium on the Dawn of Science, for Breasted has begged off, and Rostovtzeff is not back from abroad. Still, I think it's worth working on.

Breasted is not the only person to beg off, for you in your letter followed suit, and so has Sarton in his letter. I wish I could beg off from being obliged to give a presidential address, but as I can't properly do so I shall doubtless be bringing pressure on all of you to do your share on the programme. So you may expect me to be after you on your return from abroad next autumn. Your paper on tarantism would do perfectly well, if that's what you think will be most likely to be ready.

You did not give me the name of your boat, else I would have sent you a bon voyage cable; but I shall take the occasion of this letter to wish the family a pleasant trip and a delightful summer. I wish that I might look in on you at Lucerne, but that is not to be this summer, I regret to say.

Always sincerely yours,
    Harvey Cushing

James Henry Breasted (1865–1935) historian and egyptologist in Chicago. Mikhail I. Rostovtzeff (1870–1952) classical historian. George Sarton (1884–1956) Belgian-American historian of science. Tarantism: Fictitious symptoms resulting from the bite of the tarantula.

Dear Dr. Cushing:

Thanks so much for your letter. If you are in a jam with your program next winter I will, of course, be willing to help. I do not know, however, when my study on tarantism will be ready. It is an extremely complicated subject and I would not like to present it before I am really through with it. Perhaps I will find something else during the summer.

I hate to come back to the Noguchi lectures again. Dr. Edward H. Hume just wrote me that he may not be back from China in time to give his lectures during the next academic year. I therefore had to postpone them to October 1935. In other words, we will not have any Noguchi lectures next year unless you would consent to come down. I do wish you could come and spend a week with us in the Institute and lecture on any subject you choose. You, of course, need not decide now, but perhaps you will think it over during the summer.

With best wishes, I am always
    Yours very sincerely,
      [Henry E. Sigerist]

Tarantism see C. to S. of 23 May 1934. Noguchi lectures see C. to S. of 15 March 1934. Edward H. Hume (1876–1957) expert on Chinese medicine; from 1938 on a staff member of S.'s Institute.

SIGERIST to CUSHING, Baltimore ?, 22 October 1934

Dear Doctor Cushing:

Let me tell you how much I enjoyed the fragment of your autobiography published in the Atlantic Monthly. It is perfectly delightful that you will have your personal experiences presented in this way. The Institute subscribes to the Atlantic Monthly in order to have a copy of the original presentation of your memoir.

We had a very pleasant summer in Europe. I did some work in France and Belgium during June and July, spent August in Switzerland and September in Italy. I found a great deal of new and interesting material so that my mediaeval work is progressing very nicely. I also had a very pleasant week-end with Klebs. He was very cheerful, working hard on his book which, I am sure, will be a contribution of first-rate importance.

We were sorry that you did not come abroad. It would have given us great pleasure to have you visit us in our little summer house near Lucerne which proved to be extremely satisfactory. It has a garden right on the Lake and good fishing and swimming so that I had an excellent rest there.

I hope that you had a good summer, and that we may meet some day soon. May I ask if there is any chance of your coming down some time for the Noguchi lectures? You know that you will be most welcome on any date you choose.

With warmest regards, I am
  Very sincerely yours,
   [Henry E. Sigerist]

A report on S.'s work in France, Belgium and Italy (Sigerist 1934d). Klebs see C. to S. of 10 January 1927; his book on incunables (Klebs 1938). Noguchi lectures see C. to S. of 15 March 1934.

CUSHING to SIGERIST, New Haven, 24 October 1934

Dear Henry:

So happy to have your letter which was dragged out of you by the articles in the Atlantic Monthly. I was rather dubious about having them published, and of course they are only excerpts from a journal which was written with no expectation of its ever seeing the light of print.

You must have had a grand time last summer. I heard from Klebs that he had had a visit from you. He seems to have been very hard at work of late, and I hope his magnum opus will be far enough along so that he can get it in the printer's hand by the end of the year. I have a deep feeling that it is going to be a very important piece of work.

I have only just begun to pick up my lost threads and the next thing to get behind me is this History of Science meeting which I do hope will go off well.

It strikes me as a very curious organization which appears to be almost wholly in Brasch's hands for a choice of speakers and so on. Still, I suppose that's about the best we can do with such a far-flung body of people as constitute the Council with so many diverse interests. He has left no place for me on the programme to make a speech, which of course is a great relief to me, though Sarton has been pressing me to say something about science and the humanities. I wish I might tap your ventricles to know what you may think of it yourself and what I ought to say.

The Noguchi lectures, perhaps for 1935, are still in my mind, and somewhat on my conscience. I would of course greatly like to do it, but I haven't gotten around to it yet, much less giving you a definite answer.

Always with best regards and greetings to your family, I am
Sincerely yours,
Harvey Cushing

Articles in Atlantic Monthly see S. to C. of 22 October 1934. Klebs see C. to S. of 10 January 1927; his "magnum opus" (Klebs 1938). Frederick E. Brasch, secretary of the History of Science Society. Sarton see C. to S. of 23 May 1934. Noguchi lectures see C. to S. of 15 March 1934.

SIGERIST to CUSHING, Baltimore ?, 5 November 1934

Dear Doctor Cushing:

Mr. Frederick Brasch was here the other day, and we all are most anxious to have you talk at the meeting of the History of Science Society. Science and the Humanities is a splendid subject, and I am sure that nobody is better prepared to discuss it than you.

I was very much distressed to hear that John Fulton, following you [sic] example, has developed a [xxxx], but Winternitz wrote me that he is getting along very well.

I am looking forward to being in New Haven in January. Winternitz is preparing a course on Social Aspects of Medicine and wants me to give a few lectures.

With kind regards, I am
Very sincerely yours,
[Henry E. Sigerist]

Brasch, Fulton, and Winternitz see C. to S. of 24 October 1934, C. to S. of 18 November 1931, and S. to C. of 28 November 1933, respectively. [xxxx] protected health information A. M. Chesney Archives of the Johns Hopkins Medical Institutions.

Cushing to Sigerist, New Haven, 31 December 1934

Dear Henry:

It was so nice to have had a glimpse of you in Washington and I only wish that I had been young enough and vigorous enough to have kept longer on your trail Friday night.

There is one thing of which I meant to speak to you though it escaped my mind. I read with the greatest interest Professor George Hendrickson's article in your Bulletin. I find that he is tremendously interested in the whole history of guaiac and its introduction through Nicholas Pol and others. Do drop him a note (not as coming from me) and ask whether he couldn't be encouraged to persue this aspect of the subject now that he has gotten interested in Fracastorius and his times. It might pull something out of him that would be as interesting and important as the paper you have already published for him.

I saw Winternitz last night and chided him for getting ahead of me in having you and your wife as guests when you come up for your lectures. I shall nevertheless insist on sharing some of your time while here, for there are many things I want to talk over with you.

Always with warm regards, I am

Sincerely yours,

Harvey Cushing

George O. Hendrickson, Yale professor of Latin and Greek Literature; his article (Hendrickson 1934). Guaiac, a drug used against syphilis in the early modern times. Nicolaus Pol (–1546) contributed to the knowledge of guaiac in Europe by his treatise of 1517. Girolamo Fracastoro (1478–1553) Italian physician, anatomist, poet, wrote about syphilis. Winternitz see S. to C. of 28 November 1933.

Sigerist to Cushing, Baltimore ?, 2 January 1935

Dear Doctor Cushing:

It was a very great pleasure to see you in such good health in Washington the other day. I think that the meeting was a great success, and it is certainly most gratifying that the Society is developing in such a splendid way.

As I told you, I am most anxious to print your address in our Bulletin. If you could let me have the manuscript before January 15, I could place your paper at the head of the March number.

I very much hope to see you in New Haven soon, and in the meantime, I am with best wishes

Yours ever

[Henry E. Sigerist]

"Society" of the History of Science. C.'s paper (Cushing 1935).

Sigerist to Cushing, Baltimore ?, 3 January 1935

Dear Doctor Cushing:

I was very glad that you drew my attention to Professor Hendrickson's interest in the history of guaiac. I wrote him immediately and I hope that he will continue his studies on the history of syphilis.

The talk he gave us last winter was most fascinating, and I was glad to print his paper in our Bulletin. I am not quite convinced that he is right in his explanation of the word "syphilis", but it was certainly worthwhile to attack the problem from a somewhat different angle.

With best wishes, I am

Very sincerely yours,

[Henry E. Sigerist]

Hendrickson, his article (Hendrickson 1934) and guaiac see C. to S. of 31 December 1934.

Cushing to Sigerist, New Haven, 4 January 1935

Dear Henry:

Thanks for your letter. I will see if I can get the paper ready for you by the 15th. It needs much improvement, I fear, and now that I have cooled off about it I find difficulty putting my mind on it again. But your letter will spur me to do so.

Always yours,

Harvey Cushing

CUSHING to SIGERIST, New Haven, 9 January 1935

Dear Henry:

Since finishing up and getting the brief address I gave in Washington in somewhat better shape, it seems to me that it hardly deserves going into your journal and that it is the sort of ephemeral skit that had better appear in some less pretentious place. You only heard the first half of it, and the last is rather an appeal for scientists to get off their perch and to devote themselves a little more to sociological problems. This has really so little to do with the history of medicine that I feel your readers would wonder how you happened to accept it for your journal – other than through friendliness to me. Anyhow, I think I had better send it on to Cattell to look over and see what he thinks about it. I will ask him to return it promptly if he does not want it, in which case I should be able to send it on to you by the 15th.

We are all looking forward eagerly to your advent here next week, and I hope you and Mrs. Sigerist are not going to be exhausted by the programme laid out for you.

Always sincerely yours,
Harvey Cushing

C.'s address (Cushing 1935). James McKeen Cattell (1860–1944) psychologist, publisher and editor.

SIGERIST to CUSHING, Baltimore ?, 21 January 1935

Dear Dr. Cushing:

It was a great pleasure seeing you again, and in such good shape. You were extremely good to us and both Mrs. Sigerist and I greatly appreciate your hospitality.

Yale is a great University, and it is the only medical school in this country where I feel at home, besides the Hopkins.

I am so glad that we had a quiet hour in your library. You certainly have one of the most remarkable collections I know of.

The invitations to the meetings of our Medical History Club will be sent to you regularly. As you will see, I am endeavoring to make them attractive. So far, we have had quite good meetings this year.

I also ask the Hopkins Press to send you our new Bulletin which now has started its independent life. In the first number, you will find the talk of Dr. Welch which is very "Popsy".

With kind regards, I am
    Very sincerely yours,
        [Henry E. Sigerist]

Welch see C. to S. of 17 January 1929; "Popsy" was his nickname; he had died in April 1934.

CUSHING to SIGERIST, New Haven, 25 January 1935

Dear Henry:

I hope you and Mrs. Sigerist have reached Baltimore safe and sound, and hope too that you haven't forgotten your week here in New Haven. I am glad that you feel about it as you say that you do in your letter which reached me yesterday.

I have just heard from Cattell saying that he will take my paper partly read before the History of Science Society, and I hasten to write you of this so that you perhaps will not be banking on it yourself. I would have been proud to have it in your nournal [sic], but I think <u>Science</u> is the best place for it as it is something of no permanent value but merely perhaps in a way appropriate to our momentary political needs. I am afraid the scientists won't like it very much, but I shall have to take a chance on that.

    Always affectionately yours,
        Harvey Cushing

Cattell see C. to S. of 9 January 1935. C.'s paper (Cushing 1935).

CUSHING to SIGERIST, New Haven, 12 February 1935

Dear Henry:

Herewith quite a long story. A number of years ago I went to Dr. Welch's rooms with his nephew, Fred Walcott, and found them in the customary mess with a chess problem on the floor and unopened letters on the desk and all the chairs full of magazines and papers of one kind or an-other.

Across the arms of a morris chair was a long box which apparently he had started to open without avail and had simply let it go. Walcott, if I remember correctly, asked the housekeeper if she knew what it was and she said that she didn't but that it had been there for a good many months. I have a vague idea that something was said afterwards to Dr. Welch about it that day jokingly and he replied: "Oh, yes, it's a gold-headed cane that has been sent to me." I had an idea that it was a cane which had been handed on from several people.

Now Fred Walcott's son has just brought me a copy of "The Gold-Headed Cane" which was in Dr. Welch's library and which his father had given him to bring me as a memento. The book has a book-plate of Harold C. Ernst, and within it is a letter addressed to Dr. Welch from Mrs. Ernst saying that she was mistaken when she wrote previously in that the "wood of which the box is made came from the Medical School building on Boylston Street whereas Dr. Ernst had left a record to say that it had come from the old Medical School building on North Grove Street". In this letter was enclosed a sealed envelope on which she had written: "Key to box containing gold-headed cane". On the envelope, which is very much soiled and faded and looks as though it had been lying around for a long time, Dr. Welch has written: "Mrs. Ernst". The post-mark reads "Boston January 3, 1924".

Do let me know whether there is any such box that might contain a replica of the gold-headed cane or any record anywhere that has come to light among Dr. Welch's papers that such a cane had been passed on to him by Harold C. Ernst of Boston. The box to which I refer as having seen was merely a pine box which I suppose may have concealed a box holding the cane to which this is the key.

I shall be very much interested to know whether you can shed any light on this; and if you find such a box wanting a key, I shall promptly send it to you.

Always sincerely yours,

H.C.

Welch see C. to S. of 17 January 1929; he had died the year before this letter was written. Harold C. Ernst, Harvard bacteriologist. *Gold-Headed Cane* (Macmichael 1828).

Sigerist to Cushing, Baltimore ?, 15 February 1935

Dear Dr, Cushing:

I read with greatest pleasure your presidential address in Science. I agree with you that this was the better place for the publication of the address as it reaches a much larger public.

Thanks for your very interesting letter. I will see what I can find and will let you know as soon as I have a result.

Very sincerely yours,
[Henry E. Sigerist]

Address in Science (Cushing 1935).

Sigerist to Cushing, Baltimore ?, 25 February 1935

Dear Dr. Cushing:

Miss Broemer, Dr. Welch's secretary, remembers that a few years ago Dr. Welch sent the box with the cane to a friend. He passed it on. Unfortunately, we have so far been unable to find out who this friend was. The box was carried to the Express Company by one of the Library boys. This must have been between 1929 and 1932. That is to say, after the opening of the Library and before I joined the Hopkins.

We are now hunting for the friend, and as soon as I find any trace of him, I shall let you know.

Very sincerely yours,
[Henry E. Sigerist]

The Welch Medical Library of the Johns Hopkins medical institutions was opened in 1929.

Sigerist to Cushing, Baltimore ?, 13 May 1935

Dear Dr. Cushing:

I am very sorry that I will not be able to hear your memorial address on the occasion of the dedication of the Beaumont Memorial Highway.

I received a very kind invitation, but unfortunately could not accept it as we are sailing for Europe on May 25th.

I had news of you through Dr. Fulton, in Atlantic City the other day, and heard that you intend going abroad also. If you go to Switzerland, I hope that you will pass through Lucerne and will drop in to see us. Our address there will be Haus Utohorn, Kastanienbaum. I am going to Russia first, but will be in Switzerland toward the end of August.

I am looking forward to sailing soon. Eight months of daily routine without a break are a very long time.

With kind regards, I am
    Very sincerely yours,
        [Henry E. Sigerist]

CUSHING to SIGERIST, New Haven, 16 May 1935

Dear Henry:

Thanks for your letter. I wish that I might look forward to seeing you at Lebanon on June the 1st, but I would be embarrassed to see you there knowing how much better you could say something worthy of Beaumont on the occasion than I could. I wish that I might have gotten down to the meeting at Atlantic City. Fulton told me how enjoyable it was and how pleased he was to see you there.

No chance, alas, of my dropping in on you at Lucerne. I should like to do so to have a first-hand account on your experiences in Russia, but I shall have to wait until you get back for that pleasure.

Do give my warm regards to the family, and with best wishes for a profitable and interesting vacation, I am
    Always affectionately yours,
        Harvey Cushing

P.S. Do you by any possibility know of anyone who may be going to the Congress in Madrid? The Government is gunning for someone to send as a representative from this country.

Lebanon, CT, birthplace of William Beaumont (1785–1853) physician and physiologist. Madrid was the site of the International Congress of the History of Medicine.

Cushing to Sigerist, New Haven, 17 May 1935

Dear Henry:

Do you know Bergson's collection of essays called "La pensée et le Mouvant" which has gone into many editions? If you do, you will remember his essay on "the philosophy of Claude Bernard". Klebs has taken the trouble to translate this essay and to submit it to Bergson for his corrections of the translation. Both Fulton and I think that it ought to be published, to which Klebs agrees but insists that his name not appear. However, I think it might be possible to formulate a little introductory note and perhaps include Bergson's letter to Klebs.

I owe you an apology for having sent my History of Science Society skit to Science rather than to you, and I would like to make amends by sending you this translation should you care for it and think it suitable to publish in your Bulletin.

Hoping this may catch you before you get away, I am

Always yours,

H. C.

Henri Bergson (1859–1941) French philosopher; his collection (Bergson 1934). Claude Bernard (1813–1878) French physiologist. Klebs see C. to S. of 10 January 1927; his translation (Bergson 1936).

Sigerist to Cushing, Baltimore ?, 20 May 1935

Dear Dr. Cushing:

Nothing would give me greater pleasure than to publish Klebs' translation of Bergson's essay on Claude Bernard. I hope you can persuade Klebs to give it to me. It certainly should be published and the Bulletin would undoubtedly be a good place for it. You probably saw that in the last number we had a paper on Claude Bernard by Dr. Olmstead [sic], and I am sure that Bergson's essay would be most welcome to the readers of the Bulletin.

I am very disappointed that I shall not see you in Switzerland this summer. We are sailing in a few days.

Dr. Krumbhaar of the University of Pennsylvania is going to Madrid and, as he happens to be president of the American Association of Medical History, I think it would be most appropriate to appoint him official delegate to the Congress.

Wishing you a good summer, I am with best wishes
Very sincerely yours,
[Henry E. Sigerist]

Paper on Claude Bernard (Olmsted 1935). Krumbhaar, Edward B. (1882–1966) pathologist and founder of AAHM in 1929.

CUSHING to SIGERIST, New Haven, 21 May 1935

Dear Henry:

Thanks for your letter. Not knowing when the next issue of your Bulletin is to be published or who is going to represent you during your absence abroad which I suppose will be for the full summer, I am sending you a copy of Klebs' translation together with a letter from Bergson to Klebs, regarding the same. I think if you cared to write a preliminary note to say that you cherish the opportunity of publishing a translation of this essay about Bernard written by a philosopher and translated by his friend and neighbor, a medical historian, as made clear by the letter that passed between them, it would be all that would be necessary.

When Klebs first sent the translation on and it was suggested that it ought to be published somewhere, he raised no objection but requested that his name be left out of it entirely. I think with the publication of Bergson's letter Klebs' relation to the matter would be perfectly well answered.

You may, however, very possibly see him in Switzerland while you are abroad and perhaps can take up personally with him the question of using Bergson's letter.

Always sincerely yours,
Harvey Cushing

Henri Bergson and Claude Bernard see C. to S. of 17 May 1935.

Dear Dr. Cushing:

Thanks ever so much for your letter of May 21st, and the manuscript. The translation is excellent and I shall be delighted to publish it in our Bulletin.

Our July number is in print already, and during August and September we will not publish any numbers. The paper therefore will be published in the fall, and this will give me a chance to talk the matter over with Klebs when I see him in Switzerland in September. I am most anxious that the paper be published, conforming to his wishes.

With kind regards, I am
    Very sincerely yours,
      [Henry E. Sigerist]

"Manuscript" of Klebs' translation of Bergson's essay on Claude Bernard (Bergson 1936).

SIGERIST to CUSHING, Baltimore ?, 21 October 1935

Dear Dr. Cushing:

I am back after an exceedingly interesting and busy summer. I spend [sic] nearly three months in Russia, travelling all over the country as far south as Armenia and I saw and heard a great deal.

I saw Klebs twice and we were all very disappointed that you did not come abroad this year. Then I attended the International Medical History Congress in Madrid. Spain was lovely at this time of year, and the Spaniards certainly gave us a grand reception.

By the way, the Committee of the International Society of the History of Medicine was very much in favor of holding its next International Congress in 1938 in the United States. I have the impression that the formal invitation would be welcomed and accepted. Krumbhaar and I were rather hesitant as we would not like to have the Congress here unless we were sure that we could make it a success. What do you think of the scheme? You had experience with the International Physiology Congress. I wonder if it would be possible to raise sufficient funds so as to reduce the expenses of the trip for the members. Such a Congress would, of course, stimulate the interest in the subject in this country tremendously.

It occurred to me that if the Congress were postponed to 1939 when the World's Fair will be held in New York, it might be easier to obtain reductions with the steamship companies.

I would very much like to hear your ideas about the matter. The International Committee is having a meeting on February 1st in Paris and the formal invitation ought to be in their hands before that date.

May I remind you that we are still hoping to see you here as Noguchi lecturer this winter. Any date that suits you will be convenient to us. I am sending you under separate cover a copy of the last year's lectures which, I am sure, will interest you.

With kindest regards, I am
Very sincerely yours,
[Henry E. Sigerist]

In Madrid S. was awarded his first honorary degree. Krumbhaar see S. to C. of 20 May 1935. The 1938 Congress of the International Society of the History of Medicine was not held in the U.S. but in Yugoslavia instead.

CUSHING to SIGERIST, New Haven, 23 October 1935

Dear Henry:
So glad to have your nice letter of October 21st telling me something of your summer movements. I knew of course that you had seen Klebs who wrote me about his visits with you.

The Madrid meeting must have been excellent and I wish that I might have been there with you to have seen Spain in the autumn. The only time I was ever there was in the late winter of '15 when it was wet and cold.

I wish I knew what to say about the Society of the History of Medicine coming here for 1938. I think we could swing it; but your suggestion of waiting until the following year when the congressists might have better rates offered to them owing to the World's Fair in New York is an excellent one and I rather think after conferring with Krumbhaar and others I would put that up to the Committee.

I by no means have forgotten your open invitation to come and give the Noguchi Lectures. But alas, I am pretty decrepit and I don't think there is any prospect of my doing so this year. I have been working all summer on my War diary which is going to be published sometime, and have had no energy for anything else. In fact, I have been here without interruption all these months because of my decrepitude; and though it sounds rather forlorn, I have had an enjoyable time with other people who similarly have had reason for foregoing a summer vacation.

Always with warm regards and greetings to the family, I am

Sincerely yours,

Harvey Cushing

Meetings in Madrid and presumably the in U. S. see S. to C. of 21 October 1935. War diary (Cushing 1936).

CUSHING to SIGERIST, New Haven, 26 October 1935

Dear Henry:

Thanks hugely for sending me Gregory Zilboorg's book which I read with the greatest interest, having a copy of the Witch's Hammer on my shelves and not heretofore having known much about it.

It is truly a remarkable story and very well told, and I am glad to have been put on Johann Weyer's trail for he is in the class with the Tukes and Pinel and others, though it was long after his time when they saw the light.

I wish that I might put together some Noguchi Lectures for you as good as these, but I think there is small chance of that in my present decrepit state.

Always sincerely yours,

H. C.

Gregory Zilboorg (1890–1959) psychiatrist in New York, friend of S.'s; (Zilboorg 1935). Witch's Hammer (Sprenger 1487/1906), pamphlet of a dominican inquisitor. Johann Weyer (1515–1588) physician, early writer against witchcraft. William Tuke (1732–1822) early psychiatrist who founded the asylum Retreat in England. Philippe Pinel (1745–1826) French physician and psychiatrist.

SIGERIST to CUSHING, Baltimore ?, 30 October 1935

Dear Dr. Cushing:

Thanks ever so much for your two letters. I was very sorry to hear that your health was not so good, but do not say that you are decrepit; this seems a terrible exaggeration.

I am very glad you liked the little volume of Zilboorg. It has been very well received and we even have a request for a French translation. I wish we could have such a volume of yours. At any rate, you know that the invitation is always open.

I shall be in New Haven in March but sincerely hope to see you before that.

With kindest regards, I am
Very sincerely yours,
[Henry E. Sigerist]

Zilboorg see C. to S. of 26 October 1935.

CUSHING to SIGERIST, New Haven, 11 November 1935

Dear Henry:

I understand that a young man named Scott Buchanan was working with you last winter; also that he has written a book about Galen and Galenic medicine which I have been requested to read and criticise.

Before I put my nose to this task, can you tell me something about him and of the nature of his studies and how important they may be? He sounds to me rather visionary.

Always yours,
Harvey Cushing

Scott M. Buchanan (1895–1968) professor of philosophy and educator; see also S. to C. of 14 November 1935; his book on Galen not identified.

Dear Dr. Cushing:

Scott Buchanan, associate professor of philosophy at the University of Virginia, was with us during the academic year 1933 to 1934. He came on a fellowship of the Josiah Macy, Jr. Foundation. Dr. Kast wanted to know how a philosopher would look at medicine.

Buchanan spent most of his time attending lectures, courses and clinics all over the Medical School, and doing some historical research particularly on Galen, in our Department.

I found him a rather confused mind. I could never find out what he really wanted and I had the impression that he did not quite know himself. He was very interested in mediaeval philosophy, particularly in scholasticism. I was quite glad when he left as I could not do much with him.

I have heard of the book, but have not seen it yet. I wonder what it is like.

Very sincerely yours,
    [Henry E. Sigerist]

Buchanan see C. to S. of 11 November 1935. Dr. Kast not identified.

CUSHING to SIGERIST, New Haven, 15 November 1935

Dear Henry:

Thanks for your illuminating note about Scott Buchanan. I have read his dissertation with interest but at the same time with great labour. I find the lingo of the philosopher extraordinarily difficult to follow. His general thesis seems to be that we must get back to Galen, who was both a philosopher and a physician, if we really wish to accomplish anything in what he looks upon as a crisis in modern medicine.

I suppose you must have seen Hans Zinsser's jovial book about the biography of the louse, in which he impudently quotes a paragraph from Alfred Whitehead and Gertrude Stein side by side as being equally unintelligible.

My friend Northrup here, however, tells me that the philosophers regard Buchanan as one of the most brilliant and promising of their kind among the younger generation. So I take it that there is something lacking in my own make-up that I find the MS. difficult to follow.

You will remember Lincoln's reply to someone who asked him how long a man's legs ought to be. He said: "Long enough to reach from his body to the ground." I have a feeling about Buchanan that his legs aren't quite that long. But then, he is young and he may perhaps live to see them elongated.

Always yours,
Harvey Cushing

Buchanan see letters of 11 and 14 November 1935. Hans Zinsser (1878–1940) Harvard bacteriologist and epidemiologist; (Zinsser 1985). Alfred Whitehead (1861–1947) British mathematician and philosopher. Gertrude Stein (1874–1946) American writer and patron of the arts. Northrup not identified.

Cushing to Sigerist, New Haven, 3 March 1936

Dear Henry:

I am just out and around again after two long months in hospital and have come upon the bundle of papers from the Institute which you were so kind as to send me. I am delighted to have them, and they will be filed where they can be gotten at and made useful to as many people as possible. It's a most creditable lot of work for you to have sponsored.

Always with warm regards, I am
Sincerely yours,
H.C.

Sigerist to Cushing, Baltimore ?, 9 March 1936

Dear Dr. Cushing:

I was so glad to hear that you are at home again after these two long months in the hospital. We always had news about you through Miss Goodwillie.

I am going to attend a students' conference in New Haven Saturday and Sunday, and hope that I will be able to drop in at your home some time Sunday afternoon. At any rate, I shall call you up. I am staying with Winslow who is running the students' conference.

 With kind regards, I am
  Very sincerely yours,
   [Henry E. Sigerist]

Miss Goodwillie, possibly C.'s secretary. C.-E. A. Winslow (1877–1957) Yale professor of Public Health.

Sigerist to Cushing, Baltimore, 22 May 1936

Dear Dr. Cushing:

 I do not remember if I told you before that we intended to devote a special number of the Bulletin to the memory of Garrison. The number is to contain a bibliography and a number of essays illustrating the various aspects of Garrison's personality and work. I know that you used to have quite a correspondence with Garrison at the time, and I know that with your inimitable skill in portraying people, you could make a most delightful contribution. Garrison's was such a complex personality that it is difficult to do him justice; but I think that such a number in which the librarian, the historian, the musician, the man, would be portrayed by various people could convey an idea of who Garrison was. I feel that without you the number would be utterly incomplete, and I would be delighted if you would accept to contribute an essay to this number. You could make it as short or as long as you would like; you could insert passages from his letters just as you wish. There is no hurry. I would like to have the manuscripts together in October so that we could publish the number in January or February.

 I hate to impose upon you, but I know that not only I myself, but all who knew and liked Garrison would greatly appreciate a contribution from your pen.

 We are sailing Monday. It was a busy winter but it was worthwhile.

 With best wishes, I am always
  Very sincerely yours,
   [Henry E. Sigerist]

This is the only copy of a letter of S. showing the letter-head of Baltimore. Garrison see C. to S. of 9 November 1931. Garrison memorial number of the Bulletin of the History of Medicine (Sigerist 1937).

CUSHING to SIGERIST, New Haven, 27 May 1936

Dear Henry:

Thanks for your letter. I'll try to put my hand to it and see what I can do with a note about Garrison for your October number. I am glad to know that you are getting away for your annual vacation. I suppose you will be sojourning again on the Lake of Geneva and trust that you will see Klebs. I hear from him frequently and he seems to be in good fettle.

Always sincerely yours,

H. C.

Garrison see C. to S. of 9 November 1931. Klebs see C. to S. of 10 January 1927.

SIGERIST to CUSHING, Baltimore ?, 10 October 1936

Dear Dr. Cushing:

I just came back from Europe after four interesting and very delightful months spent in Russia and Switzerland.

I saw Klebs and John Fulton, and you probably heard that we had a very delightful trip together to the meeting of the Swiss Society of the History of Medicine and Science.

I am perfectly delighted that you are willing to contribute an article to our Garrison memorial number. I received some very good papers, and I hope to be able to publish the number some time in January or February. If you could let me have your manuscript some time in November, I would greatly appreciate it.

I hope that you are well and that you had a good summer, and with kind regards, I am

Very sincerely yours,

[Henry E. Sigerist]

S. refers to his second study tour in the Soviet Union. Garrison memorial number see S. to C. of 22 May 1936; (Sigerist 1937). Fulton see C. to S. of 18 November 1931.

CUSHING to SIGERIST, New Haven, 12 October 1936

Dear Henry:

So glad to have your letter, but I am horrified to think that I may have intimated to you that I could do something in Garrison's memory for the memorial number you are putting together in his honour. I alas have already booked myself up more deeply than I should have done, and this past month have begun to get my nose into a brain tumor paper that has long been overdue. To switch off from this to F.G.H. [sic] would require more nimble pen than I in my present dotage possess.

I had all his letters bound this summer, and Major Hume has been looking them over for a paper which he is writing, possibly for your same number. If that is the case, he will have stolen such thunder as I might have had. Still, I see that you give me until November so that I will mull it over and if by any possibility I can do something that I think worthy of him, I will endeavour not to fail you.

I wish that I might have been with you and Fulton and Klebs on that trip you took together.

Always with warm regards and greetings to the family, I am
> Sincerely yours,
> > Harvey Cushing

F. H. Garrison number see S. to C. of 22 May 1936. C.'s paper on brain tumors is probably (Cushing / Eisenhardt 1938). Major Edgar Erskine Hume; his paper on Garrison (Hume 1937). The Garrison Memorial Number (Sigerist 1937) does not contain an article of C.

SIGERIST to CUSHING, Baltimore ?, 15 October 1936

Dear Dr. Cushing:

Thanks ever so much for your letter of October 12th. I just found out that I can not possibly publish the Garrison number before February. This would leave time for the manuscripts up to the middle of December, and I do hope that this will leave you sufficient time to write something for the memorial number.

I just received yours and Fulton's bibliographical study on Galvani and Aldini. It is splendid and I am delighted to see it out.

With kind regards, I am
Very sincerely yours,
[Henry E. Sigerist]

Luigi Galvani (1737–1798) Italian physician and scientist. Giovanni Aldini (1762–1834) physicist, nephew and editor of Galvani. The Cushing and Fulton study on Galvani and Aldini (Cushing/Fulton 1936).

CUSHING to SIGERIST, New Haven, 13 December 1938

Dear Henry:

I shall of course wish to continue my membership in the History of Medicine Association. I believe I already subscribe [sic] five dollars for the Bulletin; and if that covered the dues for regular members, that is all to the good.

It was grand to have seen you here a short time ago looking so fit and well.

Always with regards from house to house, I am
Sincerely yours,
Harvey Cushing

The gap of two years since the last letter is likely to be due to lost letters or else to frequent contacts by visits or telephone calls. In November 1938 S. gave the three Terry Lectures at Yale which were published in book form (Sigerist 1941); S.'s progressive views on socialized medicine (social insurance) were beyond Cushing's conservative views (Fulton 1946,703).

SIGERIST to CUSHING, Baltimore ?, 20 December 1938

Dear Dr. Cushing:

Many thanks for your kind note of December 13. The Bulletin will be sent to you through the AAHM in the future and the dues to the Association cover the price of the subscription. I am glad to say that the response to my circular letter was extremely gratifying. We are receiving new applications for membership every day.

It was such a pleasure to see you the other day and I shall never forget the delightful evening at John's house.

With all good wishes for Christmas and the New Year, I am

Yours very sincerely,

[Henry E. Sigerist]

AAHM: American Association for the History of Medicine. "John" Fulton, see C. to S. of 18 November 1931.

SIGERIST to CUSHING, Baltimore ?, 7 January 1939

Dear Dr. Cushing:

I just received a letter from India from a Dr. D. V. Subba Reddy who is very interested in medical history and has written a few papers for our Bulletin. He tells me that he found in the records of Fort St. George a name, "Bernard Ozler" who apparently was in India in the 17th century. He would like to know whether this "Ozler" had any relationship with Sir William. You are the only one who could possibly know.

With kind regards, I am

Yours most sincerely,

[Henry E. Sigerist]

D. V. Subba Reddy (1899–1987) medical historian in India. Fort St. George is the name of the first British fortress in India, founded in 1639. "Sir William" Osler, see C. to S. of 2 December 1933. Cushing had written a voluminous biography of Osler (Cushing 1925).

CUSHING to SIGERIST, New Haven, 9 January 1939

Dear Henry:

Thanks for your note. I don't believe the XVIIth century Bernard Ozler could have had anything to do with W. O., though anything is possible, as I suppose Cornish people were apt to be seafaring travellers and some of them may well enough have gone to India. I did not undertake to trace the family back of his father, Featherstone, though I have a vague recollection that there were some relatives that had emigrated to another country, possibly New Zealand. Willie Francis possibly might know about this and I will send the letter on to him and ask him to answer it.

Always yours
Harvey Cushing

W. O.: William Osler, see S. to C. of 7 January 1939. William W. Francis, physician, medical historian, librarian of the Osler Library in Montreal. According to C. (Cushing 1925) Osler's ancestor, the reverend Featherstone L. Osler, emigrated from Cornwall to Canada in 1837.

CUSHING to SIGERIST, New Haven, 13 January 1939

Dear Henry:

I have just received this note from H. P. Bayon and would like to get your reaction to it before replying.

With greetings to Mrs. Sigerist and all good wishes to you both for the New Year I am

Sincerely yours,
Harvey Cushing

H. P. Bayon, medical historian.

CUSHING to SIGERIST, New Haven, 17 January 1939

Dear Henry:

Here is a pathetic appeal from Max Neuburger. Do you think that anything could be done for him through your Institute? Could he not be asked over to give some lectures? He is an unusual person and fully entitled to receive some help and recognition from us. Please return his letter with your comment.

Always affectionately yours,
Harvey Cushing

Max Neuburger (1868–1955) Professor of Medical History in Vienna. After the occupation of Austria by Nazi-Germany in 1938, Neuburger as a Jew was forced to leave his country and emigrated 1939 to England.

SIGERIST to CUSHING, Baltimore ?, 19 January 1939

Dear Dr. Cushing:

It would be splendid to have a new edition of Garrison's book and I wish ways and means could be found to achieve this. The book, however, will need a good deal of editing as it contains not a few mistakes. I personally could not do it as I disagree with Garrison's historical views in many respects, but I should think that men like Francis or Malloch would be well qualified for the job.

You probably know that Krumbhaar is translating Castiglioni's HISTORY OF MEDICINE for Knopf. This will compete with Garrison's book and yet the two are so different that there undoubtedly is room for both.

With kind regards, I am
Yours very sincerely,
[Henry E. Sigerist]

C.'s appeal for Neuburger in the last letter is answered by Sigerist in his next letter. Garrison's book (Garrison 1913); a fourth edition had appeared in 1929 and was reprinted in 1960. Francis see C. to S. of 9 January 1939. Archibald Malloch, librarian at the New York Academy of Medicine. Krumbhaar see S. to C. of 20 May 1935. Arturo Castiglioni (1874–1953) Italian medical historian, from 1939 to 1946 exiled in the U.S.; (Castiglioni 1941). Knopf, publisher.

SIGERIST to CUSHING, Baltimore ?, 25 January 1939

Dear Dr. Cushing:

I know the desperate situation of Max Neuburger and since last spring, I have tried to find some kind of a position for him, unfortunately without any success. I am afraid that there is nothing I can do for him at the Institute. We are already six teaching medical history and I have three Germans in the Institute. I cannot possibly crowd the place with refugees quite apart from the fact that our funds are very limited.

If some other university in the country would be willing to give him some kind of an honorary chair, I think it should be possible to obtain funds to provide Professor Neuburger at least a bare living.

The situation seems to be very urgent and you probably will have heard from Sir D'Arcy Power that some of us will pledge a hundred dollars a year to allow Professor Neuburger to live in England.

I am returning the letter enclosed and with kind regards, I am

Yours very sincerely,

[Henry E. Sigerist]

Neuburger see C. to S. of 17 January 1939. From his early days as a medical historian S. admired Neuburger; he actively helped Jewish refugees to obtain jobs in the U.S., but Neuburger at age 71 could certainly not claim priority. The six teachers in S.'s staff were, in addition to himself: O. Temkin, J. R. Oliver, L. Edelstein, S. V. Larkey, E. H. Hume. The three Germans in S.'s Institute were Temkin, Edelstein, and Otto Neustätter.

D'Arcy Power (1855–1841) British surgeon and medical historian. A letter of John F. Fulton to D'Arcy Power in the matter of Neuburger (1939, undated) mentions that Neuburger's son has been placed in New York and that Fulton, C., and S. are trying to do something for Neuburger; Fulton then adds: "If anything should turn up that would seem suitable for Neuburger, I will let you know at once. I sincerely hope the Society for the Protection of Science and Learning will be able to do something for him. The barbarity of the present hysteria in the Reich [Germany] transcends anything we have known since the age of Nero."

Sigerist to Cushing, Baltimore ?, 16 May 1939

Dear Dr. Cushing:

It gives me great pleasure to inform you that the American Association of the History of Medicine at its annual meeting held in Atlantic City on May 1, 1939 has unanimously elected you an

Honorary Member

of the Association. The diploma will follow in due time, but I wish to congratulate you and I hope that you will continue to take an active part in the work of the Association.

With kind regards, I am

Yours very sincerely,

[Henry E. Sigerist]

S. writes as secretary of the American Association of the History of Medicine (AAHM).

CUSHING to SIGERIST, New Haven, 18 May 1939

Dear Henry:

Nothing could have given me greater gratification than to learn from your note that I have been made an honorary member of the American Association of the History of Medicine. Little as I deserve such a tribute, I nevertheless am greatly complimented.

I heard glowing accounts of your last history week in Baltimore and wish I might have been there to participate in it. But as you are aware, I am pretty much tied to the stake here by my physical incapacitation.

With greetings to your wife, I am

Always affectionately yours,

Harvey Cushing

"History week": 2nd Graduate Week in the History of Medicine at S.'s Institute 24–29 April 1939 for postgraduate education, with 39 participants from 16 states. C.'s "incapacitation": mainly problems with an ulcer and with his circulatory system. He died of a myocardial infarction on 7 October 1939. S. being in Europe and South Africa the rest of the year, this seems to be the last letter of his correspondence with S.

2.3. Literature

Baumgartner, Leona: *Harvey Cushing as Book Collector and Litterateur.* Bull. Hist. Med. 8, 1055–1066, 1940.

Bergson, Henri: *La pensée et le mouvant. Essais et conférences.* Paris 1934.

Bergson Henri: *The Philosophy of Claude Bernard.* (Translated by A. C. Klebs). Bull. Hist. Med. 4, 15–21, 1936.

Bliss, Michael: *Harvey Cushing, a Life in Surgery.* New York 2005.

Castiglioni, Arturo: *A History of Medicine.* New York 1941.

Cushing, Harvey: *The Life of Sir William Osler.* Oxford 1925.

Cushing, Harvey: *The Humanizing of Science.* Science 81, 137–143, 1935.

Cushing, Harvey: *From a Surgeon's Journal, 1915–1918.* Boston 1936.

Cushing, Harvey: *Bio-bibliography of Andreas Vesalius.* New York 1943.

Cushing, Harvey / Eisenhardt, Louise: *Meningiomas, their Classification, Regional Behaviour, Life History, and Surgical Results.* Baltimore 1938.

Cushing, Harvey / Fulton, John F.: *A Bibliographical Study of the Galvani and the Aldini Writings on Animal Electricity.* Ann. Sci. 1, 239–268,1936.

Davey, Lycurgus M.: *Harvey Cushing and the Humanities in Medicine.* J. Hist. Med. Allied Sciences 24, 119–124, 1969.

Fulton, John F.: *Harvey Cushing, a Biography.* Springfield, IL 1946.

Garrison, Fielding H.: *An Introduction to the History of Medicine.* Philadelphia 1913.

Hendrickson, G. L.: *The "Syphilis" of Girolamo Fracastoro.* Bull. Hist. Med. 2, 515–546, 1934.

Hume, Edgar Erskin: *Garrison and the Army Medical Library, 1891–1930.* Bull. Hist. Med. 5, 301–346, 1937.

Klebs, Arnold C.: *Incunabula scientifica et medica. Short Title List.* Osiris, Bruges 4, 1–359, 1938.

Macmichael, William: *Gold-Headed Cane.* London 1828.

Olmsted, James M.D.: *The Contemplative Works of Claude Bernard.* Bull. Hist. Med. 3, 335–354, 1935.

Sigerist, Henry E., ed.: *The Seven Defensions of Paracelsus of 1564.* Leipzig 1928.

Sigerist, Henry E.: *Vorwort.* Kyklos 2, 5–7, 1929.

Sigerist, Henry E.: *American Medicine.* New York 1934a. (Translated from German).

Sigerist, Henry E.: *Medical Societies, Past and Present.* Yale J. Biol. Med. 6, 351–362, 1934b.

Sigerist, Henry E.: *On the Teaching of Medical History. A Tentative Syllabus for a Course in the History of Medicine.* Bull. Hist. Med. 2, 123–139, 1934c.

Sigerist, Henry E.: *A Summer of Research in European Libraries.* Bull. Hist. Med. 2, 559–610, 1934d.

Sigerist, Henry E.: *Garrison Memorial Number.* Bull. Hist. Med. 5, 299–403, 1937.

Sigerist, Henry E.: *Medicine and Human Welfare.* New Haven 1941.

Sigerist, Henry E.: *Harvey Cushing*. In "Grosse Aerzte", 3rd ed. München 1954, 391–400. (This chapter on Cushing is missing in the English translation "The Great Doctors" of 1958).

Sprenger, Jakob (1438–1494): *Malleus maleficarum* (Witch's Hammer). Berlin 1906.

Zilboorg, Gregory: *The Medical Man and the Witch During the Renaissance*. Baltimore 1935.

Zinsser, Hans: *Rats, Lice and History: Being a Study in Biography, …* London 1985.

2.4. Name Index

3. Correspondence
Henry E. Sigerist – Fielding H. Garrison
1923–1934

3.1. Introduction

3.1.1. Fielding H. Garrison (1870–1935)

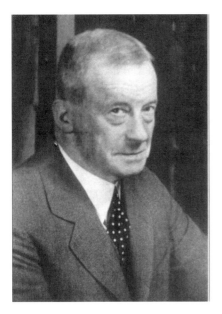

Fielding Hudson Garrison was born in Washington, DC, on 5 November 1870. In 1890 he obtained his B. A. from Johns Hopkins University in Baltimore when his teacher John Shaw Billings engaged him as assistant librarian of the Surgeon Generals's Library (now National Library of Medicine) in Washington. This library was under the direction of Billings who taught Garrison the librarian skills. Garrison started work there while studying medicine at Georgetown University, obtaining his M. D. in 1893. The Library belonging to the Army, Garrison was also obliged to start a military career. In 1909 he married Clara Brown, and in 1920/21 he served as a lieutenant colonel in Manila. Still as assistant librarian he retired at age 60 in 1930 to become director of the Johns Hopkins' Welch Medical Library and at the same time Resident Lecturer in the history of medicine, first under William H. Welch and then under Henry E. Sigerist. He became president of the Johns Hopkins Medical History Club and assumed executive duties during Welch's absence in Europe. He died on 18 April 1935 of an intestinal cancer.

Garrison was an indefatigable worker. He continued Billings' bibliographical *Index Catalogue of the Surgeon General's Library* and, together with Robert H. Fletcher, founded *Index Medicus* in 1903. He started his *Texts Illustrating the History of Medicine* (Garrison 1912) which were continued by Morton and others well into the 1990s in many new editions. At the same time he finished work on his voluminous *Introduction to the*

History of Medicine (Garrison 1913), a textbook based on his bibliographical work, that was followed by many updated editions. It was still reprinted in 1961 and for decades was the leading textbook. In addition, he wrote over 200 smaller works, among them a biography of Billings (Garrison 1915) and studies on anatomical illustration and on American medicine (Garrison 1926, 1933). There are also works on music, poetry, as well as book reviews. All this was achieved while Garrison suffered under the burden of daily bibliographical work. He was awarded honorary degrees from Georgetown University in 1917 and from Yale in 1933.

Garrison was a modest man with an impressive cultural background, knowledgable in classical and modern languages, a gifted writer more than a rhetorician. He became a propagator of medical history at his time. Yet his passion was music. The basic tragedy of his life was that "he was an artist by nature, with all the sensitivity of such, and that circumstances compelled him to spend all his life in administrative work that he loathed …" (Sigerist 1939). This made him melancholy at times and at the end of his life even bitter about his isolation. In these states of mind his wife Clara had a soothing influence.

For literature about Garrison see (Sigerist 1935, 1937, 1939), (Sigerist et al. 1937), (Kagan 1938, 1948), (Cope 1962), (Ackerknecht 1970), (Zinn 1999). A list of Garrison's works containing 235 titles (not quite complete) was prepared by (Mayer 1937).

3.1.2. The Correspondence

Unlike the other correspondences of this volume the Sigerist-Garrison corerspondence is clearly incomplete since after 1931 most of Sigerist's letters are missing. Thus, certain details in the correspondence remain unintelligible without the return letters.

Through their common friend, Arnold C. Klebs, Sigerist and Garrison may have known each other before the beginning of their correspondence. After a lone letter from Garrison of 1923 a relatively dense correspondence begins in 1926 and extends to 1934, the year before Garrison's death, with a total of 21 letters of Sigerist and 51 letters written by Garrison. In 1926 Sigerist is a young professor in Leipzig, 35 years old, while Garrison is 56, approaching the final stage of his career as a medical historian. Despite the difference in age, most of the correspondence witnesses mutual respect throughout these years.

Short as the period from 1926 to 1934 may be, one has to consider four distinct parts:

1) The letters of 1926 to 1931 show the development of the relationship first of Sigerist and Garrison and then between the Institutes of Leipzig and Baltimore.
2) In 1931/32 Sigerist is invited for a study tour in the U.S. Both correspondents are involved in the preparations and they also exchange letters during the tour.
3) Sigerist, back in Leipzig during the summer of 1932, accepts the Johns Hopkins chair offered to him, and both Sigerist and Garrison are looking forward to their collaboration in Baltimore. Garrison orders books through Sigerist in Leipzig.
4) Even though working under the same roof in 1933 and 1934, there are still seven letters by Garrison. The first two of them are completely out of tune, showing an irritated and depressed Garrison. Then he finds back to business as usual and to a harmonious cooperation.

Many topics are dealt with in these letters in addition to the history of medicine and related business. Some 30 books and other works are mentioned as well as 90 names of persons. Sigerist's letters of the early Leipzig period are written in German, a language Garrison obviously was familiar with. These German letters have been translated by the editor.

Sigerist dedicated his book on American medicine to Garrison: "Fielding H. Garrison, pioneer in medical history in the United States, co-worker and friend" (Sigerist 1933). After Garrison's death he said of his letters: "While Garrison was very reserved in personal contacts he was exuberant in his letters. His moods and whatever worried him found expression in his letters. Letter-writing was his way to free himself from oppressing thoughts and he not seldom passed harsh judgments on matters and people" (Sigerist et al. 1937). Another observer said: "His letters are revealing, full of thoughts, interspearsed with foreign language sentences, citations, confessions, and remembrances" (Cope 1962).

All of Sigerist's letters are typed, while many of Garrison's are in longhand. The letters are stored at the Archives of Yale University Library and of the Leipzig University Archive.

3.2. The Letters

GARRISON to SIGERIST, Manila, 18 August 1923

My dear Doctor Sigerist:

Enclosed herewith are the proofs of the first part of my article on "The Newer Epidemiology", for the Sudhoff Festschrift, which Dr. Singer has kindly sent me. I trust that the proof corrections will be intelligible and that I may be able to see the remainder of the proofs in due course. It was not clear from Dr. Singer's letter whether I was to send the enclosed proofs to you or to him, but I have taken the shortest path.

I want to thank you very much for the most interesting publications you have sent me, particularly the larger monograph on the recipes. They are all achieved with masterly ability and are highly illuminative of the subjects dealt with; indeed, it may please you to know that Sudhoff wrote me that he regards you as by far the most promising of all the younger medical historians of Europe, so that all I can say is: much power to your elbow in your future work. I have received several charming letters from my old friend Dr. Arnold Klebs, and think Switzerland is fortunate in having three such able medical historians as you, he and Brunner.

With kind regards and assurances of esteem, I remain

Yours very sincerely

F. H. Garrison

P.S. Please pardon the way in which the ink runs and blots in the herewith. We are now in the typhoon season, with incessant heavy rains, and the tropical humidity is such that it is impossible to write a respectable letter with pen and ink.

S. was lecturer of the history of medicine at the University of Zurich, 33 years old. G. was librarian at the Army Medical Museum in Washington, DC, on leave for military duty in Manila, 53 years old.

G.'s article (Garrison 1924) in the Sudhoff Festschrift (Singer/Sigerist 1924). Charles Singer (1876–1960) English historian of medicine in Oxford and London. Monograph on drug recipes (Sigerist 1923). Karl Sudhoff (1853–1938) German medical historian, director of the Leipzig Institute of the History of Medicine from 1905 to 1925, S.'s teacher. Arnold C. Klebs (1870–1943) medical historian in the U.S. and Switzerland. Conrad Brunner (1859–1927) Swiss surgeon and medical historian.

SIGERIST to GARRISON, Leipzig, 22 April 1926
(Original in German)

Dear Dr. Garrison,

Many thanks for your letter of March 24th. I have written to the editors of the Münchner Medizinische Wochenschrift in the matter of their fun issues. As you will see in the enclosed letter they will send you the spare issues.

Let me also thank you for your cheque for the 1926 dues.

With kind regards I am,

Sincerely yours

[Henry E. Sigerist]

Addressed to Lieutenant Colonel Dr. F. H. Garrison, Army Medical Museum, Washington, U. S. A.

S. is professor and head of the Leipzig Institute of the History of Medicine, writing to German-speaking G. G.'s letter of March 24 is missing. S. was treasurer of the German Society for the History of Medicine and Sciences (DGGMN).

SIGERIST to GARRISON, Leipzig, 28 April 1926
(Original in German)

Dear Dr. Garrison,

Many thanks for your letter of April 6th and for your interesting book review of Goldschmid. His book clearly has gaps and mistakes, yet it is most valuable as the first attempt to summarize this wide field.

You will find information on the Babylonian Suala series in Oefele, Keilschriftenmedizin, Breslau 1902, page 51. Certain parts have been published by A. H. Sayce: An ancient Babylonian Work on Medicine, in Zeitschrift für Keilschriftforschung, 1885, p. 1 ff. The whole series has been edited and translated by Friedrich Küchler: Beiträge zur Kenntnis der assyrisch-babylonischen Medizin, Leipzig 1904, S. 1f.

The enclosed card of the Verlag Lehmann in Munich concerns the fun issues of the Münchner medizinische Wochenschrift. If you like to have them, please write to the bookseller directly.

With kind regards I am
    Sincerely yours,
        [Henry E. Sigerist]

G.'s letter of 6 April is missing; his book review probably is on (Goldschmid 1925).

SIGERIST to GARRISON, Leipzig, 5 October 1926 (Original in German)

Dear Dr. Garrison,

Very many thanks for your letter of September 16th. Dr. John R. Oliver will be welcome as a member. I am pleased to see an increasing number of American members thanks to your effort.

The annual dues for next year are M 18.–

With kind regards I am
    Sincerely yours
        [Henry E. Sigerist]

G.'s letter of 16 September is missing. John Rathbone Oliver (1872–1943) psychiatrist and associate at the Institute of the History of Medicine in Baltimore, also novelist and priest. Annual dues for the German Society for the History of Medicine and Science (DGGMN). M = Marks.

SIGERIST to GARRISON, Leipzig, 8 October 1926 (Original in German)

Dear Dr. Garrison,

Many thanks for your letter of September 24th. I very well understand your point of view; my intention was just to learn about the prospect in

America. Your letter confirms that penniless doctors should not be encouraged to emigrate into the U.S. I have informed my pupil accordingly, and he now hopes to have more luck with the Dutch Colonial Office.

Again, thank you for your kind answer. With kind regards I am
Sincerely yours,
[Henry E. Sigerist]

G.'s letter of 24 September is missing.

Sigerist to Garrison, Leipzig, 23 December 1926 (Original in German)

Dear Dr. Garrison,

Many thanks for your letter of December 3rd and for the cheque of M. 18.– as the annual dues for 1927. Thank you also for your propaganda for our Society; we welcome the four gentlemen you mention, and we are pleased about the increasing number of American members.

With best wishes for a merry Christmas and a happy New Year for you and your family, I am,
Sincerely yours,
[Henry E. Sigerist]

G.'s letter of 3 December is missing.

Garrison to Sigerist, Washington, 7 January 1927

Lieber Herr Kollege:

Your kind letter of December 23rd was received and also the Paracelsus memento which I shall prize very highly.

I should like to propose for membership in your society the name of Professor William H. Welch of the Johns Hopkins University. His address is 807 St. Paul Street, Baltimore, Md. Professor Welch as you probably know has just been appointed a full professor of the history of medicine in the Johns Hopkins University. The appointment has given universal satisfaction and it will undoubtedly mean a great deal for the advancement of the subject in this country. There is no American physician who is more deserving of the honor of membership in your society.

With kind regards and cordial good wishes for the new year, believe me

Very sincerely yours,
F. H. Garrison

P. S. If you set any store by additional membership, I can get plenty and [?] worthwhile members for you at the American Med. Association Meeting next spring or at other scientific gatherings as they come to pass.

"Paracelsus memento" not identified. Welch (1850–1934) pathologist, hygienist, medical historian at Johns Hopkins University. He would be the first director of the newly created Institute for the History of Medicine in 1929.

SIGERIST to GARRISON, Leipzig, 18 January 1927
(Original in German)

Dear Dr. Garrison,

Thank you very much for your letter of January 7th. Particular thanks for Professor Welch's most welcome membership. I am very glad that a regular Chair of the History of Medicine has now been created in the United States too. This will no doubt stimulate our studies.

Every new member is most welcome.
With kind regards I am
Sincerely yours,
[Henry E. Sigerist]

William H. Welch see G. to S. of 7 January 1927.

GARRISON to SIGERIST, Washington, 12 March 1927

My dear Colleague:

Major Callender has shown me your letter of February 22nd with reference to the selection of pictures for the historical exhibit of the Army Medical Museum at the coming meeting of the American Medical Association in May. What Major Callender is after are pictures that would illustrate in a salient and arresting way the unconscious delineation of primitive plastic anatomy by prehistoric and primitive peoples, also of objects illustrating pathological changes and deformations of some provenance. What he is mainly after is a set of pictures that would be "understood by the people" as these would be utilized for exhibition purposes.

I trust you have received my draft for dues to the Society sent sometime ago. At any rate I have received the last number of the Mitteilungen.

With kindest regards, I remain
Very sincerely yours,
F. H. Garrison

Major G. R. Callender, G.'s colleague at the U.S. Army Museum. "Mitteilungen": Probably Mitteilungen zur Geschichte der Medizin und Naturwissenschaften.

SIGERIST to GARRISON, Leipzig ?, 5 April 1927
(Original in German)

Dear Dr. Garrison,

My Institute is collecting information on teaching the history of medicine in individual countries. To this end the enclosed questionnaire is being sent to the teachers of the subject. I would appreciate your information about the universities teaching the subject and by whom, since I am little informed about the situation in America. Do you happen to know how things are in Canada?

With kind regards,
Sincerely yours
[Henry E. Sigerist]

SIGERIST to GARRISON, Leipzig ?, 16 April 1927
(Original in German)

Dear Dr. Garrison,
    Would you mind giving me the exact address of Dr. M. L. Tainter? You
had been kind enough to propose him as a new member. He has already
paid the annual dues, however, without giving his address. The first issue
of the 'Mitteilungen' has been sent to Worcester but was returned as
undeliverable.
    With kind regards,
        Sincerely yours
            [Henry E. Sigerist]

M. L. Tainter, medical scientist in California.

GARRISON to SIGERIST, Washington, 18 April 1927

My dear Colleague:
    In reply to your kind letter of April 5th I am returning your enquete
[sic] filled out as you desire with data about the chairs of medical history
in this country. Apart from the Johns Hopkins University and the University of Pennsylvania none of these are full professorships, most of the teachers being either instructors like Streeter at Harvard or lecturers like Olliver
[sic] at the University of Maryland. In any case I am giving you all the
data I have at command, and if you will send copies of the enquête to the
people listed, they will send you the additional information.
    Some time ago in the collections of inaugural dissertations which we
receive annually from the University of Leipzig and other German Universities, there was included in the batch of theses for 1924 one by Horst
Fichtner entitled "Die Medizin im Avesta". Our library cards and printed
entries shows [sic] that this thesis covered 24 pages, but in sending for it to
read up on Persian medicine I found that the copy we have comprises
pages 1–16 only so that pages 17–24 are missing.
    I have gone carefully through the boxes containing these theses and
have not been able to find the missing part. If you could send me an extra
copy of this thesis for my personal use, I should appreciate it very much

and would then place it in the Library collections. I wish to study it in connection with the monograph by Fonahn on Persian Medicine.

With kind regards and assurances of esteem, believe me to be

Very sincerely yours,

F. H. Garrison

Edward C. Streeter (1874–1947) medical historian. Oliver see G. to S. of 5 October 1926. (Fichtner 1924). (Fonahn 1910).

GARRISON to SIGERIST, Washington, 7 May 1927

My dear Prof. Sigerist:

At the meeting of the International Association of Medical History at Atlantic City on May 3rd, Professor William H. Welch, recently chosen Professor of Medical History at The Johns Hopkins University, was elected President of the Historical Section and delegated to represent it at the coming International Congresses of Medical History in Europe. He will of course have the usual credentials signed by Dr. Hemmeter, the retiring president of the organization. But aside from this any courtesy you may be able to show him while in Europe will be much appreciated by me.

With kind regards and assurances of esteem, I remain

Very sincerely yours,

F. H. Garrison

Welch see G. to S, of 7 January 1927. John C. Hemmeter (1963–1931) gastroentero-logist and medical historian.

SIGERIST to GARRISON, Leipzig ?, 24 May 1927 (Original in German)

My dear Colleague,

Thank you for several letters as well as for your kindly letting me have the addresses of the American medical historians. I have sent them all the questionnaire in order to improve my inquiry.

Horst Fichtner's thesis 'Die Medizin im Avesta' appeared originally as a summary only. The full text then became commercially available. I send you a copy by separate mail.

Professor Welch's visit will be most welcome. He has already written himself, and I am looking forward to meet the highly meritorious man in my Institute.

I very much regret that it was not possible to obtain the photographs expected by Major Callender. Much as we have a large amount of pictures illustrating the history of anatomy, we lack material on primitive plastic anatomy. I am sorry I cannot help you.

With kind regards I am
    Sincerely yours
        [Henry E. Sigerist]

Fichtner see G. to S. of 18 April 1927. Welch see G. to S. of 7 January 1927. Callender see G. to S. of 12 March 1927.

GARRISON to SIGERIST, Washington, 10 June 1927

Sehr verehrter Herr Kollege:

Many thanks for your kind letter of May 24th and for the copy of Fichtner's dissertation on Persian medicine. It will be impossible to say how much I appreciate your kindness in this matter which is very timely as perusal of this book and of Professor Neuburger's chapter on Persian medicine will save me a lot of trouble. In return I am sending you a few pamphlets which you may not have seen and which may be of some use to you in your work. As soon as my fourth edition is out, I will send you a copy.

With kind regards and assurances of esteem, I remain
    Very sincerely yours,
        F. H. Garrison

Neuburger, Max (1868–1955) professor of medical history in Vienna. "Fourth edition" of (Garrison 1913).

SIGERIST to GARRISON, Leipzig ?, 21 June 1927
(Original in German)

My dear colleague,

Many thanks for your kind letter, and allow me to ask you for advice. Until last year my Institute received the Index Medicus as a gift. This was a welcome help since we are depending on gifts of the kind in view of the limited resources. Apparently the Index Medicus has now been taken over by the American Medical Association, and I fear that we are no longer on their list.

Let me therefore ask if you see a possibility that we still get a copy in the future or if I will have to subscribe. I cannot do without it, since it is the best medical bibliography.

    With kind regards I am
        Sincerely yours
            [Henry E. Sigerist]

Index Medicus, medical bibliographical series, founded by G.

SIGERIST to GARRISON, Leipzig, 6 July 1927
(Original in German)

Dear colleague,

You had been kind enough to name Dr. Herbert O. Calbery as a new member. I would appreciate your also giving me his address which is missing.

    With kind regards,
        Sincerely yours,
            [Henry E. Sigerist]

Garrison to Sigerist, Washington, 8 July 1927

My dear Colleague:

Thanking you for your kind letter of June 21st, I take pleasure in sending you the supplementary number 5 of of Volume VI of the Index Medicus, containing the valedictory statement and number 1 of the new Quarterly Cumulative Index Medicus. I will also ask the Chicago editor, Dr. Fishbein to continue to send this journal to your Institute which I have no doubt he will be glad to do.

I am very sorry that I cannot attend the conference in Holland but it will be impossible for me to get away for any great length of time.

In the same package I am sending you one or two American monographs which you may not have seen.

Trusting these will be of help and with warm greetings and assurance of esteem, I remain

Very sincerely yours,
F. H. Garrison

Morris Fishbein (1889–1976) editor of the Journal of the American Medical Association. "Conference in Holland": International Congress of the History of Medicine in Leyden and Amsterdam.

Garrison to Sigerist, Washington, 26 July 1927

My dear Colleague:

In reply to yours of July 6th, I regret to say that Dr. Herbert O. Calberry [sic] is not mentioned in the American Medical Directory. The name is probably a distortion of the name of one of the pupils of Professor Geiling of the Johns Hopkins University, but the latter is now traveling in Europe. Nevertheless, I am sending your letter to his address in Baltimore in the hope that he will be able to clear up the difficulty.

I am with assurance of esteem and regard, I am [sic]

Very sincerely,
F. H. Garrison

Calber(r)y see S. to G. of 6 July 1927. Eugene M. K. Geiling (1891–1971) pharmacologist.

SIGERIST to GARRISON, Leipzig ?, 14 September 1927
(Original in German)

Dear Colleague,

I am back in Leipzig after some traveling, and I would like to thank you for your letters of July 8th and 26th as well as for the Index Medicus and the much appreciated brochures.

We regretted your not being able to come to Holland, and I only hope that a trip to Europe will materialize next year.

With kind regards,
Sincerely yours,
[Henry E. Sigerist]

S. had attended the International Congress of the History of Medicine in Leyden and Amsterdam.

GARRISON to SIGERIST, Washington, 30 September 1927

My dear Colleague:

Thanking you for your kind letter of September 14th, I am glad to know that the publications I sent have reached you in due course. I am sorry that I cannot attend the Leyden Congress but it was impossible. Through the courtesy of Professor Sudhoff, I have received a few early dissertations of the Leipzig Institute, which I have been very much in need of and should like to ask your assistance in obtaining the subjoined which Sudhoff has suggested might be procurable in open market at 1–2 marks. If you know of any way of getting at these I should be very glad to buy them. As I am binding the most significant of these publications, will you kindly arrange to have a set of the future issues of the Leipzig ones sent me and also the historical dissertations published by the Swiss universities, particular Zurich. Those recently published on the History of Public Hygiene and Medicine in Switzerland are of unusual interest especially the one on Muralt.

Any help you can give me in this matter will be greatly appreciated. With kindest regards and best wishes, I remain
Very sincerely yours,
F. H. Garrison

Bürger (Bernhard): Jakob von Heine. Bonn dissertation, 1911.

Rau (Erich Johannes): Aerztliche Gutachten und Polizeivorschriften über den Branntwein im Mittelalter. Leipzig diss. 1914.

Rosenblum: Die medizinische Abteilung der Kataloge der Kloster-Bibliothek Alt-Zelle, Leipzig diss. 1918.

Hartmann (Friedrich): Die Litteratur von Früh- und Hoch-Salerno. Leipzig diss. 1919.

Bededict (Karl Heinrich): Die Demonstratio anatomica. Leipzig diss 1920.

Stroh (Walter): Aerztliche Bewerbungen, Berufungen etc., Leipzig diss. 1920.

Ploss (Werner L. H.): Anatomia Mauri. Leipzig diss. 1921.

Zimmermann (Isidor): Material zur Würdigung Galens. 8°. Berlin diss., 1902.

Ferckel (Christian): Zur Gynäkologie … des Joh. de Ketham. Leipzig diss. 1912.

Sudhoff see G. to S. of 18 August 1923. Muralt: Name of several important Swiss physicians of the 18th to 20th centuries.

SIGERIST to GARRISON, Leipzig ?, 8 December 1927
(Original in German)

Dear Colleague,

Thanks for your letter of September 30th. I have asked my bookseller to look for the theses you wish and to send them to you if he finds them at a reasonable price. In addition, I wrote to Dr. Wehrli in Zurich to send you his theses in the future. The works of my Leipzig Institute will be sent to you as in the past.

With kind regards,
Sincerely yours,
[Henry E. Sigerist]

Gustav Adolf Wehrli (1888–1949) Swiss medical historian.

My dear Colleague:

I should like to propose for membership in the Deutsche Gesellschaft für Geschichte der Medizin und der Naturwissenschaften Dr. Gregory Zilboorg, Bloomingdale Hospital, White Plains, N.Y., who is I think well worthy of inclusion in your society and has just completed a very excellent history of psychiatry which will be the first English work of any value on this subject.

Would it be possible to obtain any information as to the following works, whether obtainable in Switzerland or at Paris:

Conrad Gesner: Epistola ad Jacobum Avienum de Montium admiratione (in his Libellas de lacte) Zurich 1541.

/ _____ ,/ Descriptio de montis fracti sive Montes Pilati, 4°. Zurich 1555.

I am making this inquiry in the interest of a friend and any bids which antiquarian booksellers might send in as to price will be most highly appreciated.

With kind regards and assurances of esteem, believe me to be

Very sincerely yours,

F. H. Garrison

Gregory Zilboorg (1890–1959) psychiatrist in New York; his mentioned history of psychiatry could not be identified. Conrad Gesner (1516–1565) Swiss physician and scholar.

SIGERIST to GARRISON, Leipzig ?, 5 June 1928
(Original in German)

Dear Colleague,

Thanks for your letter of May 12th. It is an honor to welcome Dr. Zilboorg as a member of our Society.

As to the two books you mentioned, I shall immediately write to the most important second-hand bookseller in Switzerland, and I hope he will be able to give you the information you need.

With kind regards,

Sincerely yours,

[Henry E. Sigerist]

Zilboorg see G. to S. of 12 May 1928.

Garrison to Sigerist, Washington, 4 August 1928

My dear Colleague:

Please pardon my troubling you again about two books I am desirous of obtaining. One of these is Sudhoff's new book on ancient Teutonic medicine which I understand is already out of print. Can you inform me if this is still obtainable or when a new edition will be published? The other is a booklet of Sudhoff's listed in your very excellent bibliography at the back of the Sudhoff Festschrift called Plauderei über Medizinische Bibliotheken, Leipzig. Can you inform me if this book is still in print and if so how I might be able to obtain it. I ordered it some years ago through my importers but it has never reached me.

With assurances of esteem and regard, I beg to be believed,

Very sincerely yours,

F. H. Garrison

Sudhoff see G. to S. of 18 August 1923. For the first Sudhoff book see S. to G. of 4 September 1928; the second one is (Sudhoff 1921).

Sigerist to Garrison, Leipzig ?, 4 September 1928
(Original in German)

Dear Colleague,

Many thanks for your kind letter of August 4th. Sudhoff's book on ancient Germanic medicine has not appeared yet and it is questionable whether or not it ever will. – His work on medical libraries is the preface of a catalog of the bookseller Fock. I was able to obtain a reprint of it which I am sending you by separate mail.

Many thanks for your bibliography. I shall have it bound and available for use in our seminar room since it is of particular value for beginners.

May I suggest two works for your bibliography? These are two very valuable Swiss biographical dictionaries:

Leu, Hans Jakob, Allgemeines Helvetisches Eydgenöss. oder Schweizerisches Lexikon. 20 Bde. 1747–1765, Fortsetzungen von I. I. Holzhalb in 6 Suppl.-Bänden 1786–1795.

Historisch-Biographisches Lexikon der Schweiz, Neuchatel 1921 sequ.

The latter will be complete in a couple of years.
    With kind regards,
        Sincerely yours
            [Henry E. Sigerist]

Sudhoffs book on teutonic medicine has not appeared. G.'s bibliography (Garrison 1912), continued as Garrison/Morton and Morton up to the 1990s.

GARRISON to SIGERIST, Washington, 21 September 1928

Lieber Herr Kollege:
    Many thanks for your kind letter of September 4th and the information you have conveyed in regard to Sudhoff's book on old German medicine, also for the reprint of his valuable article on medical libraries. You take a very kind view of my slight performance on medical biography, which of course could not pretend to be exhaustive in the shape of a mere address or editorial. I want to thank you very much for the "Leu" reference which you kindly supplied.
    With kindest regards and assurances of esteem, believe me
        Very sincerely yours,
            F. H. Garrison

This letter refers to S. to G. of 4 September 1928. Leu see S. to G. of 4 September 1928.

GARRISON to SIGERIST, London, 22 August 1929

My dear Colleague:
    Passing through London, en route to the Meeting at Budapest, I hope to visit your Institut at Leipzig toward the beginning of next month and perhaps to have the pleasure of seeing you there.
    With kind regards and assurances of esteem, I remain
        Yours very sincerely
            F. H. Garrison

SIGERIST to GARRISON, Leipzig ?, 26 August 1929
(Original in German)

Dear Colleague,

Many thanks for your letter of August 22nd. I will be delighted to see you in Leipzig. Please mind, however, that on September 2nd I will depart to Budapest with 14 members of my Institute. From then on you would not find anybody here. I shall be back in Leipzig on September 18th only, because I will spend some time with my group in Vienna and Prague. Thus, I would very much appreciate it if you could manage to come earlier to Leipzig, or else after September 18th.

With kind regards,
Sincerely yours
[Henry E. Sigerist]

This would probably be the first personal encounter of S. and G. Budapest was the site of the International Congress of the History of Medicine. In 1929 the Welch Medical Library and the Institute for the History of Medicine were founded in Baltimore; head of the Institute was William H. Welch.

GARRISON to SIGERIST, Munich, 1 September 1929 [?]

In more than half of this hand-written letter the ink has faded so that only fragments are legible. The letter expresses G.'s gratitude for the reception he experienced in Leipzig by S., his wife, and the young people at the Institute.

GARRISON to SIGERIST, Carlisle Barracks, PA., 6 December 1929

My dear Professor Sigerist:

It is sometime since I have heard from you or written to you, but I have been very busy up here since October 14 and I sent from Strassburg [?] a hurried note of acknowledgment of your very great kindness to me, which I shall not soon forget. You probably know the rest of my itinerary: at Strassburg, I spent the day with Wickersheimer [,] and d'Irsay showed me what was really interesting in Paris. Sudhoff arrived in New York the day befoie I did, and I saw him in Baltimore and a good deal of him in Washington. His tour, as you know, was very successful, but he gave me no inkling of his reactions. At parting, he left with me the carbon of my translation of his Baltimore address, which is to be printed in the Johns Hopkins Bulletin, and a type-written copy of the original, but I forgot to ask him what to do with it. What I should like to know [?] is: Would it be appropriate to print it in your Archiv, and if so, shall I sound him about it (or will you?) and send it to you? I merely put this query before writing to him eventually, as it is essential to have your view of the matter beforehand. If he left it with me as a memento – O.K.

I am sorry to hear about the contretemps of the Berlin chair, but judging from what I saw of your Leipzig plant and your attractive group of pupils, who have derived their inspiration from you, I should prefer to be where you are than in the Capital of the Preussentum, but, then, I am very old fashioned in my tastes and the present world of Jazz, movies and big noise is one in which, like [?] the line in Tristan, " I would fain not dwell". There will be little chance for our subject over here, until Prof. Welch has developed a nationwide interest in it, which he is eminently fitted to do. My own statue has been like that of Dr. Reinhold Müller, a solitary outrider, like an old Army scout or skirmish-liner, making my own stuff and supplies, as I go along, and otherwise a side-issue with me, "in addition to other duties". But you probably got my viewpoint and my make-up [?] when I saw you in Germany. University developments and Seminar work will be a new departure, an interesting experiment, as didactic lecturing from a chair [?] has proved to be a total failure in this country.

I shall be here until December 15 and hope to hear from you about the above at my Washington address.

With kindest regards to Mme. Sigerist and yourself, I remain,

Yours very sincerely

F. H. Garrison

The first part of the letter refers to G.'s European tour of the summer 1929. Ernest Wickersheimer (1880–1965) French medical historian. Stephen d'Irsay (1894–1934) physiologist and medical historian of Hungarian origin, S.'s coworker in Leipzig. Sudhoff was invited to the U.S. for the inauguration of the Johns Hopkins Institute of the History of Medicine in Baltimore. "Johns Hopkins Bulletin": Bulletin of the Johns Hopkins Hospital. "Archiv" für Geschichte der Medizin. "Berlin chair": In 1930 a department for the history of medicine was created at the University of Berlin; Sigerist had been considered as chairman, but eventually Paul Diepgen was elected. Preussentum: The Prussian way.

Welch see G. to S. of 7 January 1927. Reinhold Müller (born 1882) German medical historian. "A new departure": With the creation of the Hopkins Institute of the History of Medicine and the Welch Medical Library G. was appointed as Librarian and as Lecturer of the history of medicine.

GARRISON to SIGERIST, Washington, 19 December 1929

My dear Professor Sigerist:

Having completed my course at Carlisle Barracks, I find, upon returning to my office desk, the [...] shots and other photos you had so kindly sent me. I did not know of their arrival until recently, as only letters, and no packages were forwarded to me. The pictures are not only enormously interesting to me, but will always be cherished as a delightful reminiscence of our pleasant days together. I particularly value the fine and effective portrait of yourself, which I hope to have framed eventually.

Just at present, I am tired out from the rather strenuous course of military training and am minded to rest upon my oars a bit, but I hope and believe that I shall be in fair working order before long. You will, I know, pardon this brief missive on that account.

With kindest regards and all the compliments of the coming season to Mme. Sigerist, yourself and all the students,, I remain

Yours very sincerely

F. H. Garrison

GARRISON to SIGERIST, Washington, 26 April 1930

My dear Professor Sigerist:

Here is my long-delayed compte-rendu on my European tour, which may amuse you. I will try to send copies to some of the other friends I met. Will you kindly say to them that on account of the prolonged illness of my sister (now five months in hospital), a fracture which disabled me for three weeks in January and the enormous amount of work I have had to clean up here before moving to Baltimore, I have not been able to do very much in the way of letter-writing, but in a little while

I hope to have more leisure and will then write to some of them. I received the very nice portrait of yourself sometime ago and if you want one of mine, I shall be glad to send it as soon as I can have some copies made.

Hoping all is well with you [,] and with kind regards to Mrs. Sigerist, yourself and all the young people at the Institute, I remain

Yours very sincerely

F. H. Garrison

Sigerist to Garrison, Leipzig ?, 7 July 1930 (Original in German)

Dear Colleague,

Very many thanks for your letter of April 26th and for your interesting report of your trip. I have read it with great pleasure. What you write of my Institute is very kind, indeed. I am glad you were positively impressed and, morover, that you approved of what I am aiming at.

I have heard that you will move to Baltimore, and I hope you will find more peace and quiet for work than you do now. Maybe one day I will be able to see you there. – Your photograph would please me, indeed.

With kind regards, in which my wife joins, I am

Sincerely yours

[Henry E. Sigerist]

This is S.'s last letter to G. in German.

Garrison to Sigerist, Baltimore, 3 August 1930

My dear Professor Sigerist:

Thanking you for your kind letter of July 7: I am glad the little travel sketch reached you in due course and naturally pleased that you liked it. I have also mailed to you my last editorial on medical Incunabula and will send the portrait, as soon as I can get it packed.

I was retired from active duty in the Army on May 19 and have been functioning as Librarian here since that date, finding the work very pleasant. Dr. Welch is now in California, as guest of the Huntington Library at

San Marino. It is lucky for him that he is, as the summer in this part of the country has been extraordinarily hot, so much so, in fact, that the cattle on [...] dairy farms are starving for lack of food. I had a short vacation at my seaside home early in July and hope to escape the worst heat in this climate on September 1.

I often think of my pleasant days with you at Budapest and the farewell dinner at Vienna. Will you give my best regards and greetings to all of your Leipzig group.

I wish that I could write to you in German, but alas! I have never quite recovered from the effects of tropical heat in Manila, and, in this kind of weather, it is all I can do to think rudimentarily in "United States" or what Mencken calls "the American language". I am also worried about the plight of my sister, who has been ill for nine months in Walter Reed Hospital (Washington) and has just been ambulanced over to the Johns Hopkins Hospital.

Thank you very much for the interesting reprints, which I shall read with interest.

With kindest regards and greetings to Frau Sigerist and yourself, I remain

Yours very sincerely,
F. H. Garrison

Incunabula: Early prints (before 1500). Welch see G. to S. of 7 January 1927. "Manila": see G. to S. of 18 August 1923. Henry L. Mencken (1880–1956) Baltimore writer.

Garrison to Sigerist, Baltimore, 17 August 1930

My dear Professor Sigerist:

Please regard the following as entirely confidential: Professor Sudhoff has written me three long letters about that editorial of mine on my European tour, in particular the section about the Leipzig Institute. He seems to have taken umbrage at my mention of the changes made in the museum collection, the library, the new departures in teaching and maintains that I have damaged his reputation thereby and put him in the wrong with [?] the younger people, etc. My private guess is that this is somewhat exaggerated and perhaps pure imagination, as you yourself have shown him every honor conceivable – portrait, medallion, anthology of his writings and autobiography in the Archiv, apart from your bibliography in the Festschrift, and I did not see any slightest sign of disrespect toward him at Buda-Pest, where he was the outstanding figure and seemed to be at the top notch of his being. You will readily understand, then, that it seems to me grotesque to be informed that an ephemeral, journalistic article, de jour en jour, has produced the "impression that Sudhoff's star is on the wake". This is, of course, one of the effects of advanced age – these old boys, particularly those of large physique, are apt to be boudeurs and childish if not patted on the back, like a Newfoundland or St. Bernard dog, and kept reminded of their importance every now and then. As I sensed that you are absolutely fair-minded impersonal and above professional jealousy, I want to ask, as a personal favor, that, without any intimation that you have heard from me, you instruct your personnel to keep the old fellow flattered and in a good humor, get up a dinner or banquet or something for him, see that he is as prominent and active as can be at the Roman Congress, and so on. He charged [?] up his imaginary declension in prominence and prestige to you and me, which is, of course absurd and for the rest – you understand, my little sister died in hospital on Friday morning and will be buried tomorrow, and I have been filling in a rather dreary Sunday, writing letters on this and other matters.

With kindest regards to Mme. Sigerist and yourself, I remain

Yours very sincerely,

F. H. Garrison

GARRISON to SIGERIST, Baltimore, 7 January 1931

My dear Professor Sigerist:

Thank you so much for remembering me with a copy of your wonderful book. I read the copy you sent to the Library in the evening, have nearly completed my review of it and that same night, I called up Mencken, suggesting that he get Knopf to arrange with you about an English translation. Knopf has just sailed for Europe and you will probably be seeing him about this before long. I think some one here – could – make a good translation, or perhaps you would prefer to English it yourself, which would be simpler. You have achieved a masterpiece which will fill a long felt want, namely a book for the prospective medical student and the cultivated layman, which is at once a general introduction to medicine, an outline of medical history and an orientation into medical philosophy as a rational guide to life, written in a style of the utmost simplicity. You have a remarkable feeling for the "point-counterpoint" fugato of literary composition, and I congratulate you with all my heart.

With kindest regards to Mme. Sigerist, yourself, and all the friends and pupils of the Institute, believe me

Yours very sincerely,

F. H. Garrison

S.'s book is the German original (Sigerist 1931) of his *Man and Medicine*. "Library": Welch Medical Library of the Johns Hopkins University. Mencken see G. to S. of 3 August 1930. Knopf: New York publishing house. (Sigerist 1931) was translated into English and appeared with Norton in New York (Sigerist 1932a). "Fugato": In the style of a fugue; G. has been characterized as a man of books and music.

SIGERIST to GARRISON, Leipzig ?, 21 January 1931

My dear Dr. Garrison,

Thank you ever so much for your kind letter of January 7th. I knew that my book would appeal to German readers, but I wasn't quite sure that American students would like it. So your letter gave me a very great pleasure and I thank you with all my heart for all you said about the book and for all you are doing for it.

I would be delighted to have the book translated into English, but I am afraid that I couldn't do it myself. My knowledge of the English language is to [sic] poor for it and presently I am working very hard on a new book that should come out at the end of the year so that I have practically no time. But I am sure that it wouldn't be difficult to find a good translator. I would revise several passages for the English edition, particularly the last chapter where I referred to the German conditions and where I would like to take the English and American conditions into special consideration.

With kindest regards I am

Very sincerely yours

[Henry E. Sigerist]

This is S.'s first letter to G. in English and addressed to the Welch Library. "My book":
(Sigerist 1931). English translation (Sigerist 1932a). The remark about S.'s knowledge
of English is an understatement. "New book": (Sigerist 1932b).

GARRISON to SIGERIST, Baltimore, 25 February 1931

My dear Prof. Sigerist:

Your letter of February 2 has just come and I am very sorry to hear that Knopf has declined to publish your book. The American book to which his agent refers is undoubtedly the book called "The Human Body" by Logan Clendening, a large volume written in popular vein with illustrations, which Knopf published and has now thrown upon the market at half price. I think this declination turns upon the simple fact that the publication of your book would prevent him from recouping his losses from the earlier venture. Dr. d'Irsay who has seen your letter, has kindly volunteered to write to MacMillans [sic] about the possibility of publication. If Knopf had taken hold of the proposition, I had figured that he might finance the translation over here, but from what d'Irsay says, I fancy that you could have it done at a much more reasonable figure in Germany. The cost of translating a volume of that size over here would be at least $ 500, if not more.

I am sending on my review of your book to the Academy of Medicine and will mail you a copy as soon as it is printed.

With kindest regards to Madame Sigerist, yourself and all at the Leipzig Institute, believe me,

Very sincerely yours,

F. H. Garrison

S.'s letter of 2 February is missing. (Clendening 1927). D'Irsay see G. to S. of 6 December 1929. Macmillan: International publishing company.

Garrison to Sigerist, Baltimore, 4 June 1931

My dear Professor Sigerist:

Thank you for your kind note of May 22. I am very glad to know that a good English firm is going to undertake the translation of your remarkable book. It will be sure to take hold I think. It is delightful that you are going to be with us and I shall personally look forward to your visit with pleasurable anticipation.

With kind regards to Mrs. Sigerist and yourself, believe me,
Very sincerely yours,
F. H. Garrison

S.'s note of 22 May is missing. G. has been informed of S.'s impending study tour in the U.S.

Garrison to Sigerist, Martha's Vineyard, MA, 7 August 1931

My dear Professor Sigerist:

In Dr. Welch's absence, I have been asked to prepare a prospectus of the lectures and seminar courses to be held in the Institute during the academic year 1931–2, so that this prospectus can be printed and ready for distribution before October 1. Will you kindly send me the titles of the lectures you propose to deliver and the themes of any seminar courses you might wish to hold during your residence in Baltimore. At the same time, it would be highly advantageous if you could send me the titles of any lectures you might be ready to deliver in other cities, so that we could make suitable advance arrangements. I shall be at above address (P.O.Box 1397) until after September 15, and if you will send me the above information here before that time, I will forward it to the Secretary of the Institute for incorporation in the autumn prospectus.

With kindest regards to Mrs. Sigerist and yourself, believe me
Very sincerely yours
F. H. Garrison

We are looking forward to your coming with great pleasure and interest.

G.s letter was in preparation of S.'s study and lecture tour in the U.S. 1931/32.

Garrison to Sigerist, Martha's Vineyard, MA, 28 August 1931

My dear Professor Sigerist:

Some little while ago, I received a nice letter from Frl. Margarete Meyer, acknowledging a book I sent her at Christmas. I wrote in reply to the address she gave, which was <u>10</u> Talstrasse, Leipzig, but the letter was returned, marked "unbekannt, inconnu". Will you kindly tell her that I will try to write again sometime, when I know her correct address. I was shocked to hear of the terrible auto accident she experienced and the sequels.

I wrote to you some time ago, requesting an outline of the titles of your lectures at the Institute this fall, for the customary printed circular, which is usually reprinted in the medical journals (some of them). Probably you are away, enjoying your Sommerfrische, and, if I don't hear from you in time, I will insert your name as Visiting Lecturer, with the statement: "Subjects and dates of lectures to be announced later". I am taking the same line with regard to Dr. Welch's lectures, the subjects of which he chooses as he goes along. If I can give you any assistance with regard to posting lectures for you in other cities while you are here, let me know.

With kind regards to Mrs. Sigerist and yourself, and to all I know in the Institute at Leipzig, I remain

Yours very sincerely
F. H. Garrison

Miss Margarete Meyer was a member of the Leipzig Institute at Talstrasse 38. Sommerfrische = summer resort.

Sigerist to Garrison, Leipzig ?, 1 September 1931

My dear Dr. Garrison,

I send you enclosed the titles of the lectures I propose to deliver at Johns Hopkins and the themes for a seminary [sic] course. You will find also a list of subjects available for lectures in other cities. I have already the following appointments:

Nov. 2nd:	a lecture at the German Medical Society in New York
" 9th:	a lecture on Fracastoro in Philadelphia at a meeting in commemoration of the 25th anniversary of the discovery of the Spirochaeta pallida. I have been invited to it by Riesman
" 11th:	a lecture at the Rockefeller Institute, under their auspices, those of the Charaka Club and of the Historical Section of the New York Academy of Medicine
Dec. 1st	the Sedgwich Lecture in Boston on the Origins of Hygiene
Beginning of Dec.	3 lectures at the University of Chicago
Middle of January	3 lectures at the Stanford University in San Francisco

I shall arrive in New York on the 25th of September. My address there will be: Shelton Hotel, Lexington Ave. and 49th Str. Dr. Welch asked me to wait for him in New York so that we may go together to Baltimore. I think that will be at the 10th [sic] of September or about that date.

I intend to stay six weeks in Baltimore so that I can deliver one lecture and one seminar a week. If Thursday and Friday do fit in with the scheme of your Institute I think they would be the most convenient days. It would give me the possibility to spend the week-end and the beginning of the week in other places of the East.

I am not anxious to give a great many lectures in other places, especially not in the beginning. I would not like to be obliged to travel much during October as I am looking forward to doing some work in your Institute. However, it would interest me very much to be able to visit the most important Universities of the East and some typical places of the Middle West. I am corresponding with Dr. Louis B. Wilson from the University of Minnesota who thinks that he might be able to arrange a schedule for lectures in several middle-western Universities.

With kindest regards from Mrs. Sigerist and myself believe me

Yours very sincerely

[Henry E. Sigerist]

This letter is in preparation of S.'s U.S. study tour of winter 1931/32. Fracastoro, Girolamo (1478–1553) Italian physician, anatomist, poet; wrote about syphilis. Spirochaeta (or Treponema) pallida: The germ responsible for syphilis. David Riesman (1867–1940) medical historian. Welch see G. to S. of 7 January 1927. "Your Institute": The Hopkins Institute of the History of Medicine. Louis B. Wilson, probably the Mayo Clinic pathologist in Rochester, MN.

GARRISON to SIGERIST, Baltimore, 25 September 1931

My dear Professor Sigerist:

This is the day of your arrival in New York and, as I expect to run over there on Sunday night, I would like to have you dine with me, Dr. Malloch and some others at the Army and Navy Club, 30 West 44th Street, on Monday evening, September 28 at 6.30 P.M. If Madam Sigerist is with you, I should be delighted to have her also as ladies are admitted to the dining-room of this club. I am stopping at the club and will call you up directly I arrive, either Suday night or Monday morning. I can then arrange to call at your hotel or meet you anywhere it is convenient.

I have inserted all the items for your lectures and seminar in the preliminary prospectus, which is in type, and will arrange for publicity in regard to your outside lectures after I have seen you. I have also written to Dr. Louis B. Wilson, requesting him to manage your western course of lectures, which he did so nicely in my case. I will talk to you about the other details when we meet. As Dr. Welch's ship will probably dock on Monday the 28th, I am hoping that he may be persuaded to join us at the above dinner.

With kindest regards to Mrs. Sigerist and yourself, believe me,
Very sincerely yours,
F. H. Garrison

The letter was addressed to S. at the Shelton Hotel in New York. Archibald Malloch, librarian of the New York Academy of Medicine. During S.'s 1931/32 study tour his wife Emmy remained with the children Erica and Nora in Europe. Wilson, see S. to G. of 1 September 1931. William H. Welch see G. to S. of 7 January 1927.

GARRISON to SIGERIST, Baltimore, 26 September 1931

My dear Professor Sigerist:

I find it will be impossible for me to leave here before Monday morning, however, I shall be in New York about 4 P.M. or in time for the dinner.

Hoping to see you then, I remain,
Very sincerely yours,
F. H. Garrison

GARRISON to SIGERIST, Baltimore, 1 October 1931

My dear Professor Sigerist:

Enclosed is the preliminary prospectus, in which your program has been printed as you gave it. I will take up the publicity in the next few days. I will also make arrangements about the Baltimore Club, as soon as Dr. Welch returns. Should you be coming down on October 10, I will meet you at the station. It was very pleasant and stimulating to be with you again and I am hoping that, through the contacts now made, you will have smooth sailing.

I put in a very profitable morning with Professor Marx but find that so much remains to be done, that I have arranged to spend a Sunday with him in the near future.

With kindest regards, I remain,
    Yours very sincerely,
        F. H. Garrison

S. is still in New York. Welch see G. to S. of 7 January 1927. Marx not identified.

GARRISON to SIGERIST, Baltimore, 2 October 1931

Dear Professor Sigerist:

Thanking you for your letter: It was very delightful to be with you again and I somehow feel that everything about your stay here is going to be pleasant, because you know how to "make it so", as the captain of the Pinafore observed in the opera.

In the matter of Secretaries, we have two accomplished ones attached to the Institute and both are at your service – that is what they are here for: You don't have to say them anything. One of them speakes and writes German and can take dictation in German. So you will have no trouble whatever, and I think you will be able to get away with whatever you have to do, as part of the day's work; if there is anything in Sudhoff's idea that it is unhealthy to work at night.

I think too, that you will soon acquire facility in lecturing ex tempore in English, from a few rough notes. I find that the best plan, either to speak offhand from topics or to peg it out by means of lantern slides. You

126

have then the advantage of presenting viva voce what is intended to be apprehended by the ear, which is, of course, quite different from what you write out for the eye. I never read off any Augenmusik, unless it happens to be, at the same time, Ohrenmusik. You will soon get the hang of this in English and I don't believe you will encounter any difficulty whatever, given your facility in conversing in English.

Dr. Chesney, the Dean of the Medical Faculty, is writing to you about getting placed in suitable quarters, and I will either meet you at the station or come down with you, if it can be arranged.

With kindest regards,
Yours very sincerely
F. H. Garrison

S.'s letter missing. H. M. S. Pinafore is a Gilbert and Sullivan comic opera of 1878. Sudhoff see G. to S. of 18 August 1923. Augenmusik = music for the eye; Ohrenmusik = music for the ear. Alan Mason Chesney (1888–1964) Dean of the Johns Hopkins School of Medicine.

GARRISON to SIGERIST, Baltimore, 7 October 1931

My dear Professor Sigerist:

Thanking you for yours of October 6; I am delighted that you are having such a good time and seeing things and people. We will do everything we can to make your stay here pleasant and profitable. Dr. Oliver will pick you up in the car at your Club about 9.30 of mornings, as he is nearer, and I will take you back or anywhere you like of afternoons. We shall also have plenty of opportunity to see the environs of Baltimore on Sundays, and I am arranging to motor to Washington sometime next week, if agreeable to you.

As you are coming down on the Sunday train I would suggest the following: Owing to the interruptions of the day I was with you, I am going to take a sleeper to N. Y. on Saturday night, so as to put the finishing touches to my Steinschneider Bibliographie, which is nearly completed and if you will kindly arrange to take a little later train, we can come down together. It should be much pleasanter for both, as the four hour ride is apt to be boresome without company. We could dine together on the train and could get you to the room assigned to you in the Club in plenty of time. I will call up your hotel when I get to New York on Sunday morning and arrange about meeting in the early afternoon. I feel confident that I can get away with what I want to do in the morning, as I shall arrive and begin early, by arrangement. I hope you will find this proposal agreeable and with kindest regards remain

Yours ever

F. H. Garrison

John Rathbone Oliver see S. to G. of 5 Ocdtober 1926. Moritz Steinschneider (1816–1907) published on Arabic and Hebrew Literature, (Garrison 1932).

Garrison to Sigerist, Baltimore, 25 November 1931

Dear Sigerist:

In leaving the house on Tuesday morning, I, unfortunately, left the corrected Ms. of your lecture behind me, but I managed to make another corrected copy for Miss Broemer, who is forwarding it directly to Boston. In this version I have omitted most of the insertions, which I took the liberty of adding to your original copy, for the reason that until you had gone over them and put your fiat upon them, I did not feel certain that you might want them in the copy going to Boston. You will understand, of course, that they were inserted as mere memoranda in your own copy of the lecture, to be used or not, as you see fit – more like punctuation marks than actual verbage.

I am glad you were able to get off in such good spirits and that you got something out of the evening with us. For myself, I have been, as I said in Germany, "Todesmüde", from the enormous amount of dinner eating and festivities, which were the natural concomitant of your visit. Over and above this the dank, miasmatic mists made me feel very wretched during the whole evening and, at the Club the following day, I found Dr. Welch moving around in soft shoes, with a definite attack of gout. As I told him this was the effect of the poisonous November mists, the kind that killed people in England and have been matter for poets and novelists for many generations. I am thankful to say that we do not have much of that sort of thing in this climate, but I know that they are more formidable in Baltimore than in Washington.

Here's hoping that you will have success and pleasurable experiences which you so surely deserve and here's much power to your elbow! With kindest regards, believe me,

Very sincerely yours,

F. H. Garrison

P.S.: I am asking Miss Broemer to keep the carbons, but any of the Mss can be forwarded to you, if you wish.

S. had left Baltimore en route to Boston. Miss Broemer, secretary at the Baltimore Institute. "Todesmüde" = dead tired. Carbons, copies made with carbon paper in the era before the Xerox machine.

GARRISON to SIGERIST, Baltimore, 18 December 1931

My dear Sigerist:

Thanking you for your kind letter: I am delighted to know that you have had such a pleasant and prosperous trip and feel that all the rest of it will be the same. The great West has to be seen at close range to be appreciated.

It would be difficult to convey the impression which has been left here by your lectures. People are still talking about them and my own feeling is that you have made a definite impact, in the sense of altering preconceived notions of medico-historical teaching, establishing new directives and objectives and stirring up extraordinary enthusiasm, both in the professional ranks and student body, as well as among the cultivated laity. To have accomplished all that in such a short period of time is something – "and [...] some". I am still wrestling with the Steinschneider bibliography, due to many interruptions, the complex and lengthy material and the corrections made by Dr. Marx, but I hope to be in position to 26 send it off in a few days. Incidentally, I suffer, off and on, from the myasthenia resulting from the muscle-twitch of eye-strain. I feel in despair about it at times, as the only remedy would be to knock off usage of the eyes [...] reading and writing for an indefinite period.

On Monday night, we have the next meeting of the Medical History Club, with dinner, and after that is over, I am going into winter quarters, i.e. into a temporary retirement from social activities to forestall going into a decline in the matter of Gesundheit. Like you, I have not been able to accomplish anything in the way of writing and shall have to postpone most of [?] it until the summer comes.

With warm regards from us all and wishing you a merry Christmas and a Happy New Year,

Yours very sincerely

F. H. Garrison

Should you have a moment to spare at any Haltestelle, could you give me your frank opinion of:

Rudolf Thiel [sic]: Männer gegen Tod und Teufel?

It is very readable, and seems reliable, but are all the anectdotes authenticated?

S.'s letter missing. S. is lecturing in cities in Michigan, Wisconsin, and Minnesota. Steinschneider and Marx see G. to S. of 7 October and 1 October 1931, respectively. Gesundheit = health; Haltestelle = stop (train or bus). (Thiele 1931).

Garrison to Sigerist, Baltimore ?, 7 January 1932

My dear Sigerist:

Through Dr. W., who has just returned, I am so glad to hear the good news, which, I do hope is in a way to become accomplished fact. Go to it and count upon us all for loyal support. I feel that this particular solution will resolve many difficulties and straighten out many tangles, apart from the advantage which will accrue from having a genuine self-starting, self-directing motor power in action, to drive the craft.

I am asking Colonel George Blakely, our old Adjutant General in Manila, to look you up and attend your lectures in Frisco. You will find him a very charming man, incidentally a very remarkable Goethe scholar. Ask him to show you his translation of the Charlas de café of Ramon y Cajal. I am rather neurasthenic just at present from over-usage of my eyes, probably over that Steinschneider-Bibliographie, which is just about to get off. I shall never attempt anything of the kind again; the fine print causes too much muscular imbalance. Before you sail Hawai-ward, I wish you would, out of the fulness of your knowledge, suggest a few themes [?]

that may occur to you as good for editorials of the kind I write – the Sainte Beuve type of causerie – you know. That sort of work is rather stimulating and restful, at my age.

With kindest regards, as ever, and cordial good wishes for the New Year
Yours very sincerely
F. H. Garrison

S. spent January in San Francisco and Hawaii. Dr. W. = Dr. Welch. "The good news": S. being offered the Chair of Medical History in Baltimore. Santiago Ramon y Cajal (1852–1934) Spanish histologist of the nervous system; Charlas de café (Ramon y Cajal 1920). Steinschneider see G. to S. of 7 October 1931. Charles Augustin Sainte-Beuve (1804–1869) French literary critic.

GARRISON to SIGERIST, Baltimore, 1 March 1932

My dear Sigerist:

Having been in Washington on Saturday last, I was delighted to find that our young friend, Dr. Claudius Frank Mayer, has joined up permanently with the Surgeon General's Library and has been delegated by Colonel Ashburn to be the editor of the Index Catalogue, in consequence of Dr. Allemann's retirement from active duty. Colonel Ashburn asked me to give Dr. Mayer some coaching in this work and I suggested that we could probably manage this best, if he would spend a day over here in Baltimore with me. I would like to arrange this sometime when you are here and hope that you can set aside an hour, either for a luncheon or a dinner, with Dr. Mayer and myself. I feel that he has a future before him and that whatever advice and encouragement you can give him would be most helpful.

Looking forward to the pleasure of seeing you again and with kindest regards to Mrs. Sigerist and yourself, I am,

Sincerely yours
F. H. Garrison

The letter is addressed to S. in New York. Claudius Frank Mayer, assistant librarian of the Surgeon General's Library in Washington, G.'s successor. Index Catalogue of the Library of the Surgeon General's Office, a bibliographical tool for medical historians, founded by J. S. Billings in 1880. Mrs. Sigerist met S. at the end of his tour in the U. S.

GARRISON to SIGERIST, Baltimore ?, 19 March 1932

My dear Sigerist:

Before leaving, can you spare a few moments to glance over the enclosed Thudichum article, and if you think it suitable for publication in the Annals of Medical History, will you kindly sound Hoeber about it, should you be seeing him, and return it to me in the enclosed envelope, with a brief aviso [?]. The article does cover material I have not seen before, about a London-born German physician who played a not inconsiderable part in the English medicine and pharmacy of his period, and, as it is not too long, it would be in the class of biographical sketches with which the Annals abounds. Mr. Shuler offers to translate it and, if you approve, I will submit it to Packard. Publication in the British Medical Journal, for honorarium, is, of course, out of the question. That is reserved mainly for members of the B.M.A., I have no influence there, and at my time of life, am not the least bit inclined to run errands about bootless [?] questions of that kind. I asked Dr. Chesney as to the possibility of printing it in some historical supplement of the Bulletin, but he was decidedly against it and I am inclined to agree with him in his view that such a publication, if launched, should be confined to Institute material. To let down the bars in one single instance would vitiate the policy contemplated. The rest is of course, exaggerated personal vanity and mental childishness, of the prima donna type. The green slip enclosed speaks for itself – a dreadful mutatus ab illo. Still, we must bear with the infirmities of age in this restless, chaotic period. I have asked Miss Frush [?] to mail you the catalogue of the Ilberg library which I checked in green. It seems a remarkably fine collection, but we have a great many of the medical and scientific items. Otherwise the Handapparat would be a bargin. I think this one of the best classical collections I have seen latterly and you will be able to advise us about it after seeing – or doubtless you have already seen it.

Wishing you a pleasant voyage across and with kindest regards to Mrs. Sigerist and yourself,

Yours very sincerely

F. H. Garrison

S. is at the end of his study tour in the U. S. J. L. W. Thudichum (1828–1901) German-born physician and chemist, emigrated to London. Hoeber, the publisher of the Annals of Medical History; Francis R. Packard (1870–1950) medical historian, the editor of the Annals of Medical History (this Journal existed from 1917 to 1942). Chesney see G. to S. of 2 October 1931. Bulletin of the Johns Hopkins Hospital. Handapparat = reference works. Ilberg Library, probably the library of German-speaking exiles in Great Britain. Miss Frush not identified.

GARRISON to SIGERIST, Baltimore, 23 March 1932

My dear Sigerist:

Here's hoping you got that Thudichum ms. and that it was no trouble to you. If so, I am mighty sorry to have bothered you with it. Don't mind what I said about it and just drop it in the mail before you leave. Give my best regards to everyone over the water and tell them that I will have to postpone a good deal of letter-writing until the summer, for I get dreadfully tired sometime, and then, I am past 61.

We were charmed with Mrs. Sigerist's kind letter and wish you both a pleasant voyage across and a summer which I know will be delightful.

With kind regards,
Very sincerely yours
F. H. Garrison

Thudichum see G. to S. of 19 March 1932. S. was about to return to his Institute in Leipzig.

GARRISON to SIGERIST, Baltimore, 27 March 1932

This date must be wrong; the most likely correct date is 27 March 1933, see there.

GARRISON to SIGERIST, Baltimore, 14 April 1932

My dear Sigerist:

Thank you so much for your letter of March 25. I have turned over the article to Shuler, who will translate it and then we will see what we can do about placing it. I want to thank you for the copy of the translation of your book, which came this morning and which my wife is going to read. I predict a large sale for the volume, both among the profession and the laity. I am glad to see that Dr. Welch got his preface in on time – he usually does.

I gave a lecture at Homewood on the Medical literature of England and was pleased at the receptive spirit of the students of the English classes, who are not supposed to have any interest in medicine. It is there that we shall have to look for interest and support from the student body. The subject has been practically dead in this locality [?]. Dr. Oliver has given up his regular lectures here, apparently, because none of the medical students come. The enclosed, from K. G. Koehler, Leipzig, about the Ilberg Handapparat, will explain itself. We cabled for it, and then it occurred to me that it might be merely pamphlet, material, which it apparently is, so I countermanded the order pending your decision, as you will undoubtedly have an opportunity to see the Handapparat yourself, when you reach Leipzig. From the description Koehler gives of it – few books, mainly theses, reprints and reports I doubt if it will have any selling possibilities at 1000 mks. before you arrive. In other words, Oliver and the Greek and Latin people at Homewood already have fine collections of such pamphlet material, and while the discount of 20 per cent offered is advantageous, I would rather put the $ 200 into some of the more valuable items in the Ilberg Catalogue No. 76, which you so kindly went over. Nevertheless, I have written to Koehler that I am leaving the decision about the Handapparat entirely to you and that you will place the order, if you think we ought really to possess the collection. Miss Frush has held up the items you checked in Cat. No 76 pending your decision about the Handapparat, which we assumed to include many of the items you had checked. Should you decide not to purchase the Apparat, will you kindly order from the enclosed up to $ 200?

With kindest regards to Mrs. Sigerist and yourself,
Yours very sincerely
F. H. Garrison

Shuler see G. to S. of 19 March 1932. "Your book": (Sigerist 1932a), English translation with a preface by W.H. Welch. Homewood, the Hopkins campus for the non-medical institutions. Koehler, antiquary in Leipzig. Ilberg Handapparat see G. to S. of 19 March 1932. "When you reach Leipzig": S. probably went to Switzerland before returning to Leipzig. mks. = marks, the then German currency.

Garrison to Sigerist, Baltimore, 17 April 1932

My dear Dr. Sigerist:

Beside the sum of $ 200 allowed you for the purchase of the "Hand-apparat" or of separate items equivalent of that amount, we have now an additional sum of $ 300 which we wish to apply to the further purchase of items from "Koehler's Antiquariatskatalog 76". We are enclosing a list of the items, largely of your selection, which approximate this amount and which we are ordering from Koehler today.

We are making it clear to Koehler that the bills as rendered us for the joint purchases made by you in person and by us through correspondence for the Institute of the History of Medicine must not exceed the sum of $ 500.

We are further instructing Koehler to render the bills to us for all items purchased in duplicate and not later than June 1, 1932 as the charges for same must be met out of the appropriation of the Institute for the fiscal year which ends June 30, 1932.

Very truly yours
F. H. Garrison
Librarian

Garrison to Sigerist, Baltimore, 3 May 1932

My dear Sigerist:

We are, of course, all of us delighted with the good news for which the University is as much to be congratulated as yourself, and the enclosed are for your scrap-book. I am so glad to realize that you are coming and we will, of course, do all that in us lies to uphold your hands and make the new departure a success.

Many thanks for your kind advice about Sudhoff's Thudichum paper. Will you please tell Prof. Sudhoff that Mr. Shuler is engaged in translating it and that as soon as the English version is ready, I will try to place it and will write to him about it. Due to the raw, cold spring we have had latterly (which always follows an open [?] winter in this climate), I have been suffering from right shoulder disability (probably a sub-deltoid bursitis), which is rather painful, [...] baking, and, while it lasts, engenders a strong disinclination to drive the quill [?]. As it goes away after baking or whenever we have a warm spell, I am hoping for the best, but feel very [...] about driving my car or the pen when it is on.

I had a nice letter from Hirschfeld, which I will answer today – I am glad to hear of his experiences in Greece. Please tell any friends that I will be writing them as soon as the Academic sessions are over and the warm weather is here to stay.

I gave a lecture at Homewood recently on the Medical Literature of England and am now preparing one on Persian Medicine. Until I wound into the subject I never realized what a lot more is to it – a theme we commonly dish in a few lines or dismiss from our minds. The real aboriginal Persian (Zoroastrean medicine) of the Avesta and Vendidad now obsolete except what shreds remain Yezd and Bombay, is so utterly different from the Moslem medicine which came in with the Arabic conquest, that one has constantly to be on one's guard in the matter of nuances. I gather from the travellers of the 18th and 19th centuries that the Moslemized Persian is as fanatical an adherent of Islam as the Arab and the Turk, but otherwise hates the latter as much as he does the Russian. A further complication is that the majority of self-styled Persians in Persia today are of Turkish or otherwise hybrid strain, but even the Moslem folk-medicine which all practice in the process of slow modernization by European training and spheres of influence at Teheran – very much like India, China and the Philippines.

As I understand it, you will now have plenty of money to buy books and suchlike for the Institute, apart from your 1932–3 appropriation and it would probably be well to get the bills in before July 1.

With kindest regards to Mrs. Sigerist and yourself

Very sincerely yours,

F. H. Garrison

S.'s letter missing. "The good news": S.'s accepting the call to Baltimore in April 1932 in Leipzig. Thudichum and Shuler see G. to S. of 19 March 1932. Ernst Hirschfeld, an assistant of S. in Leipzig, who in 1930 went to Berlin and later appears to have been murdered by the Nazis.

136

SIGERIST to GARRISON, Leipzig ?, before 26 May 1932 (telegram)

HAS INSTITUTE CALLISEN, SCHRIFTSTELLERLEXIKON STOP EBERT
REALLEXIKON DER VORGESCHICHTE.
    SIGERIST

GARRISON to SIGERIST, Baltimore, 26 May 1932 (telegram)

INSTITUTE HAS CALLISEN BUT NOT EBERT. GARRISON

SIGERIST to GARRISON, Leipzig ?, 27 May 1932

My dear Garrison,

    I have received your letter of April 14 and I spent several mornings
at Koehlers antiquarium. I went through the handapparat of Ilberg and
as I hesitated to buy it Koehler added 150 pamphlets dealing with medical historical subjects from other collections, without raising the price.
Under these circumstances I bought the handapparat for RM 800.–.
I saw the other books you had ordered also; they amount to about
200 dollars.

    I had a letter from Doctor Chesney the other day, telling me that the
Institute has a balance of about 2 500 dollars which can be spent till end
of June. So I bought a very fine collection of portraits and authographs
[sic] of physicians and naturalists which I found at Koehler's. The collection contains 3 800 portraits and 2 200 autographs, chiefly letters, all in all
6 000 items. Koehler wanted 5 000 RM for it, but I got it for 4 000. I think
it really is a bargain.

    I shall send all the bills in two copies to Dr. Chesney.

    I am looking forward with great pleasure to being back again soon,
and I am sure that we will have a good winter working together.

    With kindest regards, I am,
      very sincerely
        [Henry E. Sigerist]

Koehler see G. to S. of 14 April 1932. Ilberg, either a bookseller or Johannes (1860–1930) who wrote about medicine in Antiquity. RM: Reichsmark. Chesney see G. to S. of 2 October 1931. "Being back soon": in Baltimore.

GARRISON to SIGERIST, Baltimore, 1 June 1932

My dear Sigerist:

The enclosed, you will readily understand, are merely intended to help you out in spending the amount allotted to you from this year's appropriation, but apart from the less expensive items, which seem good bargains, I am not assuming to recommend anything, as you will be on the spot and can judge of the actual and prospective value of the items for research work from your own angle. As you know, if the items are to be paid for at this end out of the 1931–2 appropriation, the bills will have to be received here before July 1 proximo, otherwise the money will lapse into the general fund, and they would have to be paid for out of your new (1932–3) appropriation, which I fancy you will want to leave intact until you get around to it. That is why I am trying to help you out a bit, in view of the small amount of time at your disposal. Dr. Chesney states that you will be privileged to draw the amount allotted out of the 1931–2 appropriation, or the balance of it not already expended, and pay for the items yourself in situ, if you wish, getting receipted bills for same until the whole $ 3000 is expended[.] The more expensive items in the enclosed lists are, of course, merely submitted as "fillers", if you are in a jam to clean up your expenditures before July 1, which will probably not be the case.

As I cease to function as Acting Director of the Institute on July 1, I am arranging to have all correspondence on important details mailed for you for decision, reserving minor details until your arrival in the fall. I am delighted to learn from Dr. Chesney that Temkin will be with you, and everyone is looking forward to your arrival with pleasure. Miss Broemer has been in rather poor health latterly, in hospital in fact, and I have advised her to rest until the Academic sessions are over and Institute business will be practically nil, when she can lie on her oars and take it easy during the hot Baltimore summer. To date, we have had "toter Frühling", i. e. a cold, raw springtime, I doubt if my usual summering in New England will be viable before July 15. I should like to learn your prospective plan of

138

organization when you get it blocked out and can give you some inside information about pitfalls when we meet again. If there is anything I can do for you at this end, please let me know.

With kindest regards to Mrs. Sigerist and yourself, believe me

Very sincerely yours

F. H. Garrison

Chesney see G. to S. of 19 March 1932. Owsei Temkin (1902–2002) S.'s best coworker from Leipzig. Broemer see G. to S. of 25 November 1931. "toter Frühling" = dead spring.

GARRISON to SIGERIST, Baltimore, 15 June 1932

My dear Sigerist:

I am delighted to learn through Oliver, that you are sailing on September 9, which will probably bring you in to these shores at the end of the dreadful September heat. September 1 to 21 is apt to be the hottest part of the summer and would be perfectly dreadful for apartment hunting. We are having a very late, and sometimes raw spring, and I suspect that summer in New England will not really set in until about the end of July. We are, therefore, counting on remaining around here until about that time.

With kindest regards to Mrs. Sigerist, yourself, and all other friends in Leipzig,

Very sincerely yours

F. H. Garrison

Oliver see G. to S. of 7 October 1931.

GARRISON to SIGERIST, Baltimore, 1 July 1932

My dear Sigerist:

My duties as Acting Director of the Institute cease and determine the date and I have arranged that from to-day on, all business of consequence be submitted to you by mail or held for action until your arrival in September, which will be a great and much needed simplification. I am asking Miss Broemer to send you Institute paper and envelopes for ordering of books or any other business you may want to attend to and she has already submitted to you the skeleton form of Institute activities during 1932–3 (prospective), which had been referred to me but which would be better blocked out by you, with reference to your own prospective activities and those of Temkin, Oliver and myself. I handed Miss Broemer a tentative list of five lectures I have in mind, which is all I could possibly attend to, as I wish to concentrate more on Library activities, but I hope you will collaborate with me in some printable course on composition of medical papers, reviews, editorials, obituaries, etc., the main object of which is to get some clearing-house system for reviewing books presented to the Library and Institute via [?] the Hospital Bulletin. This course was very successful in the first year of my residence here (1930–31), but somehow fell flat during 1931–2. If you could lend the cachet of your name to it for a semester, I think it might be turned into a quasiseminar, and your dynamics would do the rest. You will realize that it ought to be attended more, as graduating dissertations are not required and the medical students, as in those of the Philosophical Faculty at Homewood, whence most of the interest in our subject has come to date. There seems to be very little interest in medical history (Oliver's lecture, for instance) on the part of the student body of the medical school, but should you put over the seminary you contemplated on the history of physiology, it will probably gather in a sufficient number from the "highways and the byways" – or possibly the history of public hygiene, with reference to the students and faculty of the School of Hygiene across the way. My only reason for referring to these two possibilities is the experience and observation of one who has been on the terrain for about two years' running. As you know, d'Irsay rode to failure in these themata, but for other reasons than the intrinsic nature or attractive potentialities of the themata themselves. The feeling of Oliver and myself is that we want to stand aside and do everything we can to uphold your hands in whatever lines you choose to function.

Until latterly, we have had a cold raw spring in Baltimore this year, but now the summer is on full force, although the weather to date has been more notable for humidity than heat. I hope to be in position to leave for vacation in about two or three weeks time, but not until I have straightened out certain personal and financial affairs, which have been sadly neglected to date. I was at Yale recently with Fulton, Winslow Winternitz and others you have meet [sic] and had a very delightful stay of a couple of days. I have never seen the New 33 Haven plant before, and was astounded at the extent of new building going on and the magnificence of the new Library.

We are sadly in need of a set of Hirschberg's extensive Geschichte der Augenheilkunde, and should you run across a good bound copy at reasonable rate or be able to order one, it would be a welcome addition to our reference apparat, if you approve. All the books ordered from Koehler arrived the other day, and in good shape. The Ilberg Handapparat and the portrait-autograph series are well worth the price of admission, particularly with regard to the amount of labor expended in arranging and indexing them so effectively. They illustrate the maxim that money is the equivalent of stored up energy.

The agent of the Luminophor process (enclosed card) was in this morning and as he said you employed it in your Leipzig Institute, I naturally referred him to you, in case you want one for the Baltimore plant. We got away with the wind-up of Library and Institute budgets famously for 1931–2, but the Library budget for 1932–3 will be considerably less by reason of the present financial stringency, although the Institute funds for 1932–3 remain intact and equivalent to the budget for 1931–2. You will, therefore, start without any depletion of your financial resources.

Looking forward to seeing you in the fall and with kindest regards to Mrs. Sigerist and yourself,

Yours very sincerely

F. H. Garrison

You will probably be president of the Medical History Club next year, unless Dr. W. wishes to continue indefinitely, but of that and many other matters, more anon.

Broemer see G. to S. of 25 November 1931. Temkin and Oliver see G. to S. of 1 June 1932 and 7 October 1931, respectively. Stephen d'Irsay (1894–1934) see G. to S. of 6 December 1929. John F. Fulton (1899–1960) physiologist and medical historian at Yale University. C. E. A. Winslow (1877–1957) professor of public health at Yale. Milton C. Winternitz (1885–1959) professor of psychiatry at Yale. Julius Hirschberg (1843–1925) German ophthalmologist and medical historian (Hirschberg 1899). Geschichte der Augenheilkunde = history of ophthalmology. Koehler and Ilberg Handapparat see G. to S. of 19 March and 14 April 1932. Luminophor, a luminescing substance. Dr. W., W. H. Welch.

My dear Sigerist:

Thank you so much for sending me the book of Bry, which I hardly expected you to remember. It is most pleasant to feel that you did remember it and I shall read it with great interest during the summer. It looks like a book of considerable originality as to content.

Miss Broemer is mailing you Institute stationary, as reported in my last letter, so that you will be in position to handle any business that may come up by way of correspondence or otherwise.

This morning I had a visitor a Professor of Philosophy from a prominent Western university, who is working up a book on the theme: Scientific Method in Greek Medicine. He is a pleasant man whom I met once before, and he wanted me to read over his manuscript critically. I advised him, however, to arrange to take a seminary course under you, with a view of shaping out his manuscript for the press, and if he can arrange the time, I think he would regard the proposition favorably. I rather fancy that these are the sort of people you would like to assemble to work under your direction and such a theme as the above would probably be interesting and would best be handled by yourself. I think that in all probability, we shall have a good many people of this kind roll in before the beginning of the academic session. Should you have time, I should be glad indeed to have your slant upon such matters.

I wish it were possible for me to get across the water this summer, but dis aliter visum, and it is perhaps just as well, for I suspect that the Bucharest Congress will not amount to much and I see that you are jumping it by the act of sailing on September 9. I am cleaning up a lot of personal business here and then expect to go North about Sept. 19–21.

With kindest regards to Mrs. Sigerist and yourself,

    Yours very sincerely

    F. H. Garrison

P.S.

In a few days you will receive a letter about a bill run up against the Institute by someone who retained some of the items as his personal property. Your own good judgement will suggest the advisability of proceeding with great firmness in the matter, which can be made a very effective barrier against future intrusion upon your personal welfare and peace of mind by said person.

The National Library of Medicine has books of three authors named Bry, one of the 18th and two of the 16th centuries. Miss Broemer see G. to S. of 25 November 1931. Dis aliter visum: The gods have deemed otherwise.

Garrison to Sigerist, Baltimore ?, summer ? 1932 or later

This undated letter, starting with "Dear Sigerist" and ending with F.H.G., scribbled in pencil with many illegible words, is likely to be G.'s last letter to S. in Leipzig before his assuming the post in Baltimore. It is given here as a summary of the contents rather than as a distorted transcription.

G. read a study of the German classical philologist, F. A. Wolf (1759–1824), whose geniality and kindness reminds one of S. Both had bully teachers.

For G. university life after more than 40 years is still somewhat new. He suggests the following notions of his duties as "Lecturer":
1. Lectures and conferences on topics to be announced.
2. To supply the director (S.) with data and information from current periodicals.
3. To continuously prepare a bibliography of medico-historical literature from medical and historical sources.
4. To prepare a catalog of classic texts.
5. To prepare a monograph on the medical periodicals of the 18th century.
6. To assist the director, if requested, in providing particular data.
7. To organize reviews of the books sent to the (Welch)Library.
8. To maintain contacts with linguistic departments.
9. To assist Institute students with bibliographic reference or other information.

G. had difficulties of adjustment because in Government service he had been on his own. He has no talent for handling classes, yet might be a good catalyzer. A journal club would be very helpful for the Institute. Administrative adjustments between Institute and Library are the responsibility of the director and G. alone.

Garrison to Sigerist, Baltimore, 27 March "1932" (probably 1933)

My dear Sigerist:

One can see, with half an eye, that you have had innumerable sources of irritation in the many responsibilities devolving upon you, the necessity of burning the midnight oil in writing and preparing so many lectures and papers, apart from your book, the adjustment to a new and sometimes disconcerting environment and the natural reactions of any selfrespecting man, who "does not suffer fools gladly" to the bored and human pests, whom the Russian novelist has likened to "those summer flies which we try in vain to brush away". If I have ever bored or irritated you, with so much pressing down on your shoulders, I'm genuinely sorry. Consciously I have done all I could to uphold your hands as director of the Institute, and if I have made any mistakes, don't forget that the environment is strange and 35 new, for me as well as yourself. One or two waspish comments on European colleagues suggest fish-hooks under your nerves, where "mediocrity is never discussed", and we've all of us "been there" in moments of mental irritation. The best way out, in my experience, is that outlined in Paragraph 5, Army Regulations, which forbids praise or blame of other officers, [...] that "good wire [?] needs no bush", and what is blameworthy has either to be ignored or handled impersonally through channels. All I ask, not so much with regard to myself as with reference to smooth-running administration in the Library, is that you will see me impersonally as an old veteran, who has suffered not a little humiliation of one kind or another during the long period of consideration of possible successors of Dr. Welch's Chair. I never applied for the position and you were the only possibility for whom I ever expressed any enthusiasm. The reward of the general world for this kind of modesty before an ideal is, as you know, a certain capitis diminutis, but in this cock-eyed period of boyish mentality, which has wrecked the financial integrity of the civilized world all I ask is a little delicacy of consideration with reference to the Horatian rule [?] – "ne trucidet coram populo juvenis senem"

Very sincerely yours
F. H. Garrison

This very strange letter after one half year of cooperation of the two correspondents is totally different from the preceding ones both in contents and style and therefore hard to explain. It is at the same time apologetic, irritated and accusing. Capitis diminutis: Loss of status. Ne trucidet coram populo juvenis senem: Nor let a youth slay the old in public.

Dear Sigerist:

A thought for your birthday and wishing you many pleasant ones ad multos annos. Huxley said: Thoughtfulness for others, generosity, modesty and self-respect, are the qualities which make a real gentleman or lady, as distinguished from the veneered article which commonly goes by the name. That is the Anglo-Saxon code of equity, fair play and "cricket" or playing the game according to the rules, in which I was bred and born, when I heard you chortle over the childish trait of shying a shoe through a Gainsborough canvas. I saw, as by flash-light illumination over a vast space, the two opposite worlds in which we were trained and when Pijeau jr. [?] told me that I am regarded in these parts as "a meek type" I had to laugh. You are […] devoid of magnanimity and generosity, far from it, but "youth has its arrogance", as the poet said and you are still young, with half of a lifetime before you. I have been so puzzled by the Hetz which has been going on in the Conferences that I really don't know what to make of it and have given up trying to understand it. Your behavior toward me at the last one (am Ende) was certainly most insulting. As between you and me personally, I figure that my cold, brooding melancholy self-possession of the Scottish order, is as a red rag to a bull to a man of your impetuous, impatient nature and you have the known physical conformation of a male shrew, apart from the fact that all schoolmasters are inclined to be schoolmasterly. I may say for myself, however, that my physical well-being, apart from my health, is of a very fragile order, in other words, I am easily depressed by ennui and at the last Conference, I was quite ill, although none of the three physicians present were observant enough to glimpse the fact – a common trait of Heilärzte welche heilen nicht. If I could offer one friendly […] on your birthday it would be: eschew, as far as possible, Rücksichtslosigkeit, Schadenfreude, Neckereien, recht zur Zeit ertheilte [sic] Hiebe, Heftigkeit, Jähzornigkeit, imponiren [sic] and all similar traits of the German professoriate, as "spiritual insults" of the kind are sure to make enemies, on Bernard Shaw's principle that if you hit a man when he is off his guard or not in position to defend yourself, he may not say 36 anything, but he will never forgive you. In this country, the social technique of men like Longcope, Theobald Smith, Howell et al.s the accepted code among gentlemen and just a little bit of all right, in my opinion, I rest my case there.

For orientation, I may say that as Librarian I am responsible solely to the President of the University, that the position connotes the rank of professor, although I attach no importance to these distinctions and have made no fuss about them; and in regard to the Institute grade of Lecturer, my instructions were that I was to be a kind of free-lance liaison officer between the Library and the Institute, in such wise that it would in no way impinge upon my duties as Librarian. The crux is there and I hope we can settle it in some way or other à l'amicale.

Yours ever

F. H. Garrison

This second unusual letter of G. shows in S.'s long-hand the comment "kept as a psychopathological document". In print S. said of G. that he was sensitive like a mimosa (Sigerist 1935).

Ad multos annos: Many returns of the day. Hetz(e) = hunt. Am Ende = at the end. Heilärzte welche heilen nicht = healing doctors who do not heal. Rücksichtslosigkeit = recklessness. Schadenfreude = malicious joy. Neckereien = teasings. Recht zur Zeit erteilte Hiebe = blows in good time. Heftigkeit = vehemence. Jähzornigkeit = irascibility. Imponieren = impress. A l'amicale: In a friendly way.

New names:

Howell, William H. (1860–1945) physiologist at Hopkins.

Huxley, probably Aldous (born 1894) English writer

Longcope, Warfield T. (1877–1953) professor of medicine and director of the Hopkins Department of Medicine

Pijoan, M. jr., disciple of G., now at Harvard University.

Shaw, George Bernard (1856–1950) Irish dramatist

Smith, Theobald (1859–1934) microbiologist and immunologist.

Garrison to Sigerist, Baltimore, 22 June 1933

My dear Sigerist:

You may perhaps have seen the enclosed. At any rate I am sending it for what it is worth. A later communication pares this down to ten percent of actual deposits payable a month from date. I thought you might like to have this information if it has not already reached you through some other channels. I fancy it will be some time before we touch one hundred percent.

I have been plugging away manfully at the revised students check list, inspite of the dreadful bouts of heat (95 degrees in the shade about two weeks ago) and hope to get it off shortly. At any rate, I am "standing by", as sailors say, until I do. I have arranged about the typography with Mr. Williams and I am trying to insure the utmost compression by paring titles down to an irriducible minimum. I fancy you will approve of this line, as I am not attempting a scholastic bibliography but a handy check list for students. I have found the MacCallum dissertations wonderfully helpful, although I am naturally only taking a few high spots in the history of diseases. As soon as I get away with the job, we shall pull out for the north.

I trust Mrs. Sigerist and you will have had a pleasant and prosperous voyage, enjoyable also to the children and naturally you will be enjoying life on the Continent, where it is so much cooler than here. You know my summer address, Oak Bluffs, Massachusetts, where we shall probably remain until after the middle of September. I hope you can find time to drop me a line now and then.

With kindest regards to Mrs. Sigerist, yourself and the children.
Sincerely yours
F. H. Garrison
Librarian

This letter is addressed c/o S.'s mother in Basel. Sigerist spent the whole summer in Europe, working in libraries in Switzerland, Italy, and France. Mr. Williams not identified. McCallum probably William George (1874–1944) pathologist and medical historian at Hopkins.

As letter-like documents one may consider an invitation of G. to S. for a dinner to meet Arturo Castiglioni of 24 October 1933, as well as one of 12 April 1934.

GARRISON to SIGERIST, Baltimore, 8 January 1934

Dear Sigerist:
With reference to my program:
If you have written, or will write to Dr. A. A. Moll, Pan-American Sanitary Bureau, arranging a conference on Latin-American Medicine, as for schedule, I could then figure as follows:
1. Medical Numismatics
2. Medical Periodicals of the 18th Century [;] at any time you think best, if you will give me (say) two weeks notice for adequate preparation.

3. Spanish Medicine: Moll's proposition [?] for a joint contribution by […] and me at the Spanish Legation in February.
4. Ditto: for the Romance language group at Homewood, as for arrangement with Chenard.
5. Medical History of Schumann family to Goethe Society, January 20.
6. Medicus Medicum odit. An inter nos conference of personnel of Institute later on, say at my […] some night.
7. Lecture to English group at Homewood on Medicine in the Spectator, Jaller and Guardian (invite them here in the late spring before you leave).

This pencil-written sheet seems to be a memo rather than a letter. A. A. Moll, probably Mexican, has published on Pan-American medicine. Spectator, Jaller and Guardian: Newspapers, see also (Garrison 1934).

GARRISON to SIGERIST, Baltimore, 14 July 1934

Dear Sigerist:

Before I leave for my vacation, I want to report very good progress on the iconography of Dr. Welch. We have already assembled a good many portraits and Robert Roy of the Waverly Press makes a very reasonable offer for a volume of about fifty plates, reproduced in the very best manner, quarto size, with a few pages of introduction, at $ 300–600. This looks very favorable to me. We have acquired a great many valuable books from Dr. Welch's estate, many of which, of course, go over to the Institute side. I am just winding up this business before I leave.

The July Bulletin containing my bibliography of periodicals is out and I understand that copies will be sent me this afternoon.

With kindest regards to Mrs. Sigerist, yourself and the family and wishing you a very pleasant summer,

Very sincerely yours
F. H. Garrison

This letter goes to S. in Switzerland again. Welch died on 30 April 1934, whereupon the Institute and the Library planned for an iconography, i. e., to publish pictures of Welch during the different periods of his life (Sigerist to Klebs of 9 October 1934a).

My dear Sigerist:

Thanking you for yours of August 4, which has been some twenty days on the way here; I am delighted to learn that you have found such a pleasant abiding place at Utohorn and that you have been able to cover so much ground in the important research work you are following up. One more year of it and I fancy you will have covered the whole existing material.

To date we have had very little summer here – mostly cool Herbstgefühl weather, with sudden changes from sunshine to clouds, fog and rain, but the swimming is as good as ever, even when the water is cold, and I am getting my weight down and my rusty muscles limbered for the winter campaign.

I am sending off an editorial on "Transvaluations and Deflations in the History of Medicine and its Teaching", which I hope will help your cause a little; and have been able to block out the framework of a few lectures. Going through the Divina Commedia is slow work, on account of the archaic Tuscan diction, which is startlingly modern in the "high spots" and "mighty lines"; but I am fairly familiar with the Inferno, having gone through the 34 cantos as a student in Baltimore in 1888. Most of the scientific material is in the Purgatorio and Paradise. The whole fabric seems a colossal repository of mediaeval science and the history of the squabbling Italian city-states of the 12th to 13th Centuries. Castiglioni's résumé of the medical phases is admirable and gives the gist of the many Italian contributions on Dante as a putative student of medicine. The total literature seems enormous but I hope to get away with the complex schema by maximum compression.

I hope you will do me the honor of collaborating on the anthology or iconography of Welch pictures, as representing both Institute and Library. If the picture you speak of is not in my collection, we can write for it later.

Miss Broemer has made a thorough, business-like arrangement of the material for Flexner – the best solution and […] resolution of that tangle.

In the Literary Supplement of the New York Times for August 12 is a review of a remarkable English novel, which illustrates your views on the deflection or isolation of the sick patient from the total rhythmus of life. It is about the effects of a gastritis, merging into ulcer or cancer, upon the social and business relations of a prosaic, efficient Scotchman – something like the floating kidney motif in Tolstoi's Ivan Ilyich. The number was hustled to our trash-barrel before I could make a note of it, but I will write to the Times eventually and get the title, if you are at all interested. The book is said to be a readable presentation of material ordinarily dry and uninteresting, except to clinicians. You probably know the Tolstoi novel – lugubrious but powerful.

We are here until September 16 and shall have at least escaped the heat of the cities, which is said to have been terrific in spots. The drought in the West and South has occasioned much misery and even starvation.

With kind regards to Mrs. Sigerist, yourself and the children
Very sincerely yours
F. H. Garrison

S.'s letter missing. Utohorn, name of S.'s summer house in Kastanienbaum, a village on the Lake of Lucerne. S.'s research in European libraries (Sigerist 1934b, c). Herbstgefühl: feeling of autumn. Arturo Castiglioni (1874–1953) Italian medical historian, 1939–1946 exiled in the U.S. Welch iconography see G. to S. of 14 July 1934. Flexner, probably Simon (1863–1946) biographer of W. H. Welch.

Garrison to Sigerist, Oak Bluffs, MA, 31 August 1934

Dear Sigerist:

Thanking you for you note of August 21 about the bibliography, which I am glad you find OK: there has been a queer tangle about the Ms. of my Spectator article, slated by you for the October number and mentioned for October on the last page of the July bibliography. Five pages of the Ms., sent by Miss Brooke to me for retouching, at my request, were returned to her on August 17 (the day I received them) but a telegram from her on August 29 states that they did not reach her. In that case, she should have wired me long before, but I have sent out a P.O. trailer and have written asking her to send the Ms. on to the printer if complete as to terminal five pages or hold it until my return, when I will complete it by my notes. I am sure the Waverly Press has [...] for getting out the October Number in plenty of time and trust you will OK this, as it would [...] matters to announce printing for October and then not print. I should feel very grateful. We have had a rather gloomy autumnal season of [...] here and the last few days have been very cold, even in Baltimore. I am

150

therefore returning earlier, as the back of the hot weather has been broken (there has been snow in the West some time ago), unless there should be one of those sudden changes of the American climate. Here's hoping you will have plenty of luck with your Mss. in Italy and with best wishes from house to house I remain

Yours ever

F. H. Garrison

S.'s letter missing. Spectator article (Garrison 1934). Helen Brooke, research secretary at S.'s Institute in Baltimore. S.'s manuscripts: S. was collecting medieval manuscripts in European libraries.

This seems to be G.'s last regular letter to S. before his death on 18 April 1935. The letter may seem to be slightly confused.

Once more the letter is followed by a document which may not be a letter. It is undated, starting without a salutation, ending abruptly, scribbled in pencil with many illegible words. It is given here as a summary of the contents rather than as a distorted transcription:

The first sentence or title reads "Sigerist's book on American Medicine", i. e. (Sigerist 1933). Thus, the document possibly is a book review. The text then deals with books on the United States and their shortcomings, with the concluding sentence "Professor Sigerist's book affords a welcome relief." The very last sentence of the first page starts with "An American, who has been a spectator of" where it abruptly ends. This may also suggest that the text is part of Garrison's Spectator article. The second and third pages review S.'s book in a highly benevolent way, ending with the sentence "All in all, the volume is a splendid piece of straight-shooting".

3.3. Literature

Ackerknecht, Erwin H.: *Zum hundertsten Geburtstag von Fielding H. Garrison.* Gesnerus 27, 229–230, 1970.

Clendening, Logan: *The Human Body.* New York 1927.

Cope, Zachary: *Fielding Hudson Garrison (1870–1935).* CIBA-Symposium 10, 98–103, 1962.

Fichtner, Horst: *Die Medizin im Avesta …* Leipzig 1924.

Fonahn, Adolf M.: *Zur Quellenkunde der persischen Medizin.* Leipzig 1910.

Garrison, Fielding H.: *Texts Illustrating the History of Medicine.* 1912.

Garrison, Fielding H.: *Introduction to the History of Medicine, with Medical Chronology, and Bibliographic Data.* Philadelphia 1913.

Garrison, Fielding H.: *John Shaw Billings; A Memoir.* New York 1915.

Garrison, Fielding H.: *The Newer Epidemiology.* In Singer / Sigerist 1924, 255–268.

Garrison, Fielding H.: *The Principles of Anatomic Illustration Before Vesalius.* New York 1926.

Garrison, Fielding H.: *Bibliographie der Arbeiten Moritz Steinschneiders zur Geschichte der Medizin und Naturwissenschaften.* Sudhoffs Arch. 25, 249–278, 1932.

Garrison, Fielding H.: *A Century of American Medicine.* In Beard's "Century of Progress". New York 1933, 325–356.

Garrison, Fielding H.: *Medicine in the Tatler, Spectator, and Guardian.* Bull. N. Y. Acad. Med. 10, 477–503, 1934.

Goldschmid, Edgar: *Entwicklung und Bibliographie der pathologisch-anatomischen Abbildung.* Leipzig 1925.

Hirschberg, Julius: *Geschichte der Augenheilkunde.* 2nd ed. Leipzig 1899–1918.

Kagan, Solomon R.: *Life and Letters of Fielding H. Garrison.* Boston 1938.

Kagan, Solomon R.: *Fielding H. Garrison; A Biography.* Boston 1948.

Mayer, Claudius Frank: *The Literary Activity of Fielding H. Garrison. With an Annotated Bibliography of his Publications Related to Medicine.* Bull. Hist. Med. 5, 378–403, 1937.

Ramon y Cajal, Santiago: *Charlas de café; pensamientos, anécdotas y confidencias.* Madrid 1920.

Sigerist, Henry E.: *Studien und Texte zur frühmittelalterlichen Rezeptliteratur.* Habilitations-Schrift Zürich. Leipzig 1923.

Sigerist Henry E.: *Einführung in die Medizin.* Leipzig 1931.

Sigerist, Henry E.: *Man and Medicine. An Introduction to Medical Knowledge.* New York 1932a (translation of Sigerist 1931).

Sigerist, Henry E.: *Grosse Aerzte.* München 1932b. (Translated: *Great Doctors. A Biographical History of Medicine.* London 1933).

Sigerist, Henry E.: *Amerika und die Medizin.* Leipzig 1933. (Translated: *American Medicine.* New York 1934).

Sigerist, Henry E. to Klebs, Arnold C. of 9 October 1934a.

Sigerist, Henry E.: *The Medical Literature of the Early Middle Ages. A Program and a Report of a Summer of Research in Italy.* Bull. Hist. Med. 2, 26–50, 1934b.

Sigerist, Henry E.: *A Summer of Research in European Libraries.* Bull. Hist. Med. 2, 559–610, 1934c.

Sigerist, Henry E.: *Fielding H. Garrison.* Bull. Hist. Med. 3, 403–404, 1935.

Sigerist, Henry E.: *Letters of Fielding H. Garrison.* Bull. Hist. Med. 5, 947, 1937.

Sigerist, Henry E.: *Kagan's Garrison.* Bull. Hist. Med. 7, 357–362, 1939.

Sigerist, Henry E. and E. E. Hume, H. R. Viets, F. L. Tietsch, M. Pijoan, A. Castiglioni, C. F. Mayer: *Fielding H. Garrison Memorial Number.* Bull. Hist. Med. 5, 299–403, 1937.

Singer, Charles / Sigerist, Henry E.: *Essays on the History of Medicine Presented to Karl Sudhoff on the Occasion of his Seventieth Birthday November 26th 1923.* London / Zurich 1924.

Sudhoff, Karl: *Medizinische Bibliotheken. Eine historische Plauderei.* Archiv für Geschichte der Medizin 21, 296–310, 1929.

Thiele, Rudolf: *Männer gegen Tod und Teufel.* Berlin 1931.

Zinn, Nancy W.: *Garrison, Fielding Hudson.* New York 1999.

3.4. Name Index

4. Correspondence
Henry E. Sigerist – Erwin H. Ackerknecht
1931–1957

4.1. Introduction

4.1.1. Erwin H. Ackerknecht (1906–1988)

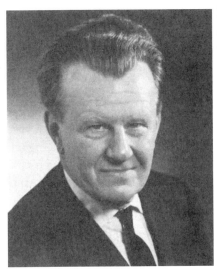

Erwin Heinz Ackerknecht was born on June 1st 1906 and grew up in the then German city of Stettin (since 1945 Szczecin, Poland). He studied medicine at the universities of Freiburg, Kiel, Berlin, and Vienna. In Leipzig (1927–1932) he was a student of Henry E. Sigerist, wrote a thesis on a topic of the social history of medicine (Ackerknecht 1932), obtained his M. D. degree and married his first wife, Helen Rother. In these years he was a communist, active in the fight against the Nazi party, and therefore left Germany to save his life after Hitler seized power in 1933. He first spent some weeks with Trotsky in Turkey. Deprived by the Nazis of his German citizenship and of his medical license, Paris became his exile home where he first was reduced to doing odd jobs but eventually completed his former studies in anthropology at the Sorbonne. He married his second wife, Lucy Krüger, who became the mother of the two daughters, Sylvia and Ellen. Gradually Ackerknecht disentangled himself from politics, disgusted by both the brown and the red form of totalitarianism. When WWII broke out he was interned in a camp, and with the German invasion of France in 1940 he was, once more, forced into an adventurous flight, taking refuge in the unoccupied zone of France, still waiting for his U.S. immigration visa. He finally was able to sail to the U.S. in 1941. After more odd jobs in New York he finally returned to medical history, becoming research fellow at the Johns Hopkins Institute for the History of Medicine in Baltimore, then directed by his former teacher Henry E. Sigerist. There he spent three productive years, guided and taught mainly by Sigerist's associate professor, Owsei Temkin. During the years 1945 and 1946 Ackerknecht was assistant curator of anthropology at the American Museum of Natural History in New York where he made use of his knowledge in ethnology and primitive medicine. The great opportunity came in 1947 when he was offered the chair of the new (second) department of the history of medicine in the U.S. at the University of Wisconsin in Madison which he headed for ten years as full professor. At that time he also became an American citizen. When in the mid 1950s his position in Madison had become less attractive to him, Ackerknecht gladly accepted the offer to fill the equivalent position at the University of Zurich and thus being able to return to Europe, not too far from his beloved Paris. In Zurich he reorganized the department and its collections, continued his research and publishing and enjoyed his success in teaching. He also made lecture tours to the U.S., combined with visits to his daughters. In Zurich he married his third wife, Edit Weinberg and retired in 1971, still remaining active and productive despite increasing health problems. He was also a Sunday painter and a collector of prints. During his decade in the Midwest he had been longing for Europe, but once living back there he realized that the U.S. "still remains my country" (Ackerknecht 1972). He died on 18th November 1988 in Zurich.

For biographical material see (Ackerknecht 1986), (Cranefield 1990), (Rosenberg 2007), (Temkin 1989), (Walser 1988, 1998). Ackerknecht's Bibliography is listed in (Walser 1966, 1976, 1986, 1988). Sketches of Ackerknecht's character, of his work and its significance can be found in the mentioned papers by Cranefield, Rosenberg, Temkin, and Walser.

4.1.2. The Correspondence

4.1.2.1. Technicalities and Explanations

There is a total of 172 letters of Ackerknecht to Sigerist and 99 letters of Sigerist to Ackerknecht, including some telegrams. A few letters mentioned in the correspondence are missing, yet there is no evidence of considerable amounts of missing ones. The missing letters are predominantly Sigerist's, in all likeliness long-hand letters of which he did not make carbon copies.

Most of the letters are in English, 9 per cent each in Ackerknecht's mother tongue, German, and in both correspondents' favorite language, French. Until 1939 the correspondence is in German; from 1941 on in English. From 1939 on there are occasional letters in French. If the original letter is in German or French this is indicated in the letterhead of this edition. The German and French letters have been translated by the editor whose intention was to maintain the unpolished style of letters, which were not written for publication, and at the same time to convey all information that they contain.

Practically all letters are dated. The majority of letters are typed. Some of Ackerknecht's letters are in long-hand, although he preferred typed letters. Sigerist liked to write in long-hand, yet he used typing in order to have his own carbon-copies made. Some of Ackerknecht's long-hand letters contain occasional illegible words which in the transcription are indicated by the sign […] or are followed by [?]. Spelling errors were transcribed as such, but are followed by the sign [sic], whereas the frequent errors in punctuation were left unchanged and unmarked as long as they did not distort the sense of a sentence. The sign [ ] was also used for Sigerist's signature which was missing on the carbon copies used. Literary works are given as, e.g., (Allen 1946) and listed in chapter 3 (Literature).

The annotations are given in small print following each transcribed letter. They are meant to help understanding the contents of the letters rather than to interpret them and are therefore kept at a minimum. They also serve as links to former letters and annotations so that persons or things can be explained once only. The term "medical historian" for the characterization of persons is used in a wide sense as, e.g., members of the American Association of the History of Medicine. A few persons sufficiently characterized and explained in the letter may not appear in the annotations. Others, most of them mentioned only once, could not be identified and are marked as such in the annotation. However, all persons mentioned in the letters are listed in the name index (chapter 4). A bibliography of all literature mentioned in the letters and annotations is also given (chapter 3).

4.1.2.2. The Correspondence

The correspondence begins in 1931 and lasts with increasing frequency all the way to Sigerist's death in 1957. In 1931 Sigerist is professor in Leipzig, 40 years old, and Ackerknecht, his doctoral student, 24 years. The first letters deal with Ackerknecht's doctoral thesis and his situation in Germany.

There follows a gap of several years until Ackerknecht, a political exile in Paris, resumes the contact with his teacher. He tells of his jobs as salesman, student of ethnology, medical librarian, painter, woodcutter, and soldier, also of his withdrawal from politics. No wonder is the physician longing for intellectual work after all these jobs outside his real interests. Sigerist's letters reappear in 1939 only, when Ackerknecht's longing for scientific work and for the U.S. immigration visa becomes outspoken and his situation at the beginning of WWII desperate. The reports of his camp life as an internee are cries of distress. He then tells of his dramatic flight before the German invaders and the additional year of waiting for the visa in unoccupied France. The correspondence then reveals Ackerknecht's lucky escape to the U.S. in 1941 and his early, rather frustrating, jobs in that year.

Then comes the fulfillment of his year-long hope: The promising beginning of historical and anthropological work at Sigerist's Institute of the History of Medicine in Baltimore in 1942. For obvious reasons there is no exchange of letters during the correspondents' three years under the same roof.

A regular correspondence then takes place during the years of Ackerknecht's career in New York (1945–46) and in Madison (1947–1957). Half of the total correspondence is between Ackerknecht in Madison and Sigerist in Pura, Switzerland, during the final decade of Sigerist's life. Sigerist, no longer the supporting former teacher, is now corresponding with Ackerknecht on an equal level and thereby also appearing in full profile. In contrast to Sigerist, Ackerknecht is very outspoken and critical of people and circumstances and is torn between Europe and America.

Ackerknecht's years at the American Museum of Natural History in New York were a crucial time. Not only did he remain in contact with Sigerist and his coworkers, but he also entered the world of ethnology and anthropology and met many of their representative scholars. Thus, the correspondence reveals his development from politics and from his thesis

162

on Virchow into ethnology as applied to medicine in the form of primitive medicine which then expanded into the general history of medicine and its social aspects – and thus back to Virchow.

Needless to say that a correspondence between two scholars with different biographies, different characters, different ages, over such a long period of time, reveals a wide array of topics. This was particularly so in the letters exchanged between Madison and Pura. Among other topics the correspondents discuss matters of the history of medicine, projects and achievements, travels, encounters, books, and persons. A total of more than 200 books and papers are discussed and over 600 persons are mentioned (see Literature and Name Index). The correspondents tell about their activities, and there is an exchange of reprints, books, and other materials. Health problems appear repeatedly in Ackerknecht's reports. The letters also tell about the correspondents' spouses and children. Both Ackerknecht and Sigerist express their worries over developments during the after-war years. Summer trips to Europe in 1953 and 1955 result in Ackerknecht's enthusiastic reports on Paris and on his encounters with Sigerist in Pura.

In this correspondence the first half of the 20th century unfolds, with its culture and convulsions, the Nazi time, the war years, and postwar Europe and America. All this is reflected in Ackerknecht's sigh "what life has done to our generation!"

This correspondence begins as one between teacher and disciple and turns into one between the colleagues and finally the friends Henry and Erwin, with an emotional side and a dramatic climax when in 1956 Ackerknecht, with Sigerist's engaged help, is fighting to obtain the chair of the History of Medicine in Zurich. After he finally had reached this goal there remained one single happy reunion of the two in spring of 1957 in Switzerland, just prior to Ackerknecht's start in Zurich and to Sigerist's death in Pura. Their hopes for frequent encounters in Switzerland were not fulfilled.

4.2. The Letters

Sigerist to Ackerknecht, Leipzig, 16 May 1931
(Original in German)

Dear Mr. Ackerknecht,

I would like to inquire about your work for the following reason. If the work could be finished as of July 1st, I could publish it in the next number of our "Kyklos". The advantage for you would be that your work would reach a wide audience at a minimum cost, since the publisher asks little for reprints. Personally I would be very glad to see your work in our year-book; it is very interesting, and its results are remarkable. Volume 4 will go to the printer and is to appear on October 1.

With kind regards I am
Yours as ever
[Henry E. Sigerist]

The letter's address is Lützenerstrasse 75, Leipzig. The work to publish was A.'s doctoral thesis (Ackerknecht 1932) which S. highly esteemed. Kyklos: The yearbook of S.'s institute in Leipzig.

Ackerknecht to Sigerist, August 1931, (Postcard, original in German)

Dear Professor Sigerist!

From my vacation I send you best greetings and good wishes for the growth of your book.

Yours
Erwin H. Ackerknecht

The picture on the reverse is a view of the beach of the island of Wollin in the Baltic near Stettin. The book mentioned is (Sigerist 1931). The postcard carries a note in S.'s handwriting that it has been answered on 14 September 1931 (see below).

SIGERIST to ACKERKNECHT, Leipzig, 14 September 1931
(Original in German)

My dear colleague,

Many thanks for your nice greetings. Enclosed find the two photographs which I made in the garden and which came out pretty well.

In the meantime I took care of the printing of your work. Unfortunately, the editor declines to bring it out as a separate publication. The people have become jittery and reserved. Thus, I will publish your work in "Archiv für Geschichte der Medizin", divided in two parts. Part one will appear in the first number of the next year on January 1st.

Let me add that it was a pleasure to have met you. I will embark in Hamburg tomorrow. In spring I shall be back, and I hope that we then meet again and keep in touch.

With kind regards I am

Yours as ever

[Henry E. Sigerist]

A.'s published thesis (Ackerknecht 1932). S. is going to spend one half year on a study tour in the U. S.

SIGERIST to ACKERKNECHT, Leipzig, 27 April 1932
(Original in German)

My dear Ackerknecht,

I have recently returned from my travels. On my desk I find your thesis, and I am very glad it has appeared. I heard favorable comments from many sides. Among others there was the enclosed letter of Beneke, a pupil of von Recklinghausen and, if I remember correctly, formerly a pathologist in Halle. Beneke also sends you the enclosed work on Virchow.

My tour was very interesting, and I will give an account of it this summer in the staff meeting. I hope you are fine, and I would be pleased to see you in the summer. I am spending my last semester in Germany since I have accepted a chair in the U.S. and will transfer in September.

With best regards I am

Yours as ever

[Henry E. Sigerist]

Rudolf Beneke (1861–1946) German pathologist. Friedrich D. von Recklinghausen (1833–1910) German pathologist. Rudolf Virchow (1821–1902) German pathologist, anthropologist, and politician. S. has been offered the chair of the history of medicine at Johns Hopkins University during his study tour in the U.S.

ACKERKNECHT to SIGERIST, Berlin, 29 April 1932
(Original in German)

Dear Professor Sigerist!

Many thanks for your letter. I was so glad to hear from you once more, but also saddened by the news that you will leave Germany. On the other hand, leaving Germany is the best one can do if one is in a position to. The outlook here is gloomy.

I am here since February, looking desperately for a job. For other reasons I am obliged to stay here as long as possible even though I don't like it and I would prefer to be in Leipzig with my wife [?], my patients, and my books. First I tried to continue historical work with Diepgen. However, I lacked both time and incentive. Now a good review in "Der Kassenarzt" brought me in contact with Julius Moses (the M.d.R.); he will see to it that I can write a pamphlet on the "freedom to heal". This seems interesting and would make sense; so I will try to do it, even if I should find a job in the near future.

My thesis I would arrange in a different way: inductive rather than deductive. Except for Moses' I have not yet seen reviews. My bad luck is that I did not have the money to have more copies printed; I am almost "sold out" by now.

Of course, I would be glad to see you, too. Should I come to Leipzig I would try to call you up. Or should I better write you in advance? In case you came to Berlin to talk about your tour I would be very glad if you could let me know it in advance.

Let me end by apologizing for my miserable typing.
Now that my thesis is printed, let me once more thank you for all your help.

With my regards and best wishes for your work
In gratitude yours
Erwin H. Ackerknecht

The radical left-wing activist A. was frightened by the rising tide of national socialism in Germany. For a short time he worked with Paul Diepgen (1878–1966), director of the Institute of the History of Medicine in Berlin; subsequently he was assistant in Berlin hospitals for internal medicine, neurology, and psychiatry. Julius Moses (1868–1953) German physician. M. d. R. not identified. A.'s doctoral thesis (Ackerknecht 1932).

In January 1933 the Nazis seized power in Germany, four months after S.'s departure for the U.S.; A. went underground and escaped in summer 1933 via Turkey to Paris. There he resumed correspondence with his former teacher in 1937.

ACKERKNECHT to SIGERIST, Paris, 21 October 1937
(Original in German)

Dear Professor Sigerist!

Today I looked into my thesis and found a letter that I had written to you four years ago but had not sent for lack of a current address. I still do not have this address but will try anyway. It can't hurt.

I have been in Paris since fall 1933. This may sound like good news, however, the whole situation of us exiles is strange. Otherwise Paris is and remains the most beautiful city in Europe, at least for people with historical or esthetic interests.

Having arrived here in possession of one worn suit, I had to find a source of income. Luckily, my wife was successful as a designer of fancy jewelry, so I could operate as her retailer. I had not been trained for this kind of activity, and one cannot precisely become rich with it. Still, we never needed help, and we did not suffer the way other emigrants did. We and our child can live decently off this income. Again I have a nice library and time to read (my former library having been "expropriated" as were my other possessions). My political activities are down, largely because these activities which one observes in the exile look rather silly.

Needless to say I have read many historical books, firstly in order to better understand this country, and secondly because reading the French historians is much more fun than reading their German colleagues.

However, I don't want to bother you with the biographical ups and downs of a former pupil. The reason of my letter is to tell you that I am living here and that, should you ever come to Paris, I would be extremely pleased to see you. It would also give me pleasure if I could help you in searching or ordering things in Paris for your Institute. On the other hand, I would highly appreciate to receive reprints of the Institute.

I do hope you had a good start in America and have met with a satisfactory environment. In view of what has happened in Germany, it was good for you to have left. I also hope your health and your family are fine.

With best regards and wishes I am

Yours devotedly

E. Ackerknecht

A. had finished his thesis with S. and obtained his M. D. in Leipzig in 1932. The stormy years of his political agitation in Germany and of his first years in exile are over. It seems likely that this is his first letter to S. since 1932. The letter has reached the addressee (see A. to S. of 8 December 1937). A. is living with his first wife Helen Rother and their daughter Ina. The letter carries the address 7. rue Vidal de la Blache, Paris XX.

ACKERKNECHT to SIGERIST, Paris, 8 December 1937
(Original in German)

Dear Professor Sigerist!

Many thanks for your friendly letter of 12 November. I was happy we have resumed contact, and even more happy that you remembered me and took the time to write a long letter. I am optimistic enough to start a new life after having been separated from people and things of my former life, yet there remains a certain vacuum, and one appreciates every bridge that can be rebuilt. My work at your department was always an oasis within my stormy existence, which was the result of circumstances rather than of intention or temperament. Maybe I can tell you more if my wish to see you next year in our old Paris shall come true.

Thanks also for the book and the reprints which arrived today. Once I will have studied the material I shall send you some remarks. It may take some time, although a [xxxx] dictates a sedentary life of reading. I admire the amount of your work, done in a relatively short time. No doubt the conditions there are much more favorable than they were in Leipzig. Compare the very load of teaching with what we had in Germany! By the way, I see that Dr. Temkin is still with you; please give him my regards. The American generosity will be helpful. It would have served the German specialists if the history of medicine would have given them a certain distance, an overview, and a sense of context. Medical history is the best, if not the only way to reach these goals.

I need not tell you how glad I am to learn that you are introducing sociological and Marxist elements into the history of medicine. This was precisely the motivation for my thesis which, unfortunately, is incomplete, not very outspoken, and written in a hurry. I tried to show, with the example already of Virchow, how fruitful such an approach can be. In France this historical approach is commonplace since Guizot, even with reactionary historians. The best along these lines seems now to be done in America. I am just reading a stimulating, if not scientific book by B. Wolfe: Portrait of Mexico. It is in America, I think, that Marxism most successfully avoids a certain dogmatic-philosophical calcification. In contrast, in Europe this is often the case, preventing the incorporation of new scientific and psychological knowledge.

Let me end with thanking you. I hope to write more in the near future. With my regards and good wishes

Yours

E. Ackerknecht

S.'s letter to A. apparently is not preserved as are the ones up to 1939. [xxxx] Protected Health Information as requested to be suppressed by the Alan Mason Chesney Archives of the Medical Institutions of Johns Hopkins University. Owsei Temkin (1902–2002) medical historian, A.'s colleague and S.'s assistant in Leipzig, S.'s collaborator in Baltimore. François Guizot (1787–1874) French historian. Bertram D. Wolfe, (1896–1977) American communist author, his book see (Rivera 1937).

ACKERKNECHT to SIGERIST, Paris, 5 May 1938
(Original in German)

Dear Professor Sigerist,

Let me first apologize to have been silent for such a long time; it was the result of work, poor health, and the ugly world events. Regarding France, the outside view may be worse and more dramatic than it is in reality. Personally I have been lucky enough to have found a minor job at a new institute for the study and prevention of professional diseases. The job is not for a living, yet it provides contact with my former profession and may even be a way out of the unattractive field of commerce. Your papers on the "Historical Background of industrial Diseases" and on "Medical Licensure" are of particular interest in view of my new activity as are all of your papers you were kind enough to send. Other papers of yours would be most welcome; I could review some of them in the "Archive" of the institute which appears at Masson's.

Among the reprints you sent I read with the greatest interest "the medical student and the social problems" and "an outline of the development of the hospital". That a rational history of modern medicine must be written with the hospital as a center-piece (hospital = site of production of modern medicine) is an old idée fixe of mine, taken over from Virchow, I guess.

I also liked "Medicine in the Tatler…" by F.H. Garrison, your "Art and Medicine", and the two fine exhibitions, proof of the intense work at your Institute.

J.R. Oliver in "spontaneous combustion" was wrong with regard to Zola's novel, but it is "Dr. Pascal" rather than "Nora"

[3 lines illegible due to faded ink]

in the quarrels that still erupt – like those about Victor Hugo or Robespierre – as reflections of new accounts,

[2 lines illegible]

I admire how much you produced in the short time and no doubt being bothered by a host of practical things.

Needless to say I have read your book with particular interest. I need not tell you either that I fully agree with the basic idea of a socialist medicine. The book is a source of so many stimuli. E.g., with regard of your old article in "Kyklos" typhoid was the […] of the Russian Revolution. However, it would not be appropriate nor useful to only praise your book without saying in a few words where I do not quite agree. The successes need to be downsized if considered as such or if compared with achievements in the Western world. This is inevitable and understandable.

[2 lines illegible]

It is better to state this fact, which you certainly mention, very clearly in order to save the "principle" or the "ideal" in view of disappointments and setbacks. For on the other hand, in real socialism there are not only individual standard achievements but rather the progress for the benefit of all the people.

170

I also disagree with your statements about democracy and its future in Russia. Constitutions, laws, and decrees are little proof for us Marxists. On the other hand, we are confronted with sad realities like the law-suits and what goes along. Of those I cannot believe one word because of my [...] own experiences with Trotzki who, by the way, stands closer to Stalin than both of them think. But then the problem of the socialist democracy (not the familiar parliamentary one) has been given a new and different meaning in recent years under Rosa Luxemburg's influence; different from what it had been in the naive years of our Bolshevist youth.

I am well aware that these lines are quite fragmentary and, in addition, have the disadvantage of touching on a subject which in our anti-rational era

[3 lines illegible]

I would have preferred to start out from subjects like abortion, free choice of the doctor, etc. rather than from generalities, and to deal in a more detailed and solid way [...] to write the book, but have not found the time to do so.

I have read two good books in English recently: Günther Reimann [?] "Germany" and B.D. Wolfe "Portrait of Mexico". There is nothing serious in German. Thomas Mann's journal "Mass und Werk" is likely to fade. So I am staying with the French historians from Guizot to Lefebre [sic] in addition to professional and psychological reading. As of recent I have suffered an attack of Balzacism, no wonder in Paris.

I do hope you have survived a busy winter and that we may see you here in the not too distant future. I also hope you won't mind my remarks on your book.

With my very best regards and wishes I am

Yours

E. Ackerknecht

In parts of this letter the ink has faded to a degree that certain lines are unreadable. (Garrison 1934). The exhibitions mentioned are likely to be the ones connected with S.'s first "Graduate Week", held as a continuation course in medical history in 1938. A.'s criticism of S.'s book (Sigerist 1937) is made at a time when A. was still a Marxist, yet had given up all political engagements and watched the Soviet purges of the 1930s with disgust. S.'s works mentioned: (Sigerist 1935, 1936 a,b,c,d).

Persons in alphabetical order:

Balzac, Honoré de (1799–1850) French novelist
Garrison, Fielding H. (1870–1935) American historian of medicine

Guizot, François see A. to S. of 8 Dec. 1937
Hugo, Victor (1802–1885) French novelist
Lefebvre, possibly Jean (16th century) French historian
Luxemburg, Rosa (1870–1919) German revolutionary socialist
Mann, Thomas (1875–1955) German novelist
Oliver, John R. (1872–1943) MD, PhD, staff member at Sigerist's Institute
Reimann, Günther (1904–2005) German/American author
Robespierre, Maximilien (1758–1794) French revolutionary
Trotzki, Leo (1879–1940) Russian revolutionary
Stalin, Joseph (1879–1953) communist dictator of Soviet Russia
Virchow, Rudolf see S. to A. of 27 April 1932.
Wolfe, Bertram D. see A. to S. of 8 Dec. 1937
Zola, Emile (1840–1902) French novelist

ACKERKNECHT to SIGERIST, Paris, 1 August 1938
(Original in German)

Dear Professor Sigerist!

Many thanks for your letter of 10 May [?] you wrote on board of a ship. Excuse me, if this will be sort of a sign of life rather than a real letter because of lack of time, yet I want you to receive this when you are in Switzerland.

Everyone being on vacation, I am quite busy at the institute. In addition, I am moving (my new address: 78, Rue Beaubourg, Paris III, Tel: Archives 7521; I can also be reached by mail or telephone at "Institut des maladies professionelles" 6, Rue de la Douane, Tel; Bolzaris 5289). On top of all, we finally suffer our notorious Paris heat which is a burden for the healthy, let alone for the semi-sick.

Thank you very much for "Science and Society" which contains many precious thoughts. For those who have the privilege to live in America it is a satisfaction, and for those who must stay in Europe it is a melancholy praise that nothing comparable exists here. In my new field of occupational medicine I also find out that the American literature is far more interesting than the European one. Part of the reason is a better organization, but also the fact that in Europe one seems to be at a dead end and in a state of total mental paralysis by the threat of war. Someone with a death sentence just waiting for his execution does not produce many ideas. This is not an intelligent attitude but it is the attitude of the people.

I do hope that you had a good return from the USSR and that your further itinerary will prove satisfactory.

I am all excited to see you soon. In the meantime I am with sincere regards

Yours

   Erwin Ackerknecht

S. spent the summer months of the 1930s in Switzerland and in 1938 once more in Soviet Russia. "Science and Society" see (Sigerist 1938). The threat of war: A. writes one year before WWII broke out.

ACKERKNECHT to SIGERIST, Paris, 27 November 1938
(Original in German)

Dear Professor Sigerist,

I have been silent for quite a while because I wanted to have straightened out certain things before writing you.

On the 1st of October I have lost my job which resulted in a couple of difficult weeks. On the 1st of December I shall have a new job (part-time) at the "Encyclopédie médicochirurgicale" with comparable tasks (analyses, bibliography etc.). It will provide the minimum to live and also time to do other things.

My affidavit of my cousin in New Orleans has arrived. On the consulate I was told it will take at least a year for the immigration visa, according to the quota. In addition, chances to find a job from here are slim. Thus, if you won't come to Paris next summer it will take quite a while until I'll have the pleasure to see you again.

Because there are better things than just making money I decided to make good use of the waiting period for the visa by studying for the diploma in ethnology. The reasons are the lack of a department like in Talstrasse and the encouragement by Professor Rivet of the Musée de l'homme. Thus, after ten years I have become a student again – a strange situation. I think it is a good decision, even if in the future I should work in the history of medicine.

All this keeps me fairly busy which is good because the political situation is not encouraging and our position in France goes from bad to worse. War has been delayed, but what a peace!

173

I should not forget to convey greetings from Walter Riese of Frankfort who used to write for "Hippokrates" and has a job here in neuro-anatomy. Except for his Kantianism he is a very pleasant fellow.

Please be kind enough to thank your wife for the friendly note she has sent me before her departure.

I hope you had a good start into the winter semester and that your book is progressing. With best regards to you and your family I am
Yours
Erwin H. Ackerknecht

Again, S.'s letter is missing. The two correspondents had met in Paris and probably discussed the possibility of A.'s emigration to the U.S. Talstrasse was the address of the Leipzig Institute of the History of Medicine. Paul Rivet, professor of ethnology in Paris. Walter Riese, a German neurologist, immigrated into the U.S. S.'s wife was Emmy Escher from Zurich. "Sigerists's book" is not identified since his last one appeared as (Sigerist 1937) and his next one as (Sigerist 1941a); it could well be his *History of Medicine*, planned since 1934 (Bickel 1997).

ACKERKNECHT to SIGERIST, Paris, 11 April 1939
(Original in German)

Dear Professor Sigerist,

I hope that not having heard from you for quite a while is no bad news. Since the beginning of my job as librarian at the Encyclopédie médico-chirurgicale half a year ago some degree of order and security has returned into my life. The job is not bad and the fact that I see 220 medical reviews is clearly positive. Much of the material pertains to the history or philosophy of medicine and some to comparative pathology of peoples and to social crises and psychoses.

The study of ethnology is very interesting. Unfortunately, I have also to do translations in order to survive. This may be as strange as is an apology of C. G. Jung by Martha Karlweis ([…] Jakob Wassermann – God save the psychoanalysts from their pupils) or even grotesque like Easter considerations of protestant-jewish ministers which reactivate biblical reminiscences of my youth.

Recently I read Leibbrand's booklet on romantic medicine which is not bad. It is rather mean that he does not cite Hirschfeld's work, of which he certainly is aware. But then where should the Germans learn to be correct? His book showed me the roots of many Marxist thoughts in the Romantic Age, among others Marx' surprising tolerance towards the Middle Ages. I see the Middle Ages in the light of recent experiences with totalitarian regimes, as the totalitarian state [...] and also, under the influence of Michelet (in whose "sorcière" there are good passages on Paracelsus), quite different from ten years ago. However, all these ideas do not bring us further because we don't have the leisure to persue them, no organ to publish them, and no receptive public.

In these beautiful Easter holidays, usually a time of hiking in the valley of the Seine, I read an interesting monograph on cholera and the rebellion of 1832 in Paris by Lucas-Dubreton ("La grande peur de 1832" Gallimand 1932). Dealing with the misery of the past may be a way to find some comfort in the present misery. All that has happened in the few months since you have been here is unbelievable. One has the pleasant choice of getting angry about the brutal meanness on the one side or of the clever cowardice on the other.

I do not know whether I shall succeed to escape from here before the war breaks out. Escape I must, because by the same iron police logic they will put me to jail (an honor, but a nuisance) if Mr. Ribbentrop comes to Paris as they will do if we go to war against Mr. Ribbentrop. And I fancy that concentration camps are equally nice wherever they are.

Much as I have an affidavit, my quota is not due before November or December. So I am desperately trying to get entrance into a country in Central or South America where I shall await the happy arrival of my U.S. visa. If, in your next letter, you could write a sentence about the desirability of my presence in the U.S. (without obligation) then I could try to convince the consul here. Unfortunately, I don't know anybody in Washington; a letter from there to the consul would be the best thing.

Enough now of these worries of a refugee. I hope your book is progressing. Will you come to Europe in summer?

[2 lines illegible]

Please remember me to your family I now have the pleasure to know. And my very best regards to you

Yours

Erwin H. Ackerknecht

This letter in long-hand again contains passages with faded ink. The last sentence shows that Ackerknecht in late 1938 had met S., his wife Emmy and daughters Erica and Nora in Paris.

Names in alphabetical order:

Lucas-Dubreton, Jean (born 1883) French historian and writer

Hirschfeld, Ernst, coworker of Sigerist in Leipzig (Hirschfeld 1930), later killed by the Nazis

Jung, Carl Gustav (1875–1961) Swiss psychoanalyst

Karlweis, Martha, Austrian writer, wife and biographer of J. Wassermann

Leibbrand, Werner (1896–1974) professor of medical history in Munich. (Leibbrand 1937).

Michelet, Jules (1798–1874) French historian and writer

Ribbentrop, Joachim von (1893–1946) Hitler's foreign minister

Wassermann, Jakob (1873–1934) German writer of psychological novels, husband of M. Karlweis

SIGERIST to ACKERKNECHT, Baltimore ?, 15 Mai 1939 (Original in German)

Dear colleague,

I wanted to write you all winter but was so extremely busy that I got far behind with my correspondence. We are being heavily involved in the fight for health insurance, and this winter I had no less than 44 lectures outside the Institue. The organized physicians here try to stem against the development, but they won't succeed here as little as they have in other countries. For the end of this month I have organized a health conference where farmers, workers, and Negroes will discuss their medical needs.

I am pleased to learn that you are working on the Encyclopédie. It certainly is a privilege to have access to such an amount of journals.

I will spend the summer mainly in South Africa where I have been invited as a professor, but I will also hit Paris sometime where I hope to see you.

I don't believe in an imminent war because war today means revolution and this is what all the governments fear. However, the threat of war will persist as well a succession of crises by which the rulers will try to remain in power.

With kind regards I am
Yours as ever
Henry E. Sigerist

This seems to be S.'s first preserved letter to A. since Leipzig 1932. S. once more was too optimistic: General health insurance was not introduced in the near future; the opposition of the American Medical Association (AMA) was still strong, and war would break out later in this year. The number of 44 lectures is not exaggerated (Bickel 1997).

ACKERKNECHT to SIGERIST, Paris, 7 July 1939
(Original in German)

Dear Professor Sigerist,

Many thanks for your letter of 5–15–38. Busy as you are, I am very glad that you took time to send a letter into my splendid isolation. I read about your many lectures with interest, and I follow the struggle for health insurance here and in the American medical literature. Hopefully, this activity has not slowed down work on your book. I enclose an Australian notice of your Soviet book.

In recent months I was busy working for my exam in ethnology which to my own surprise I have passed […]. It was my intention to start an independent work. However, since my "boss", P. Rivet, is in Bolivia and everyone here enjoys the holy vacation time, I am likely to wait until September and to spend my time reading. There is enough work to be done. But I am anxious to do productive work and not only to accumulate knowledge. For my living I still have the Encyclopédie.

Since the quota is overbooked, it will take a long waiting period to reach the U.S. on the regular way. So I hope to see you, if not there, then in Paris, provided your optimistic prognoses with respect to world peace come true. I shall be here except for the second half of July.

Best wishes for South Africa! I would love to be able to travel again. My study of ethnology has taught me that few years from now many objects may have vanished and can no longer be studied.

With best wishes and regards and hoping to see you soon
    Yours
        Erwin H. Ackerknecht

Best regards to your family too!

This was A.'s last letter before WWII broke out. "Your book" see A. to S. of 27 Nov. 1938. Soviet book (Sigerist 1937). Paul Rivet see A. to S. of 27 Nov. 1938. A.'s

Sorbonne exam provided the Certificat d'études supérieures d'éthnologie. S.'s optimistic prognosis and his plans for South Africa see S. to A. of 15 May 1939.

ACKERKNECHT to SIGERIST, St. Jean de la Ruelle (Loiret), 12 October 1939 (Postcard, original in French)

My dear teacher!

Alas, I won't be in Paris to see you this year. Also I suppose you will return from Africa directly and this after a successful time, I hope.

In July I spent relaxing days on the island of St. Marguerite in Southern France, reading, swimming and doing water-colors. In August, still working on the Encyclopédie, I finished a long article for the Institute of Social Research in New York on the development of occupational diseases during the past 20 years. On 24 August – I still could have escaped to a neutral country – I registered as a volunteer. On 6 September I have been interned together with 2000 to 3000 other refugees in Hade de Colombes of which you certainly have read in the newspapers. On 16 September I have been transported to this site, together with 200 other refugees. We are working in agriculture and building. The material conditions like food are not bad. Being expropriated and denationalized by Germany, we are officially recognized as refugees under the protectorate of the League of Nations and of France. Well, let's wait and see. Of course, I wished to be employed according to my capacities. So far there were few cases of illness and even less serious cases. Even though a mixed lot, we have organized ourselves to live under hygienic conditions and in solidarity. The morale is good. Unfortunately, there is nobody to share my interests (history, ethnology), so I am living to think of better days and hoping for the best. I keep my pre-war plans for the time after the war. My child of the first marriage is in safety in Limoges. Luckily, my second wife still lives in freedom in Paris and manages in spite of frozen bank accounts. I would be happy to hear about your present activities, since boredom is the prisoner's worst enemy.

With my sincere regards to your wife and to yourself I am

Yours

E. Ackerknecht

This is A.'s first letter after war has broken out on September 1, 1939. His adress is given as: Group 12, Collecting camp for foreigners; the meaning here is "enemy foreigners" since A. immigrated as a German, a nationality he had lost in the meantime. Daughter Ina see A. to S. of 21 Oct. 1937. Second wife: Lucy Krüger, married in 1938.

Dated 3 November, 1939 A. received the following letter from Baltimore:
Dear Dr. Ackerknecht; In the absence of Dr. Sigerist I beg to acknowledge your card of October 12. Dr. Sigerist is still in South Africa but is expected back on January 3. Please be assured that your card will be brought to his immediate attention after his return. Sincerely yours,

Virginia Davidson
Staff secretary

ACKERKNECHT to SIGERIST, St. Jean de la Ruelle, 20 November 1939 ? (Original in French)

My dear teacher,

Although Miss Davidson has been kind enough to let me know that you won't be back until January I do have to write you now. Our hope for a useful employment or to join the French army have not been successful. Thus, our situation seems pretty clear: either captivity or Foreign Legion – or else departure for the United States. However, I don't even dare to hope the latter is a real possibility even though, as you will understand, it would be my choice. I cannot expect my visa to arrive before the next 7 or 8 months, and my affidavit is of November 1938. It is therefore of vital importance for me to obtain my visa as early as possible. I would never have dared to bother you, however, under these circumstances please help me if you should have any chance to influence the American authorities there or here. I hope you will forgive my entreaty if you consider my situation.

I thank you in advance. With my best wishes for you and your family
Yours as ever
E. Ackerknecht

And in spite of all: a merry christmas and a happy new year.

A strong man's cry of distress! Miss Virginia Davidson, staff secretary to S.; see her above letter to A. of 3 November 1939.

My dear colleague and friend:

Please do not think that I have forgotten you. On the contrary, I thought a great deal of you but I was holding back with my letter because I had always hoped to be able to give you some definite answer and to offer you a position either in my own Institute or in some other university. Unfortunately I have not been successful so far. We have no vacancy on the staff just now and the regulations of the University are very strict so that I cannot give you a position without definite salary. I am, however, pursuing in my efforts and you can be sure that I shall do my best to bring you over as soon as ever possible. It is a perfect shame that a man of your talents, knowledge and ability should waste his time when he could be so useful in the United States. We have some excellent students here but the trouble with almost all of them is that they have no classical foundation and do not know languages. I shall write you soon again.

I came back from South Africa in January, much delayed by the war. I had to wait for an American ship that sails directly from Capetown to New York. But my trip was extraordinarily interesting and I wish I had had you with me. I spent five weeks in native territories making a study of health conditions and medical services, and I had opportunity to talk to several medicine men. I even consulted one in order to see what the ritual was.

Do not be discouraged. I sincerely hope that we shall see each other soon again. With all good wishes, I am

Yours very cordially,

Henry E. Sigerist

HES:T
Dictated but not signed by Dr. Sigerist

Apparently the prerequisite for an undelayed visa was a salaried position in the U. S. S. was successful in the help for immigration of several European refugees (Temkin, Edelstein, Urdang and others).

ACKERKNECHT to SIGERIST, St. Jean de la Ruelle, 31 March 1940
(Original in French)

My dear teacher,

Thank you so much for your letter of 4 March. The joy it created is hard to describe, first because of the hope you still provide, and then also as a sign of undiminished esteem. In our actual conditions, which I am not going to describe, it is difficult to maintain much of one's self. Thus, the thought of people by whom we are still favorably remembered, is a tremendous help.

Speaking of the practical knowledge you mentioned, you may remember that I went to the "Humanistisches Gymnasium" and that in addition to English and French I have a reading knowlegde of Italian, Spanish, Portuguese, Dutch, and Bulgarian.

My situation is still the same. Four weeks ago I have changed from painter to woodcutter. A tiring job. I am living with 90 men in an abandoned farm house near Orléans. The majority are recognized refugees and officially a work force of the French army. But practically we still are internees. You will understand that under these circumstances my wish to join you is undiminished.

I am continuing my excursions into history, sociology, and ethnology. It is the only thing to do in the absence of a concrete goal and of a library. I continue to read which, despite fatigue and of the noise of the crowded and boring camp life, is my only pleasure. I spent two months with Lowie's "Sociologie primitive". Having grown up with the slightly faded theories of Morgan-Engels this was extremely interesting and important.

If you are going to publish an article on your travel, I would be glad to have a copy. Thanking you for your efforts I beg you to continue remembering me since my situation is continuing to be bad. Please give my best to your family.

Yours ever sincerely

Erwin H. Ackerknecht

The German "Humanistisches Gymnasium" provided a classical education with Latin and Greek. Robert H. Lowie (1883–1957) professor of anthropology at Berkeley, expert on native Americans; A. most likely refers to Lowie's *Primitive Society* (Lowie 1919). Morgan-Engels: Their theories on the origin of the family. S. had written on his study tour in South Africa, see (Sigerist 1940).

Dear teacher,

I have the pleasure to announce that I am still alive – a fact that surprises me – and that I am even still hoping to see you some day.

The last three months were crazy and agitated, like a bad dream. I was a work soldier of the French army in the Loriet, then with the British in Brittany. They have abandoned us in the worst moment. We ran day and night for our lives. Later on there were trucks. Eventually I found myself in a French platoon in the Pyrenees. By the way, I sent a documentary of these events to my friend Eckstein in New York, and I hope he will send you a copy.

Now I have been discharged "in order to go to an overseas country", and I am doing here, next to Marseilles, all I can to obey this order which is in the best of my interest. We do not know what will further happen to us, either from the German side or from the French who may put us again in a camp. So the situation is difficult. I may have to wait for another four to six months to legally enter the United States. The consul shows an awful inertia. Would you know how to shake him? In addition, one has to make a living in the meantime. But how to do this? All my belongings are stuck in Paris for a long time. Aix, the old Roman town and capital of the Provence, the city of Cézanne, Zola, and Mirabeau, with its fountains and its tree-studded avenues, is very beautiful but for me it is a desert, since I don't know a single soul. Maybe by the accidents of life you happen to know anybody here who may be helpful? I hate to disturb you with things like that, but my situation is calling for it.

Little can be said on the general state of the country; things are too different in the individual regions. Here, e.g., where there are few refugees, one can buy nearly everything and at reasonable prices, provided one has some money. In other places like Toulouse it's quite different. Communications are poor, and unemployment is rampant. Luckily, it is summer. All has happened so quickly that nobody has found the possibility to understand what has happened, let alone to react in a sensible way.

Anyway, I hope to survive for all that, to see you sometime, and to resume a serious work after all that lost time. I'd be happy to receive an answer in my misery, and I am with my best wishes for you and your family

Yours as ever

Erwin H. Ackerknecht

The date on the letter is not clear; acording to A.'s *Autobiographical Notes* he reached Aix in July 1940. As a result of the German invasion of France in May/June 1940 there remained an "unoccupied zone" of France, comprising southeastern France which was ruled by a French puppet government. A copy of A.'s documentary of his flight is present at the archive of the Department of the History of Medicine, University of Bern, Switzerland. Eckstein, a Paris exile friend of A.'s. Paul Cézanne (1839–1906) French painter; Emile Zola, see A. to S. of 5 May 1938; Gabriel-Honoré Mirabeau (1749–1791) French revolutionary.

A. spent almost a year in Aix-en-Provence following clinical courses in the State Hospital. When he finally obtained his visa he sailed to the U.S. in May 1941. Apparently no further letters were exchanged during that time.

ACKERKNECHT to SIGERIST, New York, 20 June 1941 (Original in German)

Dear Professor Sigerist,

Many thanks for your your soothing lines of 17 June. I have consulted the time-table right away and, unless you tell me otherwise, I shall arrive <u>Tuesday, 24 June, 9:08 E.S.T. in Baltimore</u>. I am all excited, and I hope we will be able to handle the tricky problem of my future.

Again, many, many thanks and best regards to you and your family

Yours

Erwin H. Ackerknecht

Due to the war A.'s passage took six weeks. He arrived in New York on 13 June, had a letter from S. (missing) within a week, and a few days later went to see him. A.'s first job in the U.S. was as a physician in a vacation camp.

Dear Professor Sigerist,

This is the forth week of my rural exile. Thanks for the reprints which I appreciate in my state of under-activity and mental starvation. I have devoured all articles, particularly that on "Medieval Medicine" of the University of Pennsylvania Press. It is an excellent synopsis of the different forms of medieval medicine.

Let me briefly tell you about my experiences with Doctor Zilboorg. He found that P. M. is not up to my level and recommended a literary agent who passed me on to a second and a third one who then was absent for a long time. Thus, nothing came out except for an unpublished but out of date article of mine.

Here I am making my first American experiences. The hygienic conditions in this camp are very primitive – but there are many prayers to Jehova. In contrast, I am praying that no serious case of disease will occur in addition to the small stuff. The children and their counselors are very friendly, if noisy and childish. Although all the counsellors are students I have never in the past 20 years lived in such a superficial milieu of entertainment. Yet this paradise, which we Europeans will not understand, will be doomed to disappearance, which will not be fun.

Dr. Leo Kanner recommended me for a psychiatric position in Omaha. However, it is uncertain whether it is still available and will pay enough for a living. May I ask you if your budget has become transparent so that there is still hope for Baltimore, or else that I better forget it altogether. On the other hand there might be some other possibilitiy for a job in Baltimore? My desire to go to B. has so much increased and become more concrete since I have seen you and the Institute.

I hope you are having a quiet and fulfilling vacation time with your family, that it is neither too hot nor too cold, and you won't be found and disturbed.

My very best regards and wishes to you and your family
Yours
Erwin H. Ackerknecht

A.'s address is Tranquillity Camp in Earlton, NY. *Medieval Medicine* see (Sigerist 1941b). Gregory Zilboorg (1890–1959) psychiatrist in New York, friend of S.'s. PM, a progressive New York newspaper; S. published 18 short articles on group health plans in PM in 1940. Leo Kanner (1894–1981) child psychiatrist, professor at Johns Hopkins University. Being cut off from Europe as a result of the war, Sigerist spent the summer vacations 1940–1945 in several places of the rural U.S.

SIGERIST to ACKERKNECHT, Bolton Landing, NY, 11 August 1941 (Original in German)

Dear colleague,

Thank you very much for your letter. I can imagine that your camp milieu is primitive. Students here often have the level of immature high school kids. People are waking up late, if they ever do. It is a strange system that tries to delay maturity as long as ever possible.

I am terribly sorry to tell you that chances for you in Baltimore are poor at the moment. We have less money than I had anticipated. This is all the more deplorable as I would have liked you to be at the Institute right now. Next year I hope to begin work for the first volume of my *History of Medicine*, and I would have liked your cooperation for the chapter on "Primitive Medicine". Of course, I would take any chance coming up. In America one can never tell, and things can happen all of a sudden. In any case I advise you to act if a job is offered to you.

We like it much here. The landscape is charming, and the climate is a paradise compared with Baltimore. I have finished the Paracelsus volume I mentioned to you, and I am about to prepare three classics of hygiene to be printed.

In which part of New York State is your camp? I was not able to find it on the map. With many regards from all of us I am

Yours as ever

[Henry E. Sigerist]

S. and his family were vacationing in upstate New York. Once more, S. planned to begin his *History of Medicine* soon; its first chapter should be on primitive medicine. Paracelsus volume: Probably (Sigerist 1941c). Classics of Hygiene were published 15 years later (Sigerist 1956a).

ACKERKNECHT to SIGERIST, New York, 4 September 1941
(Original in German)

Dear Professor Sigerist,

I have returned to New York yesterday; my new address is 427 Walton Av., New York. If I won't find another job, I shall try to begin as a "male nurse". My camp experience ended with an uncovered check. Things one has to learn too.

I will call again on Dr. Zilboorg. And I hope that you will have more good days in Bolton Landing.

With my very best regards, to your family too
    Yours
        Erwin H. Ackerknecht

A.'s new address is in the Bronx. Gregory Zilboorg see A. to S. of 5 August 1941.

ACKERKNECHT to SIGERIST, New York, 26 September 1941
(Original in German)

Dear Professor Sigerist,

Let me announce the birth of our daughter Sylvia. She was born yesterday. I am working as a "male nurse", with little financial success to be sure. Maybe I will find a factory job in order to survive for a couple of months. My English language exam is due at the end of October.

My very best regards to you and your dear family
    Yours
        Erwin H. Ackerknecht

A. came to the U.S. with his second wife Lucy Krüger who had joined him in Aix-en-Provence.

ACKERKNECHT to SIGERIST, New York, 12 November 1941
(Original in German)

Dear Professor Sigerist,

Many, many thanks for your letter of 10 November. You cannot imagine the wonderful excitement it produced. After my camp work I have been doing nursing jobs and preparations for my exams. I would hardly have better chances for the next half year and so we would consider the activity in Baltimore as a real redeem. Let's hope nothing will interfere.

Hania Wislicka told me how busy you are. She was here three weeks ago and successfully treated our baby who grows well, makes a lot of work, but is a great joy.

I hope for a definite decision in Baltimore so that we can prepare things here and give notice for the apartment. There remains little time until the 1st of January.

With all best regards to you, your family and your co-workers
Yours
Erwin H. Ackerknecht

S.'s letter is missing. Hania Wislicka-Risemberg: Physician at Johns Hopkins.

ACKERKNECHT to SIGERIST, New York, 17 November 1941
(Original in German)

Dear Professor Sigerist!

Many thanks for your letter of 15 November. I am looking forward to 28 November full of hope. It will be a pleasure to help you with volume I, and I hope to be able to do a maximum of useful work in the six months. You cannot imagine how happy I am to finally do the kind of work I like best.

With all best regards to you, your family and your coworkers
Yours gratefully
Erwin H. Ackerknecht

Possibly the two missing letters of S. were hand-written notes of which S. had not made copies. Apparently S.'s offer was for six months only.

ACKERKNECHT to SIGERIST, New York, 2 December 1941
(Original in German)

Dear Professor Sigerist

I just received your letter of 29 December [sic] with the good news. Many thanks. So I have given notice for the 1st of January. My wife will probably go to Baltimore for two days on 18 December in order to look for an apartment. Of course, she will call. Needless to say how much we are looking forward to be in Baltimore!

    With all best regards to you, your family and your coworkers

        Yours

            Erwin H. Ackerknecht

S.'s letter missing. A.'s letter should clearly read 29 November rather than December.

SIGERIST to ACKERKNECHT, Baltimore ?, 6 December 1941

Dear Ackerknecht:

Things are sometimes moving more rapidly than you expect and I am sending you enclosed the official letter of the President of the University for your appointment.

This makes your appointment definite and all you have to do is to write President Bowman signifying your acceptance of the fellowship.

Since you may not yet be quite familiar with the style of official letters of that kind, I am sending you enclosed the draft of a letter for President Bowman. All you have to do is to copy it and mail it.

I am delighted to know that this is now all settled and I am looking forward to seeing your wife when she comes to Baltimore and to having you all here by January 1.

    Yours as ever,

        [Henry E. Sigerist]

Isaiah Bowman (1878–1950) geographer, president of Johns Hopkins University.

Dear Professor Sigerist:

Thank you very much for your letter of Dec 6, 41 and the draft of the answer to President Bowman. I copied and mailed it immediately.

We feel that we should go now as soon as possible to Baltimore and so my wife will come Monday 15. to look for an appartment [sic]. She will be very glad to see you. She will ring up at the Institute and tell you all about us.

Yours as ever

Erwin H. Ackerknecht

This is A.'s first letter written in English. After Pearl Harbor on December 7, 1941 the U.S. were drawn into WWII; on January 1, 1942 A. began work at S.'s Institute of the History of Medicine at the Johns Hopkins University in Baltimore. It was the late beginning of his professional career at age 35. As a research fellow he spent three years at what was then the best place for the study of the history of medicine. His teachers were, in addition to S., his colleagues Owsei Temkin, Ludwig Edelstein, Sanford V. Larkey, and Genevieve Miller. It was a productive time for A., resulting in many papers on primitive medicine, naval surgery, metabolism, and malaria in addition to his first book (Ackerknecht 1945). In 1942 he obtained his Medical License for the State of Maryland. In 1944 his second daughter, Ellen, was born. Of the Baltimore period one single letter exists in the archives which may not be surprising since A. and S. were living in almost daily contact.

ACKERKNECHT to SIGERIST, Baltimore, 2 August 1944

Dear Dr. Sigerist:

Here are the Galdston letters back and a copy of my answer. You bet that the Life and Time project is worthwile [sic] considering.

I guess I sounded somewhat stupid over the phone yesterday night. But the thing just sounded too good to be true. After so many bad experiences during these last 11 years of wandering I try always to keep calm in order not to be disappointed in case things eventually do not work out all right. Or in order not to be cheated (the first pay I got in this country for months of hard work consisted of cheques without provision, emanating from a millionaire!) And in order not to give up prematurely other lesser projects and demarches in favor of the one which seems so good, but may fail. But this time I did not succeed with all my golden rules. Think of going back to New York; the libraries; our friends; and Baltimore and later Yale in easy reach! Instead of going far West or to Porto Rico [sic] etc.

Yes, Porto Rico. Ruth Benedict seems to have some connections there. But frankly speaking, in my situation as an alien teaching there of all things anthropology i. e. on race, and starting again with Spanish before even my English is good enough, I hope we will be spared this. And she wrote me already that there are no libraries, of course.

The discussions with Chicago are continuing. Redfield wrote me a very nice and not all hopeless letter. But unfortunately he is leaving for China and the lieutenant of Hutchins (J.J. Schwab) I am now mostly dealing with, is not very reliable, and announces already that when it is a college position, there will be hardly any time left for research. But we will see all that.

We had three other papers this afternoon in the Institute. The plague of 1348 was almost good, Paul Bert fair, Cost of Health terrific. After more than half an hours [sic] torrent of indigested facts, Temkin stopped him fortunately, because it was past five and no hope that he would be through before another 30 minutes. We will have to take the rest tomorrow. Attendance drops in proportion to the increase in humidity. Edelstein is back, mysteriously smiling, from his mysterious trip. That is all the news I have. Baltimore summer is at its best. You do not know how happy you are.

I humbly apologize for unclean typing and uncorrect English. C'est la guerre!

      Kindest regards and best wishes also to the family
        Yours as ever
          Erwin H. Ackerknecht

A. writes to S. at his vacation address in Lewes, DE. A. in his third year at Johns Hopkins could no longer afford to live on the meagre stipend of a fellowship. In view of the filled faculty positions S. wrote letters of recommendation, praising A. as qualified to fill a chair at a good university and "I hate to see him leave because he is the best and most productive man I have on the staff (S. to Chauncey D. Leake of 27 June 1944). In turn, A. wrote Genevieve Miller on 30 May 1945: "Looking back at this occasion at my work in B.[altimore] makes me feel pretty nostalgic, because in spite of all it was an exceptionally good place to work, and there were always a few good friends around." Possibly the "thing too good to be true" was the news of a position at the American Museum of Natural History in New York which A. was indeed to fill in 1945.

Names mentioned in the letter in alphabetical order:
Benedict, Ruth (1887–1948) anthropologist at Columbia University
Bert, Paul (1833–1886) French physiologist and leftist politician, pupil of Claude Bernard
Edelstein, Ludwig (1902–1965) classical scholar, immigrated from Germany in 1934, joined S.'s staff at Johns Hopkins
Galdston, Iago (1895–1989) medical historian at New York Academy of Medicine
Hutchins, not identified
Redfield, probably Robert (1897–1958) anthropologist
Schwab, J. J., possibly John J., immigrated neurophysiologist
Temkin, Owsei, see A. to S. of 8 December 1937

SIGERIST to ACKERKNECHT, Baltimore ?, 26 February 1945

Dear Erwin,

I am sorry that I did not see you before you left although I do not consider your departure a separation. I am still hopeful that some day we again will be working under the same roof.

I wanted to show you a letter of John Fulton in which he mentions you. You will find the passage enclosed. It, of course, does not mean much because Fulton talks a great deal but it is good to know that he was impressed with your personality and work. Having done a poor job on Paul Bert himself, he should have been interested in the good job you did on the same subject.

The malaria copies have been sent out and the review copies have also been mailed. I am anxious to see what the reaction will be and will let you have whatever reviews we receive.

I had a brainstorm the other night concerning the reorganization of the Institute and I have written a memorandum on the subject that will be addressed to the Committee on Organization and Policy of the Medical School of which Dr. Week is chairman. I cannot tell you more about it now but will show you the report on some other occasion.

I expect three men from the Wyeth Company in the next few days. They want my advice for one of their stinking paintings. I, of course, will see them and will keep them warm.

I hope you are beginning to be acclimatized in New York and with warm wishes to you all, I am

Yours as ever,
[Henry]

S. writes to A. at 153 West 83rd Street in New York. John F. Fulton (1899–1960) physiologist and medical historian. Paul Bert see A. to S. of 2 August 1944 and (Ackerknecht 1944). "Malaria copies" (Ackerknecht 1945). Wyeth Institute of Applied Biochemistry, Philadelphia. S.'s hand-written signatures do not show on the following letter copies; most likely they would be "Henry".

ACKERKNECHT to SIGERIST, New York, 28 February 1945

Dear Henry:

Thank you very much for your good letter of February 26. I feel very much ashamed that I did not write you before. But this was an extremely hectic week for the both of us. We tried to make this narrow and dark place to make a place where it is possible to live in, what is not easy, and to keep our kids going. We had to do a maximum before I start working tomorrow. I am looking forward very much to doing eventually something better than tending babies and packing and unpacking things.

Though I will miss you and the Institute very much, I do not regard our departure as a true separation either. The short geographical distance between Balto and New York has already a very consolatory character. And besides I think that, even if for the time being we are not working under the same material roof, a common past, common interests and a common approach to the problem of working will always make for a certain feeling of being under a common roof.

I am very anxious to hear more about your reorganization plans. To the horror of my more "scholarly" friends I have always been very much interested in organisational problems. Of course, if one had always the right people to work with, one need not bother much about these things. But as in reality one seems to be in general rather laboring under the opposite condition, the final effect depends entirely on the way the given human raw material is organized so as to give what is the best in it.

Though I know that Fulton's compliments do not weigh too heavily, I was very glad about what he wrote to you, all the more as to a larger public he is an "authority" (and his physiological work seems to be very good indeed). I am looking forward very much to the first reactions to the malaria monograph, and I hope very much that at least from the publishers [sic] point of view it will be a success. While generally I have a certain feeling what my stuff is worth, in the case of this book I feel rather insecure,

192

as it is so far from my usual occupations and my "basic" approach. Let us hope for the best. Carter was very enthusiastic and uses the material already for teaching. But Carter is an enthusiast anyway, and a personal friend too. Thus we will have to wait for the judgement of less friendly people.

I enclose the Wyeth letters. Many ways lead to Rome, and this may be one indeed some day.

Please give my regards to Genevieve and the other Institute people, and, of course, also at home

yours as ever
Erwin

"I start working tomorrow", at the American Museum of Natural History. Fulton see S. to A. of 26 February 1945. Malaria monograph (Ackerknecht 1945). Edward P. Carter (born 1870) professor of cardiology at Johns Hopkins. Genevieve Miller (born 1914) medical historian, began her career with Sigerist from 1939 to 1947. A.'s English is still somewhat clumsy.

Sigerist to Ackerknecht, Baltimore ?, 5 March 1945

Dear Erwin:

Thanks for your letter. I quite forgot to mention that I was very pleased with the photo that you inscribed for me. I did not recognize it as my own work at first. Some day we will have to make a better one but in the meantime I have it framed on the wall in the Inner Sanctum. Please tell Lucy that I have not forgotten the pictures of her and the children. Some day she will get them but it takes some time particularly now when the Dark Room is being used by the Art Students.

I had a letter from Magnus-Levy about the manuscript that he wants you to translate. I would not advise you to undertake the job, for various reasons. One is that your English is not good enough for this kind of work and second, because Magnus-Levy is not too pleasant to deal with. He is the nagging type and would probably cause a lot of trouble.

Cordially as ever yours,
[Henry]

Lucy, A.'s wife; their children Sylvia and Ellen. Adolf Magnus-Levy (1865–1955) biochemist.

Dear Henry:

I have to ask you something technical and this gives me a most welcome occasion to have a little chat with you, as, alas, I am no longer able just to go over to your studio and to do so in a less formal way. The technical thing is: I try to get the reciprocity for my license here and have to submit my credentials. As the Gestapo doctors [sic] diploma, I have to submit again an affidavit from you that I actually doctored [sic] on Aug. 13, 1931 under your guidance. You gave already one when I applied for the Maryland Stateboard in 1942. A copy is in my file, and I would be very grateful, if you could just send me the same document, signature certified.

I have just read the little book of Stern. Though it contains absolutely nothing new to somebody who has been in your seminaries [sic], I think it is rather well done, and might be very useful to students. The little historical part is even very good. No medical man so far has dared to point out these facts. It is paradoxical that in the field of American medical history in general "laymen" (Shryock, Stern, Deutsch) have so far done a much better job than the doctors.

In the last number of Isis you will find a book review of Ashley Montague on the Pissaro [sic] letters which is a downright scandal [...]. He mixes up impressionism and neoimpressionism, and thus makes Seurat at the tender age of 6 the creator of the former. I first felt the urge to write Sarton. But I do not know him. And anyway he seems so infatuated with this miserable quack who dwells in his rear and that it probably would be of no avail. M. by the way is now lecturer of sociology at Harvard.

The Pinel meeting of the Medicohistorical society was very disappointing. Not only the attendance (20 in a center like New York) The papers of Robinson and Heaton were rather weak. Zilboorg in New York and as a president who talks more than the speakers and what a mixture of narcissm [sic] and nonsense, is simply sickening (I am sorry to say so because it is your friend; but I can not hide the bitter truth) The only brighter spot was de Saussure who not only spoke freely, but whose paper in spite of some psychanalytic [sic] flaws (Pinel was shy because he had lost his mother at the age of 14 – how the hell do these people know that this was the reason) was much better than anything I have seen from him so far.

The Academy of Medine [sic] library is unfortunately exactly as you prophesied. Fortunately our library here is very good. We have not the

194

library of Congress classification which makes for a much more comprehensible arrangement. We have for instance all the Festschriften of the last 100 years concentrated in one spot which is a great help.

I do not know whether you have seen that Pickard and Buley have just published a rather bulky history of Frontier Medicine in the Middle West. I have not yet seen it. Buley published an article on the same subject 20 years ago which is neither very good nor bad. What it will do to our malaria, I do not know. Theoretically it may influence sales favorably as well as unfavorably. I have not yet heard much concerning my book. That is I receive the usual enthusiastic "thank you" letters from the people to whom I sent it (e.g. Blegen) But that does not mean much, The fact that the old sourpuss Emerson found nothing to criticise but two printing errors, looks rather favorable. Urdang's favorable comments I value a little bit higher, though he is a friend and an enthusiast, as he at least has read the book thoroughly and has enough critical conscience not to praise things he would regard as bunk. Our director here (Parr, a Norwegian, a relatively young man in his forties, who had been a zoologist at Yale for 20 years before coming here) was very much interested, and took a copy away from me. I suppose that sales have not yet started and if they ever should come it will take some time until the thing has been properly announced by ads, bibliographies, and reviews. I have two points on the general history of malaria in the monograph (Indians ignorant of cinchona and free from malaria in precolumbian times) which might be found controversial. Should this be the case I would like to write a little note on them for the Bulletin as they seem to me of a more general interest and I have never been able to explain them in detail. Mrs. Rosen has cut out a great deal of my series, for lack of space. She asked me for propositions for another number, and I sent her about twenty, and I hope that she will find at least one suitable. I need the money badly. New York is very expensive. How I will do the number without the Welch Library is another question. But it will have to be solved.

As contacts in our department are maintained by the common lunch in which I generally do not participate, we do not have journal clubs or research conferences, and I must say that I miss it, though I used to moan about the latter sometimes. I see now that it was quite a good institution. Nevertheless with the numerous other personal contacts I have here, I make up so far pretty well for this lack of stimulation. (We do have museumwide journal clubs and research conferences. And we house the New York Academy of Science which has a very rich program every month.) Bernard de Voto was here (who writes a history of the fur trade) to look at the Catlin originals which are stocked just between my room and the one of Margaret Mead (they are much better than the reproductions) The latter drops in once in a while, and she is really as far as quick thinking is concerned one of the most amazing persons I have ever seen. I feel very much tempted to write a little pseudoanthropological paper on the still nomadic character of present American society. But I guess I better skip it for reasons of time and others.

[xxxx]. Sylvia is up again, and thus we slowly recover from this unnecessary complication of our moving troubles.

Regards to Genevieve and the rest of the department, and to Mrs. Sigerist.

> Very cordially yours as ever
> Erwin

I am almost through with the "Science of Man" and the review will be soon in your hands.

Letter-head: The American Museum of Natural History. Central Park West at 79th Street. New York 24, NY. A. was assistant curator of physical anthropology ("the best job I ever had"). The Nazis had deprived him of his MD degree and citzenship. Isis, a journal for the history of science. My book (Ackerknecht 1945). "Bulletin" of the History of Medicine. Welch Library, of the Johns Hopkins Medical Institutions. [xxxx] One sentence deleted as Chesney Archives' Protected Health Information.
    Names mentioned in the letter in alphabetical order:
Ackerknecht, Lucy and children Ellen and Sylvia
Blegen, possibly Theodore C. (1891–1969) Minnesota historian
Buley, see Pickard
Catlin, George (1796–1872) American painter
Deutsch, Albert (1905–1961) historian and journalist
Emerson, Kendall, physician at Johns Hopkins
Heaton, Claude, medical historian
Mead, Margaret (1901–1978) cultural anthropologist
Miller, Genevieve, see A. to S. of 28 February 1945
Montague, Ashley (1905–1999) british anthropologist
Parr, A. E., zoologist, director of the American Museum of Natural History in New York
Pickard, see (Pickard/Buley 1945)
Pinel, Philippe (1745–1826) French physician and psychiatrist
Pissarro, Camille (1830–1903) French Impressionist painter
Robinson, probably Victor (1886–1947) American medical historian
Rosen Mrs., Beate Caspari-Rosen, MD, wife of medical historian George Rosen.
Sarton, George (1884–1956) Belgian-American historian of science
Saussure, Raymond de (1894–1971) psychoanalyst in Switzerland and U.S.

Seurat, George-Pierre (1859–1891) painter, founder of neoimpressionism
Shryock, Richard H. (1893–1972) medical historian at the American Council of Learned
    Societies in Washington, DC, in 1949 S.'s successor at Johns Hopkins
Stern, Bernard J., author, see S. to A. of 27. March 1945. (Stern 1941)
Urdang, George (1882–1960) German-American historian of pharmacy
Voto, Bernard de (1897–1955) historian, critic, novelist
Zilboorg, Gregory, see A. to S. of 5 August 1941

SIGERIST to ACKERKNECHT, Baltimore ?, 27 March 1945

Dear Erwin:

Thanks for your letter of March 23. I am sending you enclosed the affidavit duly signed with my signature certified by a notary public who has a great name, Holbein. We still had a copy of the old affidavit so that I did not have to ponder much about the formulation of it.

I share your views on Stern's book entirely. I just reviewed it for the Journal of the American Public Health Association. There is nothing new in the book but it is an extremely useful summary that presents the widely scattered facts and figures in a most convenient way.

If the other volumes of the series are as good, this alone will justify the work of the Committee of the Academy.

It really is a sad comment that the best books on medical history are written by nonmedical men, not only in the field of American medicine. In the February number of the <u>Bulletin</u>, you will find a first-rate paper on the school of Salerno written by Kristeller, a philosopher. And I have just read for the Chicago University Press a huge manuscript on Ugo Benzi, one of the scholastic physicians who lived around 1400. It is a first-rate piece of work, by far the best such study that has been written in a long time and the author is Dr. Dean Putnam Lockwood, professor of Latin and Librarian in a small college.

I can well imagine what the Pinel meeting must have been like. [xxxx] I hear that he [Zilboorg] is writing two books but I do not know on what subjects because I have not seen him for a long time. He is becoming more and more superficial, has domestic troubles, and is so caught in the machine of New York high-priced practice that he will never be able to disentangle himself. It will take a bad end and I am sorry for him because basically he is a nice and very gifted fellow.

de Saussure just sent me an invitation to a Pinel evening that the Ecole Libre des Hautes Etudes is holding on April 18. I may be able to attend the meeting because I have to be in New York anyway some time in April. I need not say that I will look you up.

I am sending you under separate cover a copy of "The Midwest Pioneer, His Ills, Cures, and Doctors" by Pickard and Buley for review in the Bulletin. Genevieve first intended to review it but we both found that you are the man to do it since you know the subject best. If the content of the book is as good as the presentation, it should be very good indeed. Schuman would charge at least $ 20.00 for it.

We expect Schuman tomorrow. He has plans for launching a new Journal of the History of Medicine with original articles, abstracts, and foreign correspondents in every country; George Rosen to be editor. The chief difficulty is with paper and we are trying to find a formula to make the Journal a cultural project of the United Nations so that the government will give its blessing to it. There is a definite need for a second journal and Rosen has sense and experience. He is on a mission in London, by the way.

My little book of addresses and essays is going to the press next week. I wrote two additional essays for it, one – Failure of a Generation – that opens the book and one on The Social Sciences in the Medical School that I am just finishing. I wrote a short preface to set the problem and will end up with a brief outlook that will not sound too hopeful. The San Francisco Conference is going to be a big circus and I can anticipate the big speeches that will be made. The trouble is that nobody believes in this organization.

I hope that Ellen has recovered by now and that you are settled.

 With all good wishes from house to house, I am
  Yours as ever
  [Henry]

Hans Holbein (1497/98–1543) German painter. S.'s review (Sigerist 1945). Article on Salerno (Kristeller 1945). Manuscript Ugo Benzi (Lockwood 1951). Pinel, de Saussure, Genevieve Miller see A. to S. of 23 March 1945. [xxxx] One sentence deleted as Chesney Archives' Protected Health Information. Zilboorg see A. to S. of 5 August 1941. (Pickard/Buley 1945). Henry Schuman, publisher. The new journal became the Journal of the History of Medicine and Allied Sciences; its first volume appeared in 1946. George Rosen (1910–1977) medical historian, friend of both S. and A. S.'s "little book": (Sigerist 1946a). San Francisco Conference for the foundation of the United Nations.

ACKERKNECHT to SIGERIST, New York, 2 April 1945

Dear Henry:

Thank you very much for the letter, the affidavit, and the review book. So far I have had only a short look into the latter; but it seems rather good. I am looking forward with great interest to your essay-collection. When is it supposed to come out of press?

It would be really grand if old Pinel would help us to have you here. It certainly is a pity with Zilboorg, as he is a very gifted man. But as there are many ways to go to Rome, so it seems there are also many ways to go to the dogs. And while the majority of us mortals perish rather from getting down and drowned, there seems also to be a deadly kind of social high altitude sickness.

Our library here got lately a lot of books from Sweden. Two I think would also be worthwhile to be bought by the Institute and to be reviewed by the Bulletin: <u>During</u>: On Aristotle's de partibus animalium (the book is written in English); and <u>R. Stromberg</u> Wortstudien (written in German; on the names of animals, plant etc in antiquity).

We can consolate ourself [sic] that the field of medical history is not the only one to be dishonored by careless and ignorant publications. My friend Rewald just launched a magnificent attack against the increasing number of products of the Gordon-Ricci kind in his field (art-history) with the backing of the Museum of Modern Art (the criticism, not the books, is backed by this museum.

Personally I do not have much to report. The disease period is now, we hope[,] over. [xxxx]. I passed the better part of the holidays in nailing shelfs [sic] together and painting them and arranging books. Now that I have my brave little soldiers again in fighting formation I feel immensely relieved, and eager for new deeds.

Kindest regards to Genevieve and the other Institute members, I very much hope to see you soon.

As ever yours
Erwin

Review book (Pickard/Buley 1945). Essay collection (Sigerist 1946a). (Düring 1943). (Strömberg 1944). Rewald, probably John (1912–1994) art historian. Gordon-Ricci not identified. [xxxx] three sentences deleted as Chesney Archives' Protected Health Information.

Dear Erwin:

Thanks for the book review. This was quick work. I am glad you found that the book is good and I do not think that it will in any way interfer [sic] with your malaria study. The approach is different and I think that, on the contrary, the other book may help by focusing the attention on pioneer conditions in the Middle West.

I saw in <u>Science</u> recently that Dr. Faust had given a lecture on the history of malaria in America, whereupon I sent him a complimentary copy of your study. His answer is enclosed.

I will not be able to be in New York in April but have definite plans for May.

Cordially as ever,

[Henry]

Book review (Pickard/Buley 1945). Malaria study (Ackerknecht 1945). Dr Ernest C. Faust, an American malariologist.

Dear Henry:

Thank you very much for your letter and for having drawn the attention of Faust to my book. F. is a very well known malariologist, mostly statistics. I quote this part of his work. By the way, I trust you will send, or have send [sic] already the monograph to Allan [sic] Gregg, as he usually receives the Institute publications. I would, of course, be very much interested in his seeing the thing.

You do not mention your health in your letter. I very much hope that this is the expression of the fact that things are back to normal. The bad news reached us through several channels, and we were rather scared. We send you our very best wishes for a speedy recovery, and hope that you don't need them any longer at this moment. I am not going to preach you things you know yourself as well as anybody else, but I hope that the accident has had the advantage of making you slow down a little bit your murderous speed. I am very sorry that you will not be able to be with us in

April, but I hope for May. I also hope that we will then be able to give you the Koch transcriptions, we have started working on in our rare spare moments. Progress is rather slow with all the other things we have on our neck, but steady. Some of the letters are quite interesting e.g. in 1887 Koch was still not yet convinced of Laveran's discovery. He comes out as a very typical German in his letters: devoted to his work and nature, otherwise a little bit dull and not without professorial malice.

You send me the Urdang book for review. I will, of course, be glad to wade through Kremers rather dull production, be it only for dear old Urdangs [sic] sake. I suppose you know that I have no special qualifications in the history of pharmacy, and you have send [sic] me the book because you could not think of somebody else with better qualifications. In this case I will be glad to review the book as soon as possible.

Today I have to ask you a favor. Could you, in case your health does permit it to you, drop a line to Chancey [sic] Leake, and ask him whether there is any opening at his place for a teacher of anatomy? The background of the story is the following. One of my fellow anthropologists here, Earl Count, has been associate professor of anatomy for 8 years at New York Medical College, for a while even acting head of the department. The old chairholder has died, a new man has come, and they have dismissed him without any special grounds at three months notice (and after the yearly congress of physical anthropologists, where he could have looked for a job). This is in itself nothing extraordinary, as disgusting as it may be. It is the old practice in most American Medical Schools, more business schools than "Universities", to fire the scholar as you would fire a janitor. But I think that in this special case everybody of us should help Count, as he is (besides being a good teacher) one of the few real scholars I have come across here, and as on the other hand he is an extremely quiet, modest person, who has never been able and will never be able to make the necessary noise for selling himself. (What I say about C. is not only based on my personal impressions, but I have taken care to interview other people before engaging myself for him.) C. has an unusual background which probably makes him "suspect" in this country of standardisation; but in spite of these appearances he is anything but a crackpot. Son of a missionary he has grown up in Bulgaria, and gone there to a German Gymnasium. This makes him an excellent linguist. He has abandoned the traditional study of theology, in order to study zoology (he has also taught zoology) and anthropology. Though his main interest is physical anthropology (the Museum is just publishing an excellent monograph of his on mathematical problems of growth) he has also an excellent knowledge of cultural anthropology. He holds a Ph.D. from California. With his humanistic background he is very much interested in historical problems. He is just working on a book on the history of race theories, and a companion volume, a source book, covering the same field. I hope I have given you an adequate idea of the man. He will be as good a teacher of anatomy as anybody else, and he will be a real acquisition for every university who wants still to have scholars, and he should be saved from going into God knows what profession, just because he is one of these rare scholar-animals and will undoubtedly produce valuable work in the years to come. Thus, please, drop a line to Ch.L., and let me know of the results as soon as possible, as three months are a very short time, when one is looking for this kind of job, as I know from my own bitter experience.

I am still very much ashamed of my bad typing, and I know how much you dislike it. But I hope friendship will make you overlook this little human weakness, and I promise you that when I had a secretary, I would send you the most wonderful typescripts too.

Again very best wishes for your health

    Cordially as ever yours

      Erwin

Names in alphabetical order:

Count, Earle, see letter

Faust, see S. to A. of 11 April 1945

Gregg, Alan, Rockefeller Medical Sciences Director, responsible for the support of S.'s Institute

Koch, Robert (1843–1910) German bacteriologist and hygienist

Kremers, Edward (1865–1941) historian of pharmacy

Laveran, Charles Louis A. (1845–1922) discoverer of the malaria germ

Leake, Chauncey D. (1896–1978) pharmacologist and medical historian, S.'s friend

Urdang, George, see AS 23.3.45. (Kremers/Urdang 1940)

Dear Henry:

We were very sorry to hear that you are still in an unsatisfactory condition. We very much hope that with your new way of life you will soon have completely recovered.

The nephew of Plaut, the pathologist of Beth Israel here, found in Italy a little book of Aschoff on Virchow, published in 1940. He sent it to his uncle who lent it to me. It is rather well written, and interesting beyond the merely medical aspects (Aschoff tries to show that V.'s Zellularpathologie is basically still sound). In quoting Virchow abundantly on the dolichocephalic myth, the necessity of humanitarianism, freedom, internationalism etc. it is a scantily veiled anti Nazi pamphlet, and my respect for A. whom I had not liked very much, has greatly increased. At 74 he showed more courage and insight than all the Diepgen and Co. together. If you think it fits into your bookreview section I will be glad to write a short review of the book which might already be a "rarity".

I am very anxious to read the February-Bulletin of which I had a glance at Mrs. Rosen's office. As I am not yet a member of the Association (they will decide upon my application only this month) could you please have me sent a copy? (Until it is on the shelf in the Academy I am afraid I will be grandfather. They have funny customs over there)

Again our best wishes

As ever yours

Erwin

Kindest regards, of course, to Mrs. Sigerist, who gave us the first news on your health since the thing started, and to les membres de l'Institut.

Beth Israel: A New York hospital. K. A. Ludwig Aschoff (1866–1942) German pathologist, (Aschoff 1940). Virchow see S. to A. of 27 April 1932 and (Ackerknecht 1953a). Dolichocephalic: long-skulled. Paul Diepgen see A. to S. of 29 April 1932. Mrs. Rosen see A. to S. of 23 March 1945. Association: American Association for the History of Medicine (AAHM). Academy: New York Academy of Medicine.

Dear Erwin:

I am back at the office for the first time after almost three weeks and I feel much better. [xxxx] I spent 10 days there quite comfortably, and you know how things are done. I had endless tests made but the results are kept strictly confidential and every effort is made to prevent the patient from knowing what his condition is. [xxxx]. All he is told is that he should never worry.

And so, my five doctors and half a dozen nurses, nurses aids, volunteers and probably the charwoman know what my condition is, but I don't. I know, however, what I knew before, that I have to slow down. I have given up smoking entirely and I am giving up the Library on May 15. Longcope talked to the President and Dean and it was decided that Temkin would be Acting Librarian until Larkey comes back.

I plan to go to Saratoga Springs some time in June and have a regular Badekur and then will spend a few months, probably in Ithaca. I will begin volume I of the History of Medicine and will drop everything else.

I will be in New York next week. I am anxious to get rid of the <u>American Review of Soviet Medicine</u> and they have asked for a meeting of the Editorial Board. Of course, I want to see you and Lucy. Keep the evening of May 16 free. I expect to arrive in New York around 1 p.m. and will be staying at the Hotel New Yorker. I will call you up at the office as soon as I am there.

I am sending you under separate cover a short Bibliography of Industrial Hygiene 1900–1943 that we received for review. You are a specialist in the field and I would appreciate it if you could write a short review. I would also very much appreciate a review of Aschoff's book on Virchow.

I will write to Chauncey Leake concerning your friend in the next few days as soon as I catch up with the correspondence.

Looking forward to seeing you soon, I am, with good wishes to you both

      Yours ever,
        [Henry]

[xxxx] Sentences deleted as Chesney Archives' Protected Health Information. Warfield T. Longcope (1877–1953) professor of medicine and director of the Department of Medicine at Johns Hopkins. "Giving up the Library": During WWII the head of the Welch Library, Sanford V. Larkey, was in the army, and S. took over his job as an

additional burden. "President", of Johns Hopkins University, I. Bowman. Temkin see A. to S. of 8 December 1937. Badekur: bathing cure. Book on Virchow (Aschoff 1951). Leake see A. to S. of 14 April 1945.

ACKERKNECHT to SIGERIST, New York, 10 May 1945

Dear Henry:

(I apologize for writing longhand, but my typewriter broke down) Thank you very much for your letter of May 8. We were awfully glad to hear that you are now definitely better and are looking forward very much to May 16. We have already a sitter for the evening. I am very anxious to hear about your plans, and will have to tell you about a lot of details which it is to [sic] cumbersome to report in letters. (A meeting of the anthropologists here very much along the lines of your University book etc.)

I fully sympathize with you as far as the secret diplomacy of Hopkins tests is concerned. After 10 days of tests I was more nervous than ever before.

You will be interested in an article of an army physician (Kocher) in the May 14 issue of the New Republic on "Socialized" Medicine as it confirms what you have already predicted the influence of army experience on physicians would be. Thanks also for the February Bulletin. It seems a very good number and I will have to read it carefully. I was delighted to see that Olmstedt [sic] will lecture on Brown-Séquard. B-S. is extremely interesting in every respect, and I was so upset by the total absence of an adequate treatment ([…] the pitiful paper of Major in the Evans Festschrift!) that I had already started collecting material during my metabolism – and P. Bert studies. But O. will do the job much better than I could do it with all my other duties, at least for a long time to come.

Ricci offered me through Heaton to revise his book, worried by your criticism. (I think this is encouraging as far as book-reviewing goes, and in favor of Ricci's character) Unfortunately with the library conditions here and my predominantly anthropological duties I feel not able to do it, as I judge it will be an enormous job, though I could have tried [?] to do it for moneys [sic] sake. Magnus-Levy eventually dumped the translation offer. Right now I am writing a series on Eskimos for Ciba which fits in very well into my former research and actual library facilities. Then I will have to find something else. Galdston just finished a number on the history of research for them and I hear you are now writing the spas.

I will be glad to do the two book reviews for you. I have been wrestling already with the Kremers-Urdang which is of superb dullness.

The war in Europe is now over, and one should feel happier than one is able to do having a slight inkling of the future. Incidentally I picked up Schopenhauer on VE day, and his statement that life is a great penitentiary where the many expiate the crimes of the few seemed to me less old than it would have been 10 years ago. I do not think that we have much chance ever to hear of our parents, and Lucy is very depressed by the fact. The children were again sick for a week but are better now. I have to do a lot of propagandizing and "organizing" for our "Instit. of Human Morphology" and progress is slow.

Very, very best wishes for your health and à bientôt!

Yours as ever

Erwin

Regards to Mrs. Sigerist, Geneviève, the new librarian etc. etc.

"University book": (Sigerist 1946a). James M. D. Olmsted (1886–1956) biographer of Claude Bernard and others. Charles Edward Brown-Séquard (1817–1894) British physiologist (Olmsted 1946). Ralph H. Major (born 1884) medical historian. Herbert M. Evans (1882–1971) anatomist; his Festschrift (N. N. 1943). "P. Bert studies": (Ackerknecht 1944). Ricci not identified. Heaton see A. to S. of 23. March 1945. Magnus-Levy see S. to A. of 5 March 1945. Kremers-Urdang see A. to S. of 14 April 1945. Arthur Schopenhauer (1788–1860) German philosopher. VE day: Victory in Europe, 10 May, 1945. "The new librarian": O. Temkin, see S. to A. of 8 May 1945.

ACKERKNECHT to SIGERIST, New York, 23 May, 1945

Dear Henry:

Included you will find the 3 bookreviews I owe you. I apologise for having typed the Urdang-Kremers review one spaced [sic]. I hope it does not matter too much.

I would like to thank you again in Lucys [sic] name and for myself for the delightful evening we had with you. I need not go into details how much we enjoyed your company. You know it. We are now looking forward to that historic date, June 11.

Day before yesterday I had the first news from my parents (indirect ones from Switzerland) since almost three years. After a rather terrible exodus – they have of course lost everything – they had reached in March, that is shortly before the French came in, their native Wurttemberg. I am very much relieved to know them there, and think that under present circumstances that is the best news I could have. I only wish we would have once similar good news for Lucys [sic] parents.

By the way, it seems that your teacher Sauerbruch has become one of the "rulers" of Berlin. I wonder how that will end with his rather bad temper.

I forgot to ask you something rather professional. We will, of course, have to found a "Committee" for the moral and financial protection of our "Institute of Human Morphology". Could you think of any "personality" preferably in New York, but à la rigeur also outside, who would be interested enough in our problems, or interested enough in publicity, to give his name. Anatomists in this country are in general not interested at all in anatomy or morphology. But there might still be some other medical people who are. With your "nationwide" knowledge of personalities you might perhaps be able to give us a good tip.

We very much hope that your health will keep on being satisfactory. Kindest regards (also at Cloverhill and at Monument Str.) and best wishes

Yours as ever

Erwin

Urdang-Kremers see A. to S. of 14 April 1945. "Historic date June 11": S.'s next visit in New York. A.'s parents, Erwin Ackerknecht and Clara Pfitzer, had been living in Stettin in Northeastern Germany, fled before the Russians before the end of WWII. Ferdinand Sauerbruch (1875–1951) German surgeon, S.'s teacher in Zurich. Cloverhill Road: S.'s address in Baltimore; Monument Street: Address of the Institute within the medical campus of Johns Hopkins University.

SIGERIST to ACKERKNECHT, Baltimore ?, 30 May 1945

Dear Erwin:

Thanks for your letter of May 23. It was a great pleasure to see you the other day and I only regret that time was so short.

You must be glad to know that your parents are in safety. The last days of Stettin must have been pretty terrible and under Russian occupation they would be cut off from the rest of the world for a long time to come. In Wurttemberg they will be under French authority which is much more pleasant. I hope Lucy will have news of her parents soon also.

Sauerbruch somehow always manages to be on top and once Berlin is ruled by the five allied nations, the job should not be difficult because it will be easy to play one ally up against the other.

Now to the Committee of your Institute of Human Morphology. I am sorry to say that I do not know of any suitable anatomist in New York. George Wislocki at Harvard would, I am sure, be interested. He is one of the broadest anatomists in this country. Here at Hopkins, Adolph Schultz, our professor of anthropology whom you know, would undoubtedly be interested also. But this is about all I can suggest.

I am looking forward to seeing you on June 11 at Schuman's cocktail party. The Wyeth Company has called off the anesthesia meetings it was going to have in New York the same day but Schuman's party remains.

Yours as ever,
    [Henry]

Sauerbruch see A. to S. of 23 May 1945. "Five allied nations": There were only four in Berlin: US, UK, F, USSR. George Wislocki (1892–1956). Adolph Schultz (1891–1976) anthropologist. Schuman see S. to A. of 27 March 1945. Wyeth Co. see S. to A. of 26 February 1945.

ACKERKNECHT to SIGERIST, New York, 7 June 1945

Dear Henry:

Thank you very much for the cigarettes and the excellent portrait of mine which already ornates my office. It was really very thoughtful to provide me with this vital stuff I have not yet found the moral strength to renounce.

I wonder what you are going to do with your material on Rouelle, Jean? Why not write a little paper for the Philosophical Society, enlightening them about an unknown member? And what are you doing with your Zola material?

I saw Schuman yesterday. He is more upset about the Claudius Meyer [sic] business, than, I think, is warranted by the facts. I am opposed to psychopathological labeling, as you know, but ever since Meyer [sic] told me about the "persecutions" of Catholics (he, of course, included) in Horthy Hungary (!), I have made my diagnosis, and I think, that Schuman has been rather lucky to avoid an association which would have been a source of endless trouble.

We very much hope that your health situation has remained satisfactory, and are looking forward very much to meeting you Monday June 11.

Yours as ever

Erwin

Jean Rouelle (born 1751) French-American physician and pharmacist (Sigerist 1949). S. has not published on Emile Zola. Claudius Mayer at the Army Medical Library in Washington, DC. Miklos Horthy (1868–1957) regent of Hungary, brought his country into WWII as an ally of Nazi Germany.

ACKERKNECHT to SIGERIST, New York, 17 July 1945

Dear Henry:

By now you ought to be settled in Ithaca, and we hope very much that everything is going all right. I am still the curator without collection, and I feel it more than ever as I have moved into another, enormous office (new phone extension: 236), surrounded by empty cupboards. That does not mean that I am inactive. I have gone through enormous quantities of literature, am working on a little paper, and, of course, doing the eternal bookreviews. I read Olmstead's [sic] Magendie with great pleasure, and am looking forward to his Brown-Séquard, which I trust will not be inferior. By the way, we finished the Koch letters some time ago, and are waiting for your instructions how to proceed. We made one carbon of every letter, so that there would be no risk sending you the typescript in case you want to have a look at it.

Our personal life is quite pleasant. The two refugee scholars at the museum, Heine-Geldern and Weidenreich, are not only very good men in their field, but personally quite sympathetic. Heine-G. had just his sixtieth birthday, and I talked Fejos (Viking Foundation) into giving him a nice dinner in a Chinese restaurant. Weidenreich is very alert in spite of being 72 (he started with 60 a new carrier [sic], and a very successful one in China). Both his daughters had been in concentration camps and were thought to be lost, but both have reappeared. I was in medical school with one of them, and we had a very good friend in common, a biochemist at the Berlin University, one of the very few friends I still had in Germany. This one was not so lucky. I just heard from Weidenreich that he was shot in 1943. This negative selection of the "home-front" duplicating the one of the battlefields, makes prospects for a European renaissance still more gloomy, as after all the human material also counts for something in such a process.

Kindest regards to the family. Best wishes for work and health

Yours as ever

Erwin

Ithaca, NY, site of Cornell University. Olmsted see A. to S. of 10 May 1945. François Magendie (1783–1855) French physiologist and pharmacologist, teacher of Claude Bernard (Olmsted 1944). Koch see A. to S. of 14 April 1945. Three anthropologists: Robert Heine-Geldern (1885–1968) Vienna and U.S., Franz Weidenreich (1873–1948) Germany and U.S., Paul Fejos (1897–1963) Hungary and U.S.
[xxxx] Four short sentences deleted as Chesney Archives' Protected Health Information.

SIGERIST to ACKERKNECHT, Ithaca, NY, 20 July 1945

My dear Erwin,

[xxxx]

Well I have been working on THE BOOK for a whole week now and I seem to be started definitely. The thing now is to keep it going for the next twelve years, or at least as long as I live. It is a great satisfaction, of course, after all these years.The first chapter is a kind of methodology of medical history. People may yell that this is deutsche Gründlichkeit or rather, Pedanterie, but I do not care. Our field is so young that a few things have to be said that would not be necessary in e.g. the history of art. I also plan to have a number of appendices to every volume. In this one, Appendix I will be a sketch of the history of medical historiography with a critical evaluation of the various textbooks. Appendix II will be a bibliography of the various tools of medical history, reference books etc. and there will be others. I write 4 hours every morning, then I have 4 more hours for research, mostly at the library of the University, and about 4 hours for "business", correspondence, Bulletin etc. and of course, I cook dinner for the family and how!

I feel very happy in Ithaca. The house is nice and we are quite in the country, the real country with trees, and birds, and rabbits, and chipmonks. And the University is a real university, with departments for every fiels [sic], a very good library and such amenities as theatre (this week John Gabriel Borkman), concerts, a series of historical films. I recently saw "Intolerance" by Griffith, made in 1916, a remarkable film. In Baltimore, in the last three years, I was cut out from everything and I, therefore enjoy being a normal human being again, doing work that I consider worth-while.

I am glad to know that you finished the Koch letters. I will not need them here. Send them to Baltimore, or better wait until Genevieve is there in September. But send me a bill that I can sign and pass on to Hope. I think the agreement was one dollar a letter, if I remember correctly. And it might be better to make the bill out on Lucy's name. At any rate I would like you to have the money soon, and I am certainly delighted to know that the work is finished and am most grateful to you.

Best wishes to you all from us all

Yours as ever

[Henry]

[xxxx] Four short sentences deleted as Chesney Archives' Protected Health Information. THE BOOK: *A History of Medicine*, latest plan was 8 volumes history and 4 volumes sociology of medicine, one volume per year. "Deutsche Gründlichkeit" = German thoroughness. S. was an enthusiastic hobby cook. John Gabriel Borkman, a drama by Henrik Ibsen. D. W. Griffith (1875–1948) film maker. Neither S. nor A. have edited letters of Robert Koch. Hope Trebing was S.'s secretary in Baltimore.

Dear Henry:

Thank you very much for your letter of July 20. It made me really happy to hear that THE BOOK is started, and also to feel from your letter how much better you feel in the general environment of Ithaca, and after the decisive step has been done. I am very optimistic about the rest; but may I nevertheless do some carping on one point. If I am right in adding your working hours, I get 12. Now, a race over 5 km needs another economy of forces than one over 100 m. When we were cutting wood for the French, a friend of mine, who had been one of the ablest German film producers, and unfortunately was turned meanwhile into fertilizer, was often critized [sic] by the officers (not by the specialists, because he had a bigger output than anybody else) for "slowness". He used to answer: "Listen, Sir, I have only a certain amount of forces. Now, it seems this war is going to last pretty long. Thus I have to economise them, in order to get through." Why not adopt this motto as far as efforts go in your case?

My life too goes on being very satisfactory. I finished my little paper on premature children in primitive society. I was quite surprised to see that effective care of premature children starts only in the middle of the last century in France (and that when birth restriction was officially recommended) which makes my Eskimo and Bantu incubators somewhat more interesting. I am still seeing lots of people. Lowie is here, teaching summer school at Columbia, and I had a very interesting talk with him this afternoon in spite of his proverbial shyness.

I am just reading (for review in the Bulletin) "Configurations of Culture Growth" by A. L. Kroeber (the Berkeley emeritus in anthropology). It is a historic book, and in spite of the atrocious title highly interesting. The problem is the cyclic movements in different branches of culture (he analyses philosophy, science, philology, sculpture, painting, drama, literature, music, state in Egypt, Mesopotamia, China, Japan, India, Islam, Greece-Rome, and the modern European nations) It is not so sensational as Spengler and Toynbee, but therefore perhaps also more solid. I hope they have it up there in Ithaca, and you have time to have a look at it. It might be particularly interesting to you at the given moment. I would, of course, be very interested in your opinion, especially on the science chapter. He deals a lot with the Arabs, and has also a special chapter on Greek medicine. I have so far read only 250 out of the 850 pages – it is my evening lecture [sic] –

but do not regret it so far. It helps against some too easy parallelising of growth in different branches, towards which I am sometimes inclined, when one can compare the actual time relations.

We very much hope that Ithaca goes on being as pleasant as it starts.

Kindest regards from all of us to all of you

Yours as ever

Erwin

"Decisive step": The beginning of S.'s writing *A History of Medicine*, see S. to A. of 20 July 1945. Robert Lowie see A. to S. of 31 March 1940. (Kroeber 1969). Oswald Spengler (1880–1936) German philosopher of history. Arnold J. Toynbee (1889–1925) English historian. "Evening lecture", correct: evening reading.

ACKERKNECHT to SIGERIST, New York, 6 August 1945

Dear Henry:

Thank you very much for your letter of July 30, which I just found returning from a weekend up state. This certainly are [sic] hot news, and the choice must be awfully hard. Unless some details come out, which make the offer so disadvantageous that it is easy to refuse. I guess you will look at the whole thing mainly under the angle of your general plans for the next years. Whether these can be realized better here or in England, only the details will show to which I am looking forward very much. Anyway, it is good that you can show to the Chesniaks and Co. that you do not depend on them. This kind of gentlemen has always to be reminded of this fact once in a while.

I have been the last 5 days in Schenevus (Otsego Cy.) to bring out Lucy and the children. It is a very beautiful place, reminding of Southern Germany, and I am glad that they are now at least for 4 weeks out of the stench and heat of the city, with nice people, in a very nice place. I will have plenty to do meanwhile.

I am almost through with the Kroeber which is quite boring and ludicrous at times, but nevertheless gave me a lot of stimulation. I have never read the Markham. I got so disgusted with the climatologists through Ellsworth Huntington whose evidence always crumbles as soon as it is touched by somebody who knows the facts (we discussed him a good deal in the anthropo-geographical club with Carter and Albright) that I never tried another one. It does not seem as if the great civilisations in their large majority grew up in the "optimum-climate", unless it is defined after you have constructed an "average climate" from their climate which is not easy. Howells, who indeed worked here 12 years for nothing because he is a rich man, was then in Madison, and is now with the navy, is one of these chatty books in the vein of his master Hooton, and just as bad.

Weidenreich showed me today an article of the old Meinicke (82, now living as a poor refuge [sic] somewhere on the Weser) in one of these sheets the Americans print for the Germans. He emphasizes that he writes spontaneously, reminds that he was one of the last to speak publicly against "satanic" Hitlerism (2 days before the Reichstagsbrand), but honestly admits that they all became the victims not of terror alone, but the combination of terror and propaganda. He then calls for "Verinnerlichung" as the only "Ausweg". The whole thing sounds rather kümmerlich, but fits rather well into your prognostics. Though I do not think that much will come out of the whole Verinnerlichung. The Germans get too much reeducation to think of any other Verinnerlichung than the Verinnerlichung of bark, turnips and other victuals, and Hitler will soon be more popular than he has ever been at his lifetime. But I better skip this. "Politisch Lied, ein garstig Lied."

Very best wishes for the next and farther future

    Kindest regards to all of you

        Yours as ever

          Erwin

S.'s letter of 30 July is missing; it would have provided information about an offer of a chair in the history of science and the direction of a department at the University of London, offered by Charles Singer (see also A. to S. of 31 August 1945 and S. to A. of 21 September 1945). Chesniaks may allude to Allen M. Chesney, dean of the Johns Hopkins Medical School. "Up state" = upstate New York. Kroeber see A. to S. of 25 July 1945. Ellsworth Huntington (1876–1947) economist and climatologist. Carter see 28. February 1945. Albright, possibly William F. (1891–1971) anthropologist and archaeologist. William W. Howells (ca.1915–2005) anthropologist at the Museum of Natural History in New York. Ernest A. Hooton (1887–1954). Weser: a river in Germany. Reichstagsbrand: Fire of the Reichstag Building in Berlin 1933. Verinnerlichung: Internalization. Ausweg: Way out. Kümmerlich: poor, miserable. Politisch Lied, ein garstig Lied: Political song, a dirty song.

Dear Henry:

Thank you very much for the affidavit. I was already a little worried, you might not have received it, as I am leaving tomorrow for a two weeks vacation with my girls, and I wanted to send off the stuff to Albany before leaving. Now it is perfect, as the affidavit came in today.

I do not know whether I acknowledged already the cheque for Lucy which arrived with surprising speed. Comes in very handy. Thanks again for having us given this chance. I sent yesterday the letters (that is the transscriptions [sic] – the originals are still here and wait for transsportation) and a few bookreviews to Genevieve. If you disagree with the Kroeber review in important points or want to insert something, please let me know.

Métraux came back from Germany last Tuesday. I am including [sic] an abstract of what he said, which I wrote up the same evening, in order to get rid of the nightmare. It is strange, one has read all this more or less in the newspapers, but it does not impress you the same way, as if somebody comes and tells you, and, of course, gives you a wealth of details in names of places, streets, persons. But even Shapiro who heard the report too, and to whom it does not mean much, how the Königstrasse in Stuttgart looks, where my Grandmother [sic] bought me toys, and I took out my first girlfriends, or my crazy uncle, the anatomist, could not sleep either that neight [sic]. It is this forbodings for our whole civilisation which get you down, though you still rationally might hope, it might not come through. Métraux's data are besides confirmed for France and Germany by other letters and personal reports I got lately.

I had several very agreeable talks with Lowie, though also mostly about Germany. He is just writing a book on it. Ruth Benedict is going to Germany too. Anthropology seems to become a kind of Germanology.

But without me. I am going on with primitive medicine. I just finished a lecture which I am going to give here at the Academy of Sciences in October. I have two copies made, in case you arrive at primitive medicine before my lecture is published. I hope I brought out some important general points, which I had not yet published so far. On the other hand I hate the form of lectures, where you have to be dogmatic, and I contemplate to develop two special points (Primitive Surgery; and The Rational and Irrational in Primitive Medicine, where I hope I have found now a more satisfactory formulation than before) in articles where I can give the whole evidence. Especially if you should be short in manuscripts.

I spent my VJ days and a couple of Sundays translating the article of Proskauer for Schuman. Proskauer writes as you may remember "Sudhoff Deutsch". And I had to read Mommsen in order to satisfy myself that German nevertheless, even in historic treatises can be as beautiful and clear as any other language.

I heard from Temkin that you have refused the London chair. This is, of course, very good news for all your friends here, and I think for all those interested in the future of medical history here. There would not have been left much after your leaving the old USA. Temkin also sent me his book, and that is what I am going to read in my vacation. It eventually came out. Hallelujah! One can hardly believe it, that no rechecking was needed again. I guess this book is what the obstetricians call a case of protracted labor.

I hope Ithaca is still as good, and work is still progressing as satisfactorily as in the beginning, though this beginning should be rather hard, as all new started. I am sick and tired of being alone, and am glad that it will be over tomorrow.

Kindest regards to the whole family

Yours as ever

Erwin

Letters: Probably Robert Koch's, see A. to S. of 14 April 1945. Kroeber see A. to S. of 6 August 1945. Alfred Métraux (1902–1963) Swiss anthropologist; he spoke about the dismal conditions in post-war Germany. Harry L. Shapiro (1902–1990) head of Anthropology Department of the American Museum of Natural History in New York. Lowie see A. to S. of 31 March 1940. Benedict see A. to S. of 2 August 1944. VJ Day: Victory in Japan, End of WWII on 2 September 1945. Curt Proskauer (1888–1972) historian of dentistry. Karl Sudhoff (1853–1938) medical historian in Leipzig, S.'s teacher. Theodor Mommsen (1817–1903) German historian. Temkin see A. to S. of 8 December 1937, his book (Temkin 1945). London chair see A. to S. of 6 August 1945.

SIGERIST to ACKERKNECHT, Baltimore, 21 September 1945

Dear Erwin:

I have not written you for a long time but first I was busy with my book and then I knew that you were leaving soon for your vacation. We came back to Baltimore last Saturday. It was a very pleasant drive through the hills of Northern Pennsylvania. Of all the landscapes I have seen on the East Coast, this looks perhaps most like Europe and I can understand that the German settlers felt very much at home here.

Ithaca was very pleasant to the end. I left with 250 pages text and 75 pages footnotes, with notes for 16 pages of illustrations. I finished the chapter on The Antiquity of Disease or Paleopathology and came to some quite interesting conclusions. Now I have a short chapter on History and Geography of Disease that I am completing at the end of next week and this will complete the introductory part. The next will be primitive medicine and, of course, I am anxious to discuss my outline with you. I have about 30,000 words available for that section which is not too much but still infinitely more than you find in any history of medicine.

Now, I am going to tell you a secret that you must not reveal to anybody, namely that I will in all probability spend a couple of weeks in New York in October. Much as I dislike it, I have to interrupt my book for one month in order to complete the new edition of the Soviet book. I just had news from France that Payot wants to bring out the French edition as soon as ever possible. A publishing house in Bombay wants to bring out a special edition for India. A Portuguese, Italian and German edition (the latter made in Switzerland) are also agreed upon and so I am afraid I have no choice but must bring the book up to date. I will need the libraries of the American-Russian Institute and of the American-Soviet Medical Society and so I have no choice but to go to New York. But it must remain unknown otherwise I will be so swamped with engagements that I will not be able to do any work and on November 1, I must write page 1 of the chapter on Primitive Medicine. I will take advantage of the opportunity and will complete my bibliography on paleopathology in your Museum. I have a few gaps but I am sure that I will be able to fill them in New York.

The memorandum you sent me, Métraux's report, was extraordinarily interesting. It confirms much that I heard from other sides but conditions seem to be worse than one could possibly imagine. By the way, do you remember Ludwig Englert? He must have been at the Institute at the time when you wrote your dissertation, a tall Bavarian who was a classical philologist and was studying medicine. I received a letter from him from Lubeck and I am sending it enclosed because it will amuse you, the typical letter that I expected from this kind of people.

Yes, I refused the London chair. It would have been a still bigger administrative job. They have very ambitious plans for a department that will cover the entire history of science with a large staff of specialists in the history of mathematics, chemistry, physics, biology, philosophy of science, etc. The head of such a department will obviously be Mädchen für alles. Besides, I would have had to take over some old staff members who have been there for a long time, one of them a shell-shocked veteran of the first World War. But for a while it sounded quite tempting because London has incredible libraries and is only a few hours from Paris. Still, I am afraid that I would haver [sic] have written my History if I had yielded to this temptation.

 With kind regards to the whole family, I am

  Yours as ever,
   [Henry]

New edition of the Soviet book (Sigerist 1947). Payot, a French publishing house. Métraux and his report see A. to S. of 31 August 1945. Ludwig Englert, a staff member at S.'s Institute in Leipzig. London chair see A. to S. of 6 August 1945. Mädchen für alles = maid-of-all-work.

ACKERKNECHT to SIGERIST, New York, 31 October 1945

Dear Henry:

 I enclose the promised "key" for the bibliography. Thanks again that you gave us two of your evenings. We enjoyed it tremendously. It is sad that you are gone now again. I hope you did not mind Sylvias [sic] freshness. She was so tired [?] and exalted. And after all she is American. Chewing gum included.

 Very best wishes
  Yours as ever
   Erwin

SIGERIST to ACKERKNECHT, Baltimore ?, 3 November 1945

Dear Erwin:

 Thanks ever so much for the "key". It will be most useful indeed. I greatly enjoyed seeing you and the family and having a chance to talk

218

primitive medicine with you. I will have many more specific questions a month from now. At this time, I was anxious to know whether you approved of my general plan.

Railway Express is so slow that my trunks have not come yet and I have not been able to continue my work on the Soviet book. And so to fill in the time, I have been translating a paper by Semashko on Erismann who was the pioneer of hygiene and public health in Russia. He was a Swiss from Zurich and when he had to leave Russia for political reasons, he became health commissioner of Zurich. His two children went to the same school as I in 1901 and I remember them very well. He was a real pioneer of the Pettenkofer school, and since he is very little known here, I thought to publish this article in the Bulletin.

Tell Sylvia that I have not forgotten the buttons nor the chocolate or the chewing gum and that she will get them in the next few days.

My love to you all.

As ever yours,
[Henry]

Soviet book (Sigerist 1947). N. A. Semashko (born 1874) Russian hygienist. Friedrich H. Erismann (1842–1915) Swiss hygienist. S.'s translation (Sigerist 1946b). Max von Pettenkofer (1818–1901) German hygienist.

ACKERKNECHT to SIGERIST, New York, 12 November 1945

Dear Henry:

Thank you very much for your letter of Nov. 3. Thanks a lot for the buttons and chocolate for Sylvia too. Erika, whose short visit we enjoyed today very much, can testify to the fact that she appreciates them very much.

The great sensation of the last week for us has been the first letter of my parents since 1939. My father is "Kulturreferent" in Ludwigsburg, and though starting from scratch at 65, and liberated from all his earthly goods through bombing, flight, and French liberators, very courageous. It sounds much better than I had dared to hope (though he too is very positive [?] about the millions to die this winter, and pretty sad about the little understanding of the catastrophy by his countrymen). Guttentag also found at least an aunt of Lucy who could tell him that her parents are still alive, and even not bombed out. (They live so far out of the city that he could not yet meet them). Unfortunately both our sisters have disappeared. Mine in Kärnten, and Lucy's on her way to Franconia. But we hope they will turn up, more or less safe, now that postal relations in Germany are reestablished. Lucy is now, of course, very busy with sending packages, we both with letters etc.

I have thought over your suggestion of bringing out my collected articles on Primitive Medicine, and think it is a most excellent one. I could easily put together a 50,000 word volume. The next time I see Schuman I will make a "feeler". If you meet him, it might not be so bad, if you talk with him about this item too. Do you ever see Fulton? If he (or other people who talked about similar projects) ever seriously contemplated to create for me a medicohistorical situation at Yale, they should not wait too long. I still think that a medicohistorical position would allow me to produce more than my present job, as much as I like it otherwise. But if Shapiro really succeeds in endowing my Institute with 1 ½ Million Dollars, as he tries, and when I have been there for a number of years and become tied up with these problems, it will be very difficult for me to back out. (The best for me [?] would be, if somebody somewhere endowed an Institute for Primitive Medicine. But so far I have not yet met somebody to whom I could sell this idea.) Well, this is all Zukunftsmusik. For the time being I am with my bones, and write my article for Merck. Thus the article for the Bulletin has still to wait a little. But it will come!

Not much happened since you left. I was in a completely cockeyed seminary of French anthropologists. Deeply impressed by the "success" of the physicists, which indeed has generalized Bevinés [?] famous slogan "Wir Kommunisten sind alle Tote auf Urlaub", they trie [sic] to remodel anthropology along physicists [sic] lines. I think we will hear more of this craze, which is very appropriate to replace psych[o]analysis with those eager for new sensations.

Semashko's paper on Ehrismann [sic] ought to be very interesting. There have been so many interesting personalities among the "Kulturdünger" which went to Russia from Europe during the 18. and 19. century, and they are little remembered, as they fit so little into the patterns of their old or their new countries.

I enclose a short review of the little book on Fredericq. Shall I send it back right now, or keep it together with the Koch-letters? I would like to review for the Bulletin, if you can get them:

Ellis E.S., Primitive Anaesthesia and Allied Conditions. William Heinemann, London 1945.

Simmons L.W. The role of the aged in primitive society. Yale University Press 1945.

Very best wishes for your work and health

And very best regards from all of us to all of you

As ever yours

Erwin

Erica, S.'s elder daughter (1918–2002). Kulturreferent: Officer in charge of cultural affairs. Ludwigsburg, a town near Stuttgart. Otto Guttentag (1900–1991) physiologist. Kärnten: Carinthia. Fulton see S. to A. of 26 February 1945. Shapiro see A. to S. of 31 August 1945. Zukunftsmusik: Dreams of the future. Merck, probably the pharmaceutical company. Beviné not identified. "Wir Kommunisten …": We communists all are dead men on leave of absence". Semashko and Erismann see S. to A. of 3 November 1945. Kulturdünger: Cultural fertilizer. Fredericq, possibly Léon (1853–1934) Belgian physiologist.

SIGERIST to ACKERKNECHT, Baltimore ?, 12 November 1945

Dear Erwin:

I am just making plans for the January and February numbers of the Bulletin and I would like to inquire when I may expect your manuscript. I would like to have it for the January number if you could send it soon.

Cordially yours,

Henry E. Sigerist

ACKERKNECHT to SIGERIST, New York, 14 November 1945

Dear Henry:

Thank you for your line concerning the manuscript. As I wrote you yesterday, I am afraid, I will not be able to finish the article soon. As a matter of fact I think it will not be before the end of January, as we will have a meeting of the Am. Anthrop. Ass. in December.

As ever yours
Erwin

P. S. Albright got only [xxxx] removed.

Albright see A. to S. of 6 August 1945. [xxxx]: Alan Mason Chesney Archive, Protected Health Information.

ACKERKNECHT to SIGERIST, New York, 5 December 1945

Dear Henry:

I have not heard from you for quite a while. I hope that that just means that you are all right and busy. Through Gottman I just came across a book of René Leriche (the great French surgeon and holder of Bernard's chair at the Collège de France) La Chirurgie à l'ordre de la vie. La Presse Francaise [sic] et Etrangère. O. Zelnek Editeur. Paris-Aix les Bains 1944. I think the Institute should buy it and the Bulletin review it (Temkin?). It is "philosophical", contains among others a very nice piece on Halstedt [sic], written in 1913. In case you cannot get it, I will be glad to write at least a review for the Bulletin.

Thanks a lot for the review book on the Am. Indian and small pox. I had not heard of it yet. And that is just the kind of stuff I like to read and to have for my library.

In the last number of the Bulletin of the New York Academy of Med. is an article on trichinosis which you should read. It is a first rate illustration of "medieval" public health conditions in this country. I wonder whether the man could not write an article for the Bulletin. His introductory historical remarks are promising.

Bios, October 1945, has a symposium on premedical education. You might like to keep the reference.

Margaret Schlauch [?], refering to you, asked me to give a lecture on medieval medicine. I accepted, as I know nobody better here, and will try not to talk nonsense in sticking to what I know (e.g. psychopathology) and avoiding what I do not know (philology).

I submitted to Schuman a plan for a volume of essays, following your suggestion, and hope very much it will work out.

Carter probably told you, that Sauer, the geographer of Berkeley, well known for his acid judgements, made very laudatory remarks on my malaria, whereupon it seems to have dawned even upon Bowman that I might have been not so bad in spite of being a foreigner and your pupil.

I am very busy with my collection, the rational-irrational article (I go over the whole field again to make it "solid"), anthropological meetings (there is a lot of unrest and attempts to make us appendices of government and business, special reflections of the general tendency to make science as cheep as possible and as rotten as our society) book reviews, packages and letters for Germany etc. I very much hope, everything is all right with you. Emmy's letters sound rather optimistic.

Kindest regards and very best wishes to all of you

Yours as ever

Erwin

Gottman, possibly a bookseller. Claude Bernard (1813–1878) French physiologist. René Leriche (1879–1955) French surgeon. Temkin see A. to S. of 8 December 1937. William S. Halsted (1852–1922) surgeon at Johns Hopkins University. Margaret Schlauch, probably the mid-20th century New York expert on medieval English literature. Volume of essays on primitive medicine. Carter see A. to S. of 28 February 1945. Carl O. Sauer (1889–1975). Bowman see S. to A. of 6 December 1941. Emmy Sigerist, S.'s wife, see A. to S. of 27 November 1938.

Sigerist to Ackerknecht, Baltimore ?, 18 December 1945

Dear Erwin:

Yes, it is true that I have not written you for a very long time. It was not only my fault [xxxx]. I had not the courage to start a letter in longhand. At the moment, I am working on three books simultaneously, writing a new one (the History), patching up an old one (the Soviet book still) and reading page proofs and making an index of the Essays and Addresses that Schuman is publishing.

I can well imagine what a relief it must have been for you to hear that your parents are safe. It is a pity that they are not in the American sector because Hania's husband is now in charge of cultural activities in Bavaria and whatever part of Swabia is occupied by the Americans. Through him it would be very easy to keep in close touch with your father. I hope that in the meantime Lucy had had good news about her parents and that your sisters have turned up.

I had a number of letters from Germany too, sad ones and others that seem rather funny. You remember Margarita Blank who worked on case histories of Boerhaave at the Institute, a little woman from the Baltic Provinces. Her sister has studied theology and had married Bersing who was assistant in the Indic Department. They lived in Planitz in a cottage that they had built with their own hands. Well, I had a letter from Bersing telling that his sister-in-law, my old student, had been executed by the Nazis in February, 1945. She was arrested on the basis of an anonymous denunciation. Bersing and his wife are well. They are in the Russian sector in Berlin, he as curator of the Indian and Chinese collections of the Museum of Ethnology and she with an administrative job in the health department. Another letter I received from Max Lange, the doctor who had married Irene Zygoures, the Greek medical student whom you certainly remember. He is a prisoner of war in France. They were completely bombed out in Leipzig. His apartment as well as his office seemed to have been destroyed to the last objects but they had a cottage in Hiddensee where the wife and the two children seem to be at the moment. From him I heard that Sabine Hirschberg, the daughter of Hans Hirschberg, the obstetrician that you certainly knew, had committed suicide in 1943.

But the most whimsical letter I received from Heinz Zeiss, the father of geomedicine, a Nazi of the first hour who was in Moscow for a number of years in charge of the Pasteur Institute but probably as a spy also. He writes that both he and Diepgen had so much hoped that I would turn up in Berlin, that my presence would be highly desirable, etc. etc. He then adds that we should send all possible American books, scientific and others, to Berlin since Germans are so responsive to cultural propaganda. A filthy scoundrel. He is a. D. but still writes on paper of the Hygiene Institute of Berlin, still attends faculty meetings, in other words he is still going strong. A real scoundrel.

[xxxx] Half a sentence deleted as Chesney Archives' Protected Health Information. The letter is continued two days later on 20 December. Hope Trebing see S. to A. of 20 July 1945. "Essays and Addresses (Sigerist 1946a). Hania Wislicka see A. to S. of 12 November 1941. M. Blank, I. Zygoures, and H. Hirschberg were students of S. in Leipzig. Diepgen see A. to S. of 2 May 1945. a. D.: ausser Dienst = retired.

Dear Erwin:

I just want to finish the letter. I was interrupted on Monday because we had the meeting of the Johns Hopkins Medical History Club. It was a good meeting. The three papers were very good and substantial and gave a good picture of Rush. Gwinnie has become an expert exhibitionist [sic] and has put up a very good Rush exhibit quite independently without my doing anything to it. Rosen had come from Washington and Whitfield Bell from Dickinson College. Temkin gave a little dinner at the Hopkins Club and so the whole evening was most pleasant except that the attendance could have been better.

I just received the prospectus of the Journal. It looks very impressive and I am sure that you and Rosen will make a very good job of it. I wish that you and Rosen and I and a few others could come together some day to discuss the future of medical history in this country. There is a lot to worry about and a lot that could be done.

I began the chapter on Primitive Medicine with a discussion of the prehistoric material. I had to stick it in somewhere since my book is not only a history of medicine but also a kind of history of civilization seen from the medical angle. I said that we knew, so to say, nothing about prehistoric medicine but I had to mention whatever material is available. Is there any recent monograph on neolithic trephined skulls, and has anybody ever attempted to make an atlas indicating where such skulls have been found? If not, this would be a very worthwhile undertaking because the material on the subject is widely scattered.

The more I read the 4 volumes of Déchelette, the more I appreciate him. I did not know that he had been killed in the beginning of the first World War. I have a rather vitriolic editorial in the press to open the January number and I plan a much stronger one for the June number which will be published under some such title as "Toward a Robot Civilization." This is what Vannevar Bush, Bowman, and other such people are leading us to and the trend is becoming overwhelming. I think it must be opposed by all means because it will either destroy us or force people to an escape into mysticism which would be about just as bad.

With all good wishes for a Happy Christmas and New Year to you all, I am

Yours as ever,
[Henry]

Benjamin Rush (1745–1813) Pennsylvanian physician, writer, teacher. Gwinnie: Gwynneth A. Gminder, S.'s research secretary, made several exhibits at the Institute. George Rosen see S. to A. of 27 March 1945. Whitfield J. Bell, medical historian and biographer. "Journal": Journal of the History of Medicine and Allied Sciences, launched in 1946 with George Rosen, Ackerknecht, Fisch, Fulton and Trent as successive editors; the journal was welcomed by S. (Sigerist/Miller 1946). Joseph Déchelette (1862–1914) French archeologist. S.'s January editorial (Sigerist 1946c) was a plea for the freedom of research and for more research in the social sciences. His planned June editorial did not materialize. Vannevar Bush (1890–1974) influential science administrator during WWII and the Cold War. Bowman see S. to A. of 6 December 1941.

ACKERKNECHT to SIGERIST, New York, 21 December 1945

Dear Henry:

Thank you very much for your letter. I hope you are not working too hard again, and that this story with the three books sounds more terrifying than it actually is. All our good wishes for you in 1946 will not help much, if you will not stick to the line of moderation in matters of working which you adopted so successfully this spring.

I read your accounts of the different people with intense interest. Poor Margarita. There have been so many to go this way. And the Zeisses and Diepgens are all the more vocal. This impudence of the fellows is really amazing, though you prophezied it long ago. What are you answering in such cases?

I am talking about Primitive Surgery at a dinner conference of the Viking Foundation at March 22. Fejos would be very glad to invite you and to cover your expenses. I think it would not be worthwhile for you, and too tiring, to displace you exclusively for the occasion. But if you have business in New York at that time anyway, it might come in handy. They are rather generous in allowances.

Radin wrote an article about primitive medicine for Schumans [sic] book on medicine and music. I was rather scared, when I heard of it and that he polemizes [sic] abundantly with me. But as it stands it is rather good publicity for me. He treats me "respectfully", and I think that my theories, faulty as they might be, are still closer to the truth than his. (He deals in a pseudo-marxist way with primitive medicine as an invention of the medicine man for more gain and influence).

226

I had another long letter of my father. As a matter of fact, the place, where he is now, is no longer French, but American (Ludwigsburg, Stuttgarter Str. 85) I hope we will soon get more European books. He writes me e. g. of a book of Theodor Heuss (the present Kulturminister of Swabia) on "Anton Dohrn in Neapel", published in Switzerland (Atlantisverlag?) in 1940, on which he collaborated, and which should be interesting for historians of science and art. – We have also received news from Lucys [sic] parents and sister, and are very happy, and very busy writing letters and sending packages. Only my sister, who was in Carinthia, has not yet shown up.

From Dec. 27–29. I will be in Philadelphia for the annual meeting of the American Anthropological Association, and we hope that Emmy will realize her plan, to visit Lucy during this time (and how long afterwards she likes to). Here in the Museum is a lot of discussion about the relative merits of the Magnusson-and Kilgore bills. The Magnusson people have tried to get a blanco approval of the scientists here. So far without success.

I guess that is all the news. Very best wishes for the holidays, where unfortunately we can not make our traditional visit this time, to the whole Sigerist family.

As ever yours
Erwin

Margarita, Zeiss, and Diepgen see S. to A. of 20 December 1945. Fejos see A. to S. of 17 July 1945. Paul Radin (1883–1959) anthropologist. Theodor Heuss (1884–1963) became president of the Federal Republic of Germany. Anton Dohrn (1840–1909) German zoologist. Emmy Sigerist see A. to S. of 27 November 1938. Magnusson-Kilgore bills for the support of science, predecessor of the National Science Foundation.

ACKERKNECHT to SIGERIST, New York, 22 December 1945

Dear Henry:

Thank you very much for the second installment of your letter, which I received today, and let me answer it immediately. I am not so optimistic about the Schuman Journal. It will all depend on how much time Rosen will be able to spend on it, whom else we can get in as real collaborators, and how far we will be able not to be mixed up with the Schuman business interests and philosophy. (Though as far as the latter point is concerned Schuman so far has shown all the necessary tact and discretion. But he is himself in a state of transition towards the quantitative, that is the cheap, which is anyway the tendency of our culture, and God knows where that will carry him). I think to have a little meeting between Rosen, you and me, and a few other people on the future of the history of medicine, would be very good. If Rosen is discharged [?], maybe we combine it with the Viking meeting?

I think it is perfectly logical to say something about the prehistoric material in your history. I do not know of any monograph on trephining, more recent than the French one of Guiard (?) which we have at the Institute. To my knowledge there is no map either of trephining, prehistoric or other. As a matter of fact I started one, when I did one on skull cults, but never finished it. I have to take up trephining any way in my Viking paper (which at the same time, of course, will go into the Schuman book, if it comes out), and might then be able to tell you more about the whole thing. I have right now gone through a great deal of material for the Bulletin article, material I had studied years ago, and it is astonishing, how much [sic] new things one finds in rereading, when the eye has been opened for new problems. To my knowledge there are only two great centers of prehistoric trephining, the neolithic one in France, and the Peruvian one, the latter going back far beyond the Incas, and having a great marginal area of dispersion. Shapiro first described trephined skulls in the North American Southwest, and now a few have been found even in Canada. This occurrence of isolated trephings [sic] far from the centers of the custom, where they are very numerous – as a matter of fact the percentage of trephined skulls is more numerous in Peruvian collections than anywhere else and they go back at least to the beginning of our era, while all the high cultures in that region are much younger – is very puzzling from a technical point of view. I do not know of anything similar from Europe where trephining seems pretty much limited to neolithic France that is a given period and region. Nelson, our emeritus archeologist does not know either of any publication on such marginal trephinings in Europe, and MacCurdy (1924) also lists only French findings.

I am looking very much forward to your editorial. As I wrote you, in spite of much propaganda the Bush-Bowman-Magnusson approach makes people feel uneasy here in the museum. But the Kilgore thing does not inspire more confidence either, rather less as it gives the scientists still less influence in the whole development.

Very best wishes yours as ever
Erwin

228

Schuman Journal: Journal of the History of Medicine and Allied Sciences, see S. to A. of 20 December 1945. Rosen see S. to A. of 27 March 1945. Viking Foundation see A. to S. of 21 December 1945. (Guiard 1930). Shapiro see A. to S. of 31 August 1945. Gareth J. Nelson, anthropologist at the American Museum of Natural History, New York. (MacCurdy 1914). Bush, Bowman, Magnusson-Kilgore see A. to. S. of 21 December 1945.

Sigerist to Ackerknecht, Baltimore ?, 4 January 1946

Dear Erwin:

Thanks for your letters of December 21 and December 22. Emmy came back from New York most enthusiastic, singing the praise of your daughters.

I should be very glad to come to New York for the meeting on March 22. I always like to listen to you and having read so much on the subject in the last few months, I begin to feel like an expert on primitive medicine myself. It is a very interesting subject indeed. I have re-read all your papers and I am sure that they would make a very attractive little volume.

Guiart's [sic] book on trephining is rather poor and his bibliography, although quite useful, is still full of gaps. Like many Frenchmen, he does not know the American literature sufficiently. I still think that somebody should some day make an inventory of all Neolithic skulls found in Europe and North Africa with a map that would be revealing. There is no doubt that France and particularly certain sections like the Lozère, was the centre but some Neolithic trephined skulls have been found in Scandinavia, Poland, Russia, Switzerland, Austria, Italy, and Spain so that there has been a certain diffusion that a map would indicate very graphically. If ever you have somebody with the disposition of Baby Jean, this would be a most appropriate piece of work.

The Kilgore Bill is by no means perfect but I find it better than the Magnusson Bill, the purpose of which seems to be to preserve patents for private industry. I also do not like the idea of having a scientific foundation run by a small clique of dollar-a-year scientists.

I was glad to hear that you are going to give a paper to the mediaevalists. Margaret Schlauch is a splendid person for whom I have a great respect and admiration. I did not accept the invitation because I have refused all lecture engagements this year with very few exceptions. Travelling is so complicated that I do not want to wear myself out and rather preserve my energy for the book.

A Happy New Year to you all and I hope that you will have news of your sister.

Yours as ever,
[Henry]

Guiard see A. to S. of 22 December 1945. Lozère: Mountains in Southeastern France. Baby Jean not identified. Magnusson-Kilgore Bills see A. to S. of 21 December 1945. Margaret Schlauch see A. to S. of 5 December 1945.

ACKERKNECHT to SIGERIST, New York, 7 January 1946

Dear Henry:

Thank you very much for your letter of January 4. I also acknowledge reception [sic] of review copies of "Science and Scientists in neth. Indies" and "The Aged in Primitive Society". God knows, how I will do all these things, having just lost a week [xxxx] after 3 days of this perfectly insipid anthropological meeting. But what a wonderful art gallery in Philadelphia. But I will do them.

I am very glad that you will come to the Viking meeting in March. I only hope that Rosen will be here by that time. Now or never medical historians should go out and get a few new thoughts in universities or foundations for their discipline. Otherwise the whole thing will soon be nothing than a hobby and an appendix of the old books [sic] trade, but can never become (or become again) a science or part of a science.

In bed I read a lot – when my pains allowed me to read – for that medieval talk. I reread a few of your old German papers (e.g. the one in the Sudhoff Festschrift) with great pleasure, and feel they are still very "aktuell", and splendid starting points for your history.

Guiart's [sic] book is poor, and he does not know the American literature – but the Americans unfortunately are just as ignorant of the European one! This Simmons, for instance, a Yale man and not bad, writes a book on the aged in primitive society and ignores the thorough book of Koty of 1934 in German on the same subject!

Kindest regards and best wishes
Yours as ever
Erwin

230

Netherlands Indies: Today's Indonesia, (Honig / Verdoorn 1945). The Aged ... (Simmons 1945). [xxxx] Half a sentence deleted as Chesney Archives' Protected Health Information. Rosen see S. to A. of 27 March 1945. Sudhoff Festschrift (Singer / Sigerist 1924). "aktuell" = up to date. Guiard see A. to S. of 22 December 1945. (Koty 1934).

Sigerist to Ackerknecht, Baltimore ?, 8 January 1946

Dear Erwin:

Just a line to tell you that you should not be astonished if you receive an invitation to give a historical lecture at the Cooper Union. I was invited but I am not accepting any lecture invitations this winter, and I have recommended you. I do not know whether they will accept the suggestion but the lecture pays $ 50.00 which is never to be despised.

Cordially as ever,

[Henry]

The Cooper Union for the Advancement of Science and Art, in New York.

Sigerist to Ackerknecht, Baltimore ?, 12 February 1946

Dear Erwin:

I was very sorry to hear that you had all been sick and I hope that you have recovered entirely by now. What a city New York is where even cauliflower tried to murder you.

I have not written for a long time because I was very busy with the book. I have been progressing quite well and expect to be through with primitive medicine by the end of the month or early in March. I will be very anxious to have your opinion but it will take some time to have the manuscript typed.

I just had an idea and I wonder what you think of it. In the chapter on Prevention, I, of course, mentioned the inoculation of smallpox as having been invented and practised by primitives. I never felt quite easy about it because it seems so strange that such a measure should have developed in the magic-religious atmosphere of primitive medicine. It then occurred to me that variolation might be an Arabic invention that would have been spread to East and West with the Arabic conquest and particularly with the very extensive Arabic slave trade. I think it would be worthwhile to examine the matter some day. Inoculation is still practised by Mohammedan tribes all over North Africa and in Central Asia; it is also in the hands of Mohammedan groups. The Arabic influence upon the negroes of Africa was very strong as is evidenced in many folk tales and actually many other ways too. This is not more than a guess but it might lead somewhere.

Your bibliography was very useful to me. I consulted and used Clemens extensively but I think he has rather wild ideas tracing certain treatments back to the paleolithic and attributing others to the neolithic. A book I came to like very much is Mackenzie. I had never read it entirely before but now I find that it contains an enormous amount of information and some very good ideas.

Now I have just read Koty and Simons [sic] and also your book review for which, by the way, I thank you very much. I am not impressed with Simmons' statistical methods and his total disregard of any non-English literature is rather strange, but I agree with you that it is a good book. For my own purposes, I got more out of Koty because he does not limit himself to the aged but includes the sick and his use of literature is extremely broad, including even Russian publications that seem to be totally unknown to American ethnologists. I also think that Koty has a few very good points.

Now I am just beginning the chapter on the Medicine Man that is relatively easy because there is so much literature on the subject including your own paper. I think I am going to handle the chapter in such a way that I will describe more or less in detail the medicine man of half a dozen totally different tribes, one Siberian, American Indian, Bantu, Australian, etc. and then discuss at the end some traits that they have in common.

I am in touch with the Oxford Press and I am inclined to let them have the book. I think they or Macmillan are best prepared to handle this kind of book.

I am going to Mount Holyoke College tonight just to earn a few damned guineas but I do not mind going because it is a college where I have not been before and usually you get a much better reception and response in such a college than in the large universities. On March 1, I am giving another lecture to the medical students at the University of Rochester but this is merely an excuse to spend a weekend with Nora in Ithaca thereafter.

With kind regards to you all, I am
    Yours very cordially,
      [Henry]

P. S. You probably saw in the last number of the Bulletin, p. 562 that Maurice Arthus died last February at the age of 83. No wonder that we could not find any obituaries before he had died.

S. used to write his manuscripts in long-hand and have them typed. Clemens is likely to be (Clements 1932). Mackenzie is likely to be (McKenzie 1927). Koty and Simmons see A. to S. of 7 January 1946. Possibly S. means Mount Holyoke College in Massachusetts. University of Rochester in upstate New York. Nora Sigerist (born 1922) younger daughter of S., was studying Russian language and literature at Rochester, NY. Maurice Arthus (1882–1945) physiologist in France and Switzerland.

ACKERKNECHT to SIGERIST, New York, 13 February 1946

Dear Henry:

Thank you very much for your letter of February 12. I fully appreciate your reasons for not writing more often; but on the other hand I am always so very happy to have one. It is a poor substitute for the talks to which we had become so used. But it is better than nothing. And quite apart from the personal, I need some medico-historical "Gedankenaustausch". For this, New York is about as poor as Baltimore was for anthropology. Drabkin is too noncommittal. The only good man, George Rosen, is still away.

I have had the same guess, as far as Arabic origin of small-pen [?] inoculation in Africa goes, all the more as other clearly Arabic operations like needling of cataract have diffused e.g. far into Liberia, and as it also would provide the most satisfactory explanation for the strikingly rational traits (surgery and medicine) in Arab influenced East Africa. But to substantiate this would demand an enormous amount of work (on the early history of Arab medicine too) which so far I have not been able to put in; and it is even doubtful whether with the material at hand any positive conclusion could ever be reached. As far as surgery goes I will have to touch the problem in my March talk. (Diffusion of the Avicenna tradition would not have been very conducive to spread of surgery!) In case inoculation is Arab, it would be another fact of the Africans, and primitives in general, taking much easier to Islamic than to "Christian" traits. The American Indians could never be persuaded to adopt voluntarily vaccination which is even more harmless and effective than inoculation. Whereever [sic], even today,

233

in Asia or Africa Mohammedan and Christian missionaries are in competition, the latter ones come always through only second best, in spite of official backing (or partly because of?). It is on the other hand not entirely impossible that the Africans worked out inoculation all by themselves, and theoretically even the Arabs could have gotten it from them. The idea of inoculation can be very easily conceived in magical terms (sympathetic magic: similia similibus). Proof: <u>the inoculation against snakebite</u>, very widespread not only in Africa, but also among other primitives e.g. South American Indians. There is also a fundamental technique of drug application through cuts in the skin, found everywhere in connection with scarification (magic rites), but particularly developed just in Africa, which to a certain extent could have suggested inoculation.

I feel like you that Clement [sic] is useful – for the mere fact that nobody else has ever done this job – but needs some thorough critical revision, all the more as some of his statements are based on data, which are no longer valid. I like the Mackenzie [sic] very much too, and praise him at every occasion, as for instance when such chaps as Gordon come and try the same thing. He shows that a "non-professional" (he was or is a Nose-ear-throat man) can do a good job, if he has some brains and knowledge. On the other hand he has, of course, his limitations. In taking in so much classic and folklore material, the primitive "kommt zu kurz", and gets entangled in a lot of things which have nothing to do with primitive medicine properly speaking. It is my feeling that most of primitive magic (what I call primary magic) is rather different from folklore or medieval magic ("secondary magic"). But this confusion of both things is very common, even among anthropologists. Proof: the "classic" treatise on magic (in the Année sociologique VII, 1902) by Hubert and my teacher Mauss. I fully agree with your judgement on Koty and Simmons. Koty obviously was of Russian origin – in a footnote he quotes his own wildhood experiences. Inde [?] his knowledge of Russian material. God knows what became of him. He was probably Jewish too. (John stands for Jonas with Eastern Jews) It is extremely regrettable that we have so little access to the Russian material, and the excellent summary of Czaplicka, and the fact that Bogoras, Jochelson, Klements, Sieroszewski, Pilsudski (the brother), Sternberg, Shirokogoroff have at least sometimes published in English. German or French is but a poor Ersatz.

Thanks for recommending me to the Cooper Union. Unfortunately they have not shown up. I hope that the medievalists were satisfied with my talk. I had the feeling that they were. I did a great deal of reading for it, which momentarily was annoying, but which in the long run I do not regret. I also realized that I had learned quite something just incidentally in our seminaries [sic], research conferences, and informal talks. My whole trouble is that I am running around with a great "tumor" of medicohistorical knowledge, and have so little opportunity to use it, and God knows whether I will have ever one.

I had a letter of this urologist Benjamin from Rochester, the most confused and illiterate thing I have seen in a long time. Another one who would do better to leave medical history alone, but probably cultivates it for "social reasons", not being very interesting in his own field. He wanted me to tell him whether there were "plasmodium falciparum" (!) infections around Bologna in 1270 or not!!!

Yes, I saw the note on M. Arthus – and with all due respect for the deceased had a good laugh. How simple sometimes explanations are. Perhaps is Jean Rouelle still alive too? With these Frenchmen one never knows.

I hope you get the book of Leriche for review for Temkin, and for the Library. If not, my offer still stands to write a little review for the Bulletin. It is so important that it should be at least on record, like mutatis mutandis the Aschoff was.

Last Thursday Leona Baumgartner gave a very good report on her enquète on child health in France in the Medical History Club here. Assistance miserable as usual. She was truthful enough to say that not all misery seen in France now is due to the war, but also to be a bad tradition, and fair enough to warn Americans to abstain from throwing the first stone (though she felt the itch herself). This was of no help to Zilborg [sic] who opened up a sickening orgy of American selfrighteousness. He might be a delightful companion for a good meal. As the president of a medicohistorical club he is a pain in the neck. I certainly have every reason to feel bitter about the French. But if I see these poor people scolded by these well fed "veinards" who think that good luck is a merit, I feel like defending them with teeth and claws. That people in Europe after the last 30 years are not full of pep and initiative, is all too well understandable. That they have still some left, that is the true miracle.

I hope you enjoy your trips to Mount Holyoke and Rochester, and am looking foreward very much to meeting you here in March. If there are any questions on primitive medicine please let me know. The article for the Bulletin should now be finished in 2 weeks. These 2 diseases since December, and other troubles with the collection set me back so much.

The following reference is nothing particular, and the article is not extremely solid in all points. But he brings up at least a good new approach for dental paleopathology: Klatsky M.: Function versus nutrition as a controlling factor in dental health. J. of the Am. Dent. Ass. 32: 1416, 1945

With kindest regards from all of us to all of you
Yours as ever
Erwin

Gedankenaustausch: exchange of ideas. Clements and McKenzie see S. to A. of 12 February 1946. "Kommt zu kurz": is neglected. Koty and Simmons see A. to S. of 7 January 1946. Cooper Union see S. to A. of 8 January 1946. Plasmodium falciparum: One of the strains of micro-organisms causing malaria. Arthus see S. to A. of 12 February 1946. Rouelle see A. to S. of 7 June 1945. Leriche see A. to S. of 5 December 1945. (Aschoff 1940). Zilboorg see A. to S. of 5 August 1941.

New names in alphabetical order:
Avicenna (980–1037) Arabic physician, scientist, philosopher
Baumgartner, Leona (1902–1991) commissioner of New York City Department of Health, hygiene propagandist, child health and medical historian
Benjamin, urologist
Bogoras, Waldemar, anthropologist
Czaplicka, Maria A. (1886–1921) Polish anthropologist
Drabkin, Israel E., S.'s staff member for Graeco-Roman science
Gordon, probably Andrew J., medical anthropologist
Hubert, probably Annie, medical anthropologist
Jochelson, Vladimir I. (1855–1937) Russian anthropologist
Klatsky, M., dentist/anthropologist
Klements, Dmitrii C. and D. A., Russian anthropologists
Mauss, Marcel (1872–1950) French anthropologist and sociologist
Pilsudski, Bronislaw P. (1866–1918) Polish cultural anthropologist
Shirokogoroff, S. M., Russian anthropologist
Sieroszewski, Waclaw, Polish anthropologist
Sternberg, Lev Y., Russian anthropologist

Dear Henry:

Could you please do the following two things for me: 1) let me have one of the Institute copies of Max Bartels: "Die Medizin der Naturvölker" on a loan. Oh shame, we do not have it in the museum. In general I do not use it, because so much of its sources are outdated. But now I would like to have it for some comparisons. 2) return the manuscript of my Academy lecture on primitive medicine, as it is the only copy which I have, and I would like to submit it to Schuman. You will have an almost complete reprint soon.

I am including [sic] references to a very interesting Vesalius volume of the Basler naturforschenden Gesellschaft, in case you do not have it yet. Also reference to an article in "Science" which you might have overlooked, and which shows more intelligence and medicohistorical knowledge than the average. I sent to this fellow Dieuaide my Malaria, and a letter, because I am always interested in anybody, who shows some medicohistorical knowledge, and does not belong to the usual crowd of booklovers, but did not succeed so far in eliciting more of a response than a polite "thank you" letter. That is the rule with any men.

I am working like hell, butchering ("dissecting") most of the day a lot of cadavers for maceration for my collection. It is not very pleasant and very tiresome. I hope to finish (because I have to finish) my article for the Bulletin till March 1. The point of it will not be so much [sic] new ideas, than a rather abundant and recent documentation for some of my pet theories. I am now finishing my first year here. In spite of a lot of personal troubles (moving, diseases) and mercenary work (translations, abstracts) and work on my collection I have written 9 papers and some 30 book-reviews, and do not feel too dissatisfied. Only I am looking forward for some rest in summer. Thanks for the beautiful invitation for the Noguchi lectures. I felt sorry that I could not assist.

It was a pleasant surprise to hear that Temkin is coming out with an article, and menacing to write some more. Alice Marriott's "Ten Grandmothers" is a very delightful collection of short stories on Plains Indians. I had to read it for review and for once I am glad I had to.

Lucy was out all these last Sundays and holidays (and I alone with the kids – they had also a mild flu) hunting for summer quarters around here. It seems she found something yesterday on Long Island. We had the first letter of her sister this week, a quite long one 18 pages, and well written, and were sick for a couple of days. She plucks her husbands [sic] beard as they have no water, soap, and blades. We will make the paleolithicum, as Heine-Geldern uses to say. I do now understand a lot of things better, for instance about feeling "guilty". She does not feel so anyway, as she worked against the Nazis even during the war. The average German has not seen the murder of millions of innocents in the East, and just as little imagination as anybody else. But he has seen, everyone of them, thousands of just as innocent women and children burned alife, crushed or scalded or starved to death in the sealed cellars as a consequence of "strategic bombing". So at best he feels even. According to the letters I have seen so far, typhus must have been very common among German soldiers in the East in 1942 and 43. Now almost everybody we once knew, seems to have tuberculosis, and mostly (this is already the case among the French children) the more rapid and virulent forms.

Well, this is no pleasant subject. And I have to go back to my article anyway.

Kindest regards and very best wishes from all of us to all of you
Yours as ever
Erwin

(Bartels 1893). Andreas Vesalius (1514–1564) Renaissance anatomist. Dieuaide, probably Francis R. (1892–1977) physician and medical historian in New York. "My Malaria": (Ackerknecht 1945). Noguchi Lectures: a lecture series at S.'s Institute. (Marriott 1945). [xxxx] Half a sentence deleted as Chesney Archives' Protected Health Information. Heine-Geldern see A. to S. of 17 July 1945.

SIGERIST to ACKERKNECHT, Baltimore ?, 4 March 1946

Dear Erwin:

I have just spent a week-end in Rochester where I gave a lecture to the students and in Ithaca where I went to see Nora. In order not to delay matters, I had the book of Bartels and your manuscript sent before I left (March 1, Railway Express). I hope you have received them safely. I am looking forward to seeing the manuscript in print because I have quoted it several times. I also liked your article on incubators and taboos very much. It is a strange taboo and strangely scattered over the primitive world. Volume 1 of the new Journal looks splendid and very substantial. I had it with me on the trip and read it with much pleasure.

Any reference to European medico-historical publications you can send us will be very welcome. It is incredible how out of touch we have become in a few years only. I heard today that the Swiss have published a new edition of the main works of Paracelsus in 5 volumes of which I had never heard. I am going to carry all such titles in the Bulletin until we can secure review copies. Since I have no idea when we can get the book of Leriche, I would greatly appreciate it if you could send me a review.

F. R. Dieuaide was professor of medicine at the Peiping Medical College so that he should have first-hand experience.

With kind regards, I am

    Yours as ever,

      [Henry]

Rochester and Ithaca, NY, Nora see S. to A. of 12 February 1946. Bartels see A. to S. of 23. February 1946. A.'s article (Ackerknecht 1946a). New Journal see A. to S. of 22 December 1945. Book of Leriche see A. to S. of 5 December 1945.

ACKERKNECHT to SIGERIST, New York, 5 March 1946

Dear Henry:

Thanks for your letter, and the manuscript and the Bartels, which arrived safely yesterday. I am glad that you liked my article and the "Journal". Fulton raised some fuss about the technical side of it. Important as that may be, I am primarily concerned about the contents of publications. From this point of view it does not look too bad.

Besides butchering I am now preparing my lecture for March 22. (Friday) on Primitive Surgery. Are you staying over the weekend? I hope it will be one, where Rosen is here from Boston. (He usually comes only every second Sunday) so that you can see him. Will there not be a meeting of the Association this year?

I have finished the article for the Bulletin (Natural Diseases and Rational Treatment in Primitive Medicine) and it is now being typed. It should have about 10,000 words. I will write a <u>short</u> review of Leriche. If you actually get it, and Temkin feels like, that will not preclude his writing one too.

Kindest regards from all of us to all of you

Yours as ever

Erwin

Bartels see A. to S. of 23 February 1946. "Journal" see A. to S. of 22 December 1945. Fulton see S. to A. of 26 February 1945. Association: American Association of the History of Medicine (AAHM). Leriche see A. to S. of 5 December 1945.

SIGERIST to ACKERKNECHT, Baltimore ?, 14 March 1946

Dear Erwin,

Thanks for your letter of March 5. In the meantime you will probably have received a postcard announcing that the Annual Meeting of the Association will take place in Atlantic City On May 26–27. I very much hope that you will come. Schuman was here and we had a short glimpse of him. He seems very enterprising. If the Journal maintains the standard of the first number, it will be splendid. The illustrations could be better but this seems to be a sore spot in all American journals, and I am only too well aware that ours are sometimes very poor also.

I am looking forward to receiving your paper. It will go to the press as soon as I receive the manuscript. The February number is already in page proofs and should be out soon. The March number is just going into page proofs and with your paper, I would like to open the April number. The press is now working quite well and our chief difficulty is the bookbinder who delays finished numbers sometimes by three weeks.

I hope to be through with my section on Primitive Medicine very soon. I reread with much pleasure your article on Psychopathology etc. The Siberian shaman and the Bantu inyanga are really strange phenomena but it occurred to me that we have a certain parallel in our own society. How many neurotic individuals become psychiatrists and particularly psychoanalysts. This seems to be a somewhat related adaptation mechanism.

I am looking forward to hearing you next week. I plan to arrive in New York on the 21st because I have a meeting of the Medical Advisory Council of the UAW-CIO that day. Unfortunately I will have to go home on the 23rd. I have so much work pending that I cannot stay away longer.

With all good wishes, I am
  Yours as ever,
    [Henry]

Association see A. to S. of 5 March 1946. UAW-CIO: United Automobile Workers – Congress of Industrial Organizations.

ACKERKNECHT to SIGERIST, New York, 18 March 1946

Dear Henry:

This is only to thank you for your letter of March 14. As far as "Gedankenaustausch" goes, I am looking forward very much to next Friday. Your parallel between shamans and psychoanalysts is very good though they will not like it very much. The manuscript will be mailed tomorrow.

Kindest regards
  Yours as ever
    Erwin

Gedankenaustausch = exchange of ideas.

ACKERKNECHT to SIGERIST, New York, 3 April 1946

Dear Henry:

Thank you very much for your letter. You will have received mine meanwhile. I thus answer today only the Castiglioni question. It would be a lie, if I would pretend that I am looking forward with particular pleasure to reviewing it. But I am an old soldier, and if you think that I am the one who has to empty the calice [sic], please pass it around.

It seems that Rosen comes home today from the army for good. I hope to see him soon.

Lucy is still rather tired. And so am I.

Kindest regards

Yours as ever

[Erwin]

Arturo Castiglioni (1874–1953) Italian medical historian, from 1939 to 1946 exiled in the U.S.

ACKERKNECHT to SIGERIST, New York, 12 April 1946

Dear Henry,

Enclosed another bookreview. I certainly enjoyed doing this. Perhaps you can get more from Glasser for the Bulletin. He seems to be very good.

Let me thank you again that you came for my lecture, which was certainly a great help to me. We had a nice weekend with Carter. He was rather disappointed with the anthropologists. He knew how bad the historians and geographers are, and had hoped the anthropologists might be better. I am sorry that I had to drag you into this crowd. Well, they are all alike. I forgot to tell you about Fulton's lecture on Cushing here. Technically it was good. And contained some very interesting and important points. But that Cushing could make somersaults, that he wanted to give up medicine when his anesthesia case died, and that he scribbeled little designs in his notebook, as all students do, was all equally important, and, of course, great. (Cushing was certainly a great man – so was probably even Osler. But this kind of worship provokes one into a position of utter disgust with the subject matter. I desperately try to keep out this stuff from Schuman's Journal.) I wonder how the "Fulton on Cushing" will be, the book. I am afraid it will equal "Cushing on Osler". Of the latter I once heard an American say in praise that you could read the whole thing without ever realising that the book was written by somebody. Well, to me that is just the bad thing, this collecting of facts without any discriminatory point of view.

I read a delightful book of Giraudoux on Lafontaine. Kerillis on de Gaulle seems to be not based on facts, but suspicions. K. is very suspicious. At the end of the month I am giving a lecture in Philadelphia (in the Anthropol. Society) Is there anybody or anything worthwhile to be seen (except the Museums)? Lucy came home from the hospital Sunday, and is still rather weak. I feel lousy. Worked too hard, and had no relaxation so far. Well, it will all come out with the washing.

    Kindest regards from all of us to all of you

      Yours as ever

        Erwin

Otto Glasser wrote on Roentgen (Glasser 1945), reviewed by A. Carter see A. to S. of 28 February 1945. Fulton see S. to A. of 26 February 1945. Harvey Cushing (1869–1939) neurosurgeon and historian of medicine. William Osler (1849–1919) professor of medicine at McGill University, Johns Hopkins, and Oxford, England. Fulton's Cushing (Fulton 1946). Cushing's Osler (Cushing 1940). Giraudoux on Lafontaine (Giraudoux 1943). Kerillis on De Gaulle (Kerillis 1945).

ACKERKNECHT to SIGERIST, New York, 15 April 1946

Dear Henry:

    You will understand that I was very excited, when today I read in a Swiss bibliography the following reference:

    Georg Buschan: Ueber Medizinzauber und Heilkunst im Leben der Völker

    Berlin 1941 (816 pp. Bibliogr. Of 32 pp.)

The late Sanitätsrat Buschan was practising gynecology and fornication in my late hometown of Stettin (beg your pardon: Sczeczin [sic]). I thus know rather well what he was worth and what not. It is not very likely that as far as outlook goes he had more than the late Sanitätsrat Max Bartels, but as a compiler he was very strong (see "Buschan's illustrierte Völkerkunde" etc.) And that is something too. Will we ever see this book? Or was the whole edition among the 40 million books burned in Leipzig? (what a retail man in book burning was Goebbels from the behavioristic point of view). I still hope against hope that you will find a copy, and buy, steal, liberate or whatever, in Switzerland. I also wrote immediately to my father to look around.

    By the way the book I got the reference from should also absolutely be bought by the Welch Library. It contains, besides a great deal of tropical medicine, a great amount of ethnographical, historical, and bibliographical information (the latter covering just the war years for Germany, Switzerland and France!) The reference is:

Acta tropica edited by Geigy, Gison and Speiser, Verlag für Recht und Gesellschaft, Basel. Vol. I, 1944, Vol. II, 1945.

A book, which, I am afraid, medical historians will have to have a look at too, is C. G. Jung

Psychologie und Alchemie

Zürich 1944

Jung (who by the way jumped the bandwagon in time and is now thundering on German guilt) has developed the whole history of psychology from – alchemy. Well, as far as he and his crowd is concerned, he is probably even right.

George Rosen started work in the Health Department today. I saw him twice this week (thanks heaven I got another Ciba Nr. on my old hobby "the Doctor as a statesman and politician") He will be in Atlantic City on Saturday May 25 too.

Kindest regards

Yours as ever

Erwin

Georg Buschan (1863–1942) German physician and anthropologist (Buschan 1941). Sanitätsrat: Health councillor. Stettin on the Baltic Sea was A.'s hometown which in 1945 became Polish, the correct Polish spelling being Szczecin. Bartels see A. to S. of 23 February 1946. Josef Goebbels: Hitler's propaganda chief. Welch Library of the Johns Hopkins Medical Institutions. Carl Gustav Jung (1875–1961) influential Swiss psychologist.

Sigerist to Ackerknecht, Baltimore ?, 25 April 1946

Dear Erwin:

Just a line to tell you that Emmy will be arriving in New York Tuesday morning. Unfortunately I cannot accompany her because I have my last Seminar that same evening. It is the end of the course and I therefore felt that I could not call the Seminar off. I had planned to take a night train so as to be in New York Wednesday morning when Emmy sails but she insists that I should not do it since visitors are not permitted on board ship and probably not even to the pier. So there actually is not much sense in my coming, but I would be very grateful to you if you would see that Emmy gets off safely.

I have to thank you for a letter and will answer it in a couple of days.

　　With kind regards, I am
　　　　Yours as ever,
　　　　　[Henry]

In this first year of public transatlantic traffic after WWII Emmy was sailing in April, while S. and the daughters took a plane in July.

ACKERKNECHT to SIGERIST, New York, 4 May 1946

Dear Henry:

Enclosed the Castiglioni review. It was a torture as I tried to remain honest and to be polite in the same time. In German it would have been very easy to review the piece in two words: Italienischer Salat.

We enjoyed Emmi's visit greatly. [xxxx]. I saw her off to the station; I could not wait for the rest, but I trust everything worked out all right.

There is a rumor that you will be in town next week. Would be nice to see you. I do not think that anything worthwhile happened since my last letters. The official mail, at least with the American Zone, works now very satisfactorily. I had already two letters from my father. From letters and oral reports one gains the impression that the Nazis are having a pretty good time in all four zones. Not very encouraging.

Rosen, der Schlauberger, has passed the Castiglioni review to de Saussure, who will like it, bacause there is so much talk of the "unconscious". Merton wrote politely in the NY Times bookreview that it is rotten.

Day before yesterday I had to discuss a (lousy) paper on Iroquois medicine at the Annual Meeting of the New York State Medical Society. The other paper on folklore was given by Harold Thompson of Cornell, a nice chap, who quoted you with reverence, and also spoke very warmly of your stay in Cornell 5 years ago.

　　Kindest regards
　　　　Yours as ever
　　　　　Erwin

Castiglioni see A,. to S. of 3 April 1946; his book (Castiglioni 1946); "Italienischer Salat": Italian hodge-podge. [xxxx] One sentence deleted as Chesney Archives' Protected Health Information. "American Zone" of occupation in Germany. "Schlauberger": artful dodger. De Saussure see A. to S. of 23. March 1945. Harold W. Thompson (1891–1964) historian, folklorist.

ACKERKNECHT to SIGERIST, New York, 5 May 1946

Dear Henry:

I herewith take the liberty to recommend to your good graces our French colleague Dr. M. David. She is a survivor of Oswiecim [?], and tries to learn what can be learned in Baltimore before returning to France, and I thus thought she should meet you, though I know how busy you are.

As ever yours

Erwin

Perhaps Temkin can show her around?

Oswiecim, Polish for the German name Auschwitz in Poland.

SIGERIST to ACKERKNECHT, Baltimore ?, 14 May 1946

Dear Erwin:

It was awfully good of you to look after Emmy in New York the other day. I had a telegram that she had arrived in Paris last Thursday and today I just received an airmail letter written last Friday at the Gare de Lyon while she was waiting for the train to Switzerland but this is the last I have heard and I am beginning to worry. I just sent a telegram to Basel and hope to have an answer tonight. Travelling conditions in France must be perfectly awful, trains sold out days in advance, no time-tables held, luggage stolen if you do not sit on it, etc. American cigarettes seem to be the only currency that has any value and Emmy fortunately had a supply with her.

I am deeply buried in ancient Egypt at the moment. I just tried to figure out whether health conditions were better 3,000 years ago than they are now. Herodotus found that the Egyptians were the healthiest people on earth while today they are about the most rotten with disease on earth. I am inclined to believe that the ancient Egyptians were in better health and [sic] the present ones. The population of the country was about 7 million in antiquity and is 16 million today. In other words, the same land area has to feed twice the population. The agricultural methods used today are the same as in antiquity and most of the delta is used not for the growing of export crops, particularly cotton. Modern medicine and public health might have compensated for this but with 1.6 physicians and 2.6 hospital beds per 10,000 population, modern medicine is non-existent outside of Cairo and Alexandria.

Herodotus came from a malaria region and was probably impressed by the fact that Egypt had no or very little malaria. It seems to me that under the Turkish domination, the entire economy of Egypt went to pieces and as a result poverty and the incidence of illness must have increased considerably.

I do not know if I wrote you that I thought your review of Castiglioni's book was a real masterpiece. Whoever can read between the lines knows what it is all about and Castiglioni will be delighted because he will notice only the sentences in which he is praised. He found the review in the New York Times excellent. And so, everybody is happy including the editors of the Bulletin.

I was in New York last week but only for one evening and night for that dinner of the American Russian Institute.

Artelt wrote two letters, one to me and one to Temkin. He has lost his chair in Frankfort because he joined the Nazi party in 1941 to save medical history from the SS, as he says. He hopes that the matter will be reconsidered. It seems, although he is not too clear about it, that the libraries of the Berlin and of the Leipzig Institutes have been taken by the Russians so that I will probably find them in Moscow on my next trip. Diepgen and von Brunn have both kept their chairs because they were not Party members but they have nothing to work with.

Well, I hope to see you in Atlantic City soon and with kind regards, I am

     Yours as ever,
       [Henry]

Gare de Lyon: A railroad station in Paris. S.'s mother and sister lived in Basel. Herodotus (ca. 500–424 B. C.) Greek historian. The Turkish domination of Egypt ended in 1918.

The book is likely to be (Castiglioni 1946). Walter Artelt (1906–1976) German medical historian. Part of the library of the Leipzig Institute was taken by the Russians and apparently never showed up. Diepgen see A. to S. of 2 May 1945. Walter von Brunn (1876–1952) German medical historian, S.'s successor in Leipzig. Atlantic City, NJ, was the site of the 1946 meeting of the American Association for the History of Medicine (AAHM).

ACKERKNECHT to SIGERIST, New York, 16 May 1946

Dear Henry:

Thank you very much for your letter. I was very happy to see that you hadn't yet forgotten me entirely. We are very glad to hear that Emmy arrived safely. We had a letter of hers mailed in Le Havre. It seems that the specimens of Homo sapiens Helveticus she was with on ship, came rather as a shock to her. I hope she does not get too much shocktherapy in general, and in melancholic states in particular, though it is very fashionable now.

I was very interested in what you wrote about Egyptian pathology. It seems to make good sense. This question of the actual occurrence of disease is one of the very hardest. I am struggling with it as far as my primitives go for years now; but my material is so contradictory that I still do not dare to publish it. One of the greatest difficulties is, as I have always emphasized, that "disease" is a matter of convention and social definition. What might have looked to be a very healthy population to somebody a hundred years ago, is none according to our present standards. And vice versa. You make the point with Herodotus who was "conditioned" to malaria. Did you have a look on that slightly cockeyed and yet very stimulating English book by Pearse and Crocker on the Peckham experiment? According to P. and C. only 10 per cent of their sample is "healthy". But a hundred years ago it would probably not have been even one percent. So what is health? And are we entitled to look at human history as a long disease, which only now clears a little up (for a short interlude)?

Egyptian medicine is, of course, also very important to me as a "primitivist", as it seems to offer a look on an important stage in the formation of medicine from primitive to rational, being one type of what Temkin once called archaic medicine. (Another one, better known to me, is Peruvian). One of the outstanding characters of primitive medicine is "speciali-

248

sation", that is atomization of knowledge. In Egypt we seem to assist to the process of organising the dispersed parts into one body. And it might be possible that the mere increase in quantity makes for a change in quality (I am in general no friend of Hegelianism, but here the formula seems to make sense)? I don't know whether I make myself sufficiently clear. One of the most difficult problems is the genesis of the rational in medicine. One of the possible hypotheses seems to me that the piling up of practices mostly understood magically, or not understood at all, opens the eyes for certain "Gesetzmässigkeiten". Take for instance surgery. The trephiners just know to trephine and nothing else. So do the amputators, or the boil-openers, or the bonesetters etc. But when, as in Peru, all practices are concentrated, that should open a new outlook. I once discussed this problem with Wittfogel, the economic historian, and he has a parallel concept to "archaic medicine" in economics, which he calls "Oriental Society" (and where he unduly emphasises one aspect: irrigation) But here he too argues that the new society is not so much different by its elements which can all be found in primitive societies, but by the addition of all these elements.

I am inclined to think that some truth is contained in Artelts [sic] statements. And it is typical that he is dismissed though to my knowledge he has never written anything half as disgusting as Mr. Diepgen, nor has he spyed international conferences like D., but A. is out and D. is in office. Perhaps you can buy some of the books the Russians "liberated". The Russians can not have much use for them, as their writing of the "history" of science, for the time being at least, seems to consist in claiming Russian priority for all and sundry. They have gotten a "priority" complex which seems even bigger than the Italian one. In this respect one of the funniest books I ever read is Arcieri's recent book on Cesalpino. Though he has a pretty good case, he succeeds in spoiling it. And what a language!

At present Kroeber is in town, on his way to California, back from London where he gave the Huxley lecture. He called me up, and I am seeing a good deal of him, and having a wonderful time. He is 70, and though he had a [xxxx] two years ago, in full vigor.

In the last number of the Journal of American Folklore is quite a nice article of Mark Graubard. He invented (for experimental reasons) PCT (Psycho-Catalytic-Therapy) as an "improvement over psychanalysis" [sic] – in his mind a sheer nonsense, but he was struck by the facility with which he could put it over on most people.

I hope you have not overlooked the announcement of a great new periodical to come out next September. Name: AMERICAN CULTURE". Contents: Exclusively advertising.

A bientôt

Yours as ever

Erwin

P.S. Just one silly question: how do you account for the <u>increase in population</u> in Egypt, in spite of worse health conditions? Any factors which could have brought improvement in one particular field in spite of general health decline? E. g. infant mortality, more people attaining old age, disappearance of certain epidemics, less wars and accidents, or famines? What does Albright think about it? EA

<u>Another P. S.</u> This sacré Schultz has made another discovery which he should publicise [sic] and try to stir up some trouble. Of course, again he ignores what he has at hand: Gorillas have yaws. Oh, I think I told you that one. EA

P.S. No. 3 (Pfui) : Jago [sic] sent me today Dr. Antonio Requena, Museo de Ciencias Naturales, Los Caobos-Caracas, Venezuela. The fellow who made the sensational discoveries on Precolombian tuberculosis down there. He makes a very excellent impression (English trained) and his stuff looks serious. He prepares a big book on Paleopathology. The Institute should absolutely ask him for reprints. EHA

Herodotus and Artelt see S. to A. of 14 May 1946. (Pearse/Crocker 1943). Hegel, Georg Wilhelm F. (1770–1831) German Philosopher. Gesetzmässigkeit: In accordance with theoretical principles. Karl August Wittfogel (1896–1988) anthropologist and economist. Diepgen see A. to S. of 2 May 1945. (Arcieri 1945). Andrea Cesalpino (1519–1603) Italian botanist and philosopher. Kroeber see A. to S. of 25 July 1945. [xxxx] Chesney Archives' Protected Health Information. Mark A. Graubard (born 1904) historian of biology. Albright see A. to S. of 6 August 1945. Schultz see S. to A. of 30 May 1945. Iago Galdston see A. to S. of 2 August 1944.

Sigerist to Ackerknecht, Baltimore ?, 30 May 1946

Dear Erwin:

Your paper was splendid but it is a crime that there was no chance for discussion. What about the publication? I know, of course, that you are publishing an extensive paper on primitive surgery in the <u>American An-</u>

thropologist but it might be advisable to publish a short paper in the Transaction number of the Association, that is the July number of the Bulletin, pointing out primarily the contradictions that were the major theme of your paper. There may be some repetition, of course, but I think it would be good for you to be represented among the papers of the Association if it were only with a few pages.

We both thought that Bilikiewicz must be dead but contrary to expectation, he survived as well as his wife and two children and he is now Professor of Psychiatry and of the History and Philosophy of Medicine at the University of Gdansk (Danzig). It seems, however, that the rest of his family was wiped out and he says that what he went through is indescribable. He is building up an Institute of the History of Medicine and I am going to send him all our publications.

With good wishes, I am

Yours as ever

[Henry]

Tadeusz Bilikiewicz was a Polish staff member at S.'s Leipzig Institute and a colleague of A. around 1930.

ACKERKNECHT to SIGERIST, New York, 7 June 1946

Dear Henry:

Thank you very much for your letter. I had some doubts what to do with the "Contradictions". I will, of course, follow your advice, and write a few pages, refering the interested to my "comprehensive" and more documented paper. You will get the short paper sometime next week, when our typist is back.

Dr. Paul Fejos, Viking Fund, 14 East 71 Str., New York 21, N. Y. wants to subscribe the Bulletin for their library. Please have him the necessary prospectus etc. sent.

Last Saturday night Otto Guttentag dropped in on his way back to California (on a troop train – 5 days). It was extremely pleasant, and intensely interesting, as, apart from the general things one knows already, he had a lot to tell on medical conditions, personal as well as scientific.He was in close contact with Sauerbruch and Vollhardt, and might go back for 6 months as an adviser for reorganisation of the medical curriculum (he took away from me your reprint on a new medical school). V. and S. think that under the emergency conditions no longer everybody can be admitted to the study of medicine, and that the curriculum has to be modernized. According to G.s impression the younger generation is not very good (the Germans speeded studies up since 1935!) But in some fields very good research has been done (dis. [?] of bloodvessels, auscultation and percussion on an objective basis etc.) He also feels that there is better understanding for clinical problems than here. Typical for American attitudes is that, while a lot of English people watch Sauerbruch operating, and the Russians have a regular team of 8 watching him every day, no American ever showed up. As French, English, and Russian officers are still forbidden to have venereal diseases, he had an extensive practice amongst them, and has a very flowery letter of a russian [sic] General for having cured him with penicillin in a week. Well, it would go too far to tell all his anecdotes. I proposed him to have all the minor stuff mimeographed, and to write a real article on medical science in G. on the basis of all the books he brought back. I think this would fill a real gap.

I hope everything is all right with you, and the meeting did not tire you too much. I enjoyed very much meeting you, though, of course, meetings are not very conducive to long talks.

Will we see you before you leave for Switzerland? (Please don't forget to look for the Buschan in Switzerland). The children were in bed for a week with a cold, but are o.k. again, and Lucy hopes to go to the country definitely a week from now, and I will go with her for the first five days, to help her fixing the house a little. Then I will start writing my Ciba papers to streighten [sic] out the budget.

Kindest regards from all of us
    Yours as ever
      Erwin

Fejos, Guttentag see A. to S. of 17 July 1945 and 12 November 1945, respectively. Vollhardt, probably Franz Volhard (1872–1950) German professor of medicine. Sauerbruch see A. to S. of 23 May 1945.

Dear Erwin,

I have not written you for a very long time but I have kept all your letters religiously and will answer them now.

It seems a long time since we were in Atlantic City and a good deal has happened here. The chief event in my family probably is that Nora became engaged to a Canadian doctor, Kenneth Ingham, and is going to marry in the autumn. It all began with the Cooperative Commonwealth Federation in Canada winning the elections in Saskatchewan. Since they won on a platform that promised the people a complete system of free medical services, they invited me, as you know, to make a survey and draw up a plan. There I met a Captain Sheps who was once in Washington, came to a cocktail party to the house and brought a friend of his, another Captain, and he's the man. He is a very nice boy, son of a doctor in Ontario, 28 years old, very liberal, was three years in the Army and is not quite sure yet where he will be next winter. Nora, of course, will continue with her studies in some way or other. She is at home at the moment and will come with us to Switzerland while her fiancé is taking a post-graduate course in California.

Emmy seems very happy in Switzerland. She is visiting with all her relatives all over the country, aunts, great aunts, first, second, third, and fourth cousins. Switzerland is so small that everybody seems to be related somehow. I am only glad that I need not see all these people.

Our plans for the summer are still unchanged. If everything works out properly, the girls and I will be flying to Geneva on the 23rd of July. My mother and I will spend the first three weeks together in St. Moritz "taking the waters." I seem to have reached the point where I will need another such treatment and St. Moritz combines the waters with the high altitude quite apart from being one of the most beautiful spots of Switzerland. Later, we will probably spend a few weeks in the Tessin where a Swiss friend of ours who lives in California has a house that we may use. And September I plan to spend in Zurich doing some work at the Library trying to find out what has been published in Europe during the war. I have also been invited to attend the annual meeting of the Schweizerische Naturforschende Gesellschaft that will be held in Zurich and that will at the same time commemorate the 200th anniversary of the foundation of the Zurich Naturforschende Gesellschaft. I have been a member of both for many years and I am sure that I will find all my old colleagues and friends there.

I just had a letter of my old German publisher, Bruno Hauff, the owner of Georg Thieme Verlag, a most typical letter. He is a man of humble origins that he always tried to conceal, very intelligent and very ambitious. He married the daughter of a lawyer at the Reichsgericht in Leipzig who was a little Jewish, not very much, just about 50 per cent but was, of course, baptized and had money. When Hitler came, he divorced his wife "to save the firm". The publishing house has been completely destroyed with all the stocks but Hauff moved to Wiesbaden, reopened shop, the Deutsche Medizinische Wochenschrift is coming out again and at the moment he has 30 scientific books in the press. He wants to bring out new editions of my books because, as he says, there is a great interest in them among the German physicians and also, says he, among the Americans in Germany. It all sounds like a joke but you can't kill these people. They always come back.

Strange things do happen. In the same mail, I had a letter from a book dealer in Buenos Aires who wrote that he had sold over 200 copies of my Soviet book in a few days and that he would like to have an autographed copy for his private collection. By the way, have you a copy of "The University at the Crossroads"? If not, let me know and I will send you one. I do not know if I ever told you that an Islandic [sic] edition was being made of "Civilization and Disease", probably for the herring fishers of Iceland.

Now to your last letters. We are trying desparately to get a copy of Buschan's book. I am obviously also very anxious to see it. It will be hard to find the book but I will try in Switzerland. I have also written to the Library of Congress because I was told that they are taking entire stocks of German publishers and are selling the books for $ 1.00 a piece to other libraries. I hear that the price of the books is deducted from the cost of the occupation of Germany.

The Acta Tropica we have here in the Welch Library. Jung's "Psychologie und Alchemie" has been ordered and is probably here already.

I have written to Dr. Antonio Requena and am anxious to see his publications.

The Egyptian population problem is becoming more and more complicated. I found that around 1800 the population had dropped to 2 million 500 thousand, probably as a result of the Turkish regime while it was

254

7 million in antiquity. By 1897 the population had increased to 9.8 million and it was 14.1 million in 1927. The whole problem needs further investigation. I found another interesting figure, however, in one of Ruffer's best papers, the one on the consanguineous marriage of the Egyptians. There he states that the average age of the Ptolemys, not counting the few who were murdered, was 64 years which is quite a respectable age for those days.

How do you like the cottage on Long Island and how is the family? I am sure they enjoy being away from the city. We have had a marvelous summer so far and I only hope it will continue like this. So much for today.

Yours as ever,

[Henry]

Nora Sigerist's planned marriage with K. Ingham did not materialize; she later married the composer and Columbia professor of music, Jack Beeson. Schweizerische Naturforschende Gesellschaft = Swiss Academy of Sciences, which comprises the Swiss Society of the History of Medicine. Bruno Hauff (born 1884). Deutsche Medizinische Wochenschrift = German Medical Weekly, the predominant journal of general medicine in Germany. Soviet book (Sigerist 1937), University at the Crossroads (Sigerist 1946a), Civilization and Disease (Sigerist 1943). Buschan's book and Jung's Psychologie und Alchemie see A. to S. of 16 April 1946. Requena see A. to S. of 16 May 1946. (Ruffer 1921).

Ackerknecht to Sigerist, New York, 1 July 1946

Dear Henry:

Thank you very much for your long letter which I appreciated and enjoyed very much.

First of all let me congratulate to Nora and to you at the occasion of her engangement. Marriage is in our society still the most promising carrier [sic] for women. "Socialized Medicine" got you into all kinds of troubles. For a change it got you into matchmaking.

I envy you most wholeheartedly for your going to Europe. First of all for sentimental reasons. But this being the hottest day so far experienced (and my typing and contents unfortunately seem to reflect this fact very strikingly) here this year, also for very plain climatic reasons. It must be a great blessing to live once again in a country where summer is not a curse.

Bruno Hauff's Maerchen amused me greatly (because what's the use of getting sick). This seems to be a whole category of gentlemen. My friend Hermann Hesse printed a little letter for them, which might interest you (please return).

I have not yet a copy of "University at the Crossroads". I am so glad that you are looking for the Buschan too. Egyptian vital statistics turn out to become another "Rouelle". Too bad that you have no candidates for the doctorate who could do the spadework. Because one would have to go through the rich history of epidemics, and also perhaps the history of nutrition in Egypt. You have no time to go off on such sidelines. If I had only more time. But I have this collection and these bookreviews, and I am hardly through with "Suggestion in Primitive Society", and plunged in another Ciba Nr. (The Doctor as a politician), and then I have still to fix the book for Schuman (Selected Essays) before the summer is over. What I gain in time by the absence of the family, I loose through the weekends out there. But they are happy, and it is a nice place, if you go in for this countrystuff.

We also try with Rosen to get the Society of Medical History, which after the war and one year of Zilboorg-Bain is in bad condition, back to its feet.

We get now lots of letters from home. Mostly not too encouraging. My father had rather abruptly to leave for the country. The terrible load of work and mental strain had been too much for his bloodpressure. He is 66 after all.

I was quite amused of getting lately a frantic call from Ruth Benedict. She had to review a book of a certain Castiglioni for the Herald Tribune, and could I not give her at least one point of the book which she could praise. She had not been able to detect one. Well, I know what she had been through. The rather revolting thing is that Arturo seems to think of the Schmarrn as a masterpiece. De Saussure had reviewed it as tactfully as possible for the Journal. A.C. got hold of the manuscript of the review by some error, and made De Saussure such a scene over the phone that the latter withdrew his review. He is now in Italy, and in case he comes back he better does not try this trick with me. I would withdraw my review too, but only to replace it by another one, where there would be no euphemisms left. This history of quinine is another headache. This woman is a very good writer. And she has looked into a lot of books. The trouble is that she seems unable to read. Why don't these people write streight [sic] fiction. Well, I will try to take it as easy with her as possible, too.

I still have a faint hope to see you before you leave.

    Kindest regards and best wishes

      Yours as ever

        Erwin

Hauff see A. to S. of 26 June 1946. Maerchen = fairy tale. Hermann Hesse (1877–1962) German poet and novelist. Buschan, Rouelle see A. to S. of 15 April and 13 February 1946, respectively. New York Society of Medical History, probably under the leadership of Zilboorg and D. C. Bain. Ruth Benedict, Arturo Castiglioni see A. to S. of 2 August 1944 and 3 April 1946, respectively. Schmarrn = rubbish. De Saussure see A. to S. of 23 March 1945. "Journal" of the History of Medicine and Allied Sciences. History of Quinine and its author not identified.

SIGERIST to ACKERKNECHT, Baltimore ?, 18 July 1946

Dear Erwin,

This is the last letter before I leave on the 23rd, if we leave because you probably saw that all Constellation planes have been stopped. They had dozens of accidents particularly fires and René Sand, the professor of social medicine in Brussels who was here for two days last week, told me that the whole French delegation to the U.N. Health Conference had almost been killed in such a machine. I still hope that they have enough other planes to take us over in time.

Thanks for your letter and the two book reviews and also for the beautiful letter of Hermann Hesse that I am returning enclosed. It is a splendid document, very human and just the right words.

I had a letter from Illing who is a physician in a sanatorium at Partenkirchen. He was in the Army throughout the war, fortunately, as he says, on the Southern front in Italy and Africa. He writes that Plügge has become an excellent internist at the Municipal Hospital at Darmstadt. That Sprockhoff has been killed in the war, you probably knew. The three of them spent several years with Weizsäcker in Heidelberg.

I do not remember if you knew Baensch, the professor of Roentgenology at Leipzig, a very nice fellow. His wife popped up in Baltimore a few days ago. She is American-born, was able to get an American passport, came here with her children and is now trying to get her husband over because somebody must support the children although he is a German and although he was, against his will I am sure, a member of the Nazi party. At the moment he is in Zurich working with Schinz. With her American passport in hand, she was able to smuggle her husband and Bruno Hauff into the American zone.

I am sending you a copy of my little book under separate cover and with all good wishes for you and yours for a good summer,

I am

Yours as ever,

[Henry]

René Sand (1877–1953). Hermann Hesse see A. to S. of 1 July 1946. Wolfram Illing, Herbert Plügge, and Helmut Sprockhoff were members of S.'s Institute in Leipzig, associates of Weizsäcker, probably Viktor von Weizsäcker (1886–1957) promotor of psychosomatic medicine. Willy Baensch (1893–1972) radiologist in Washington, DC. Schinz, Hans Rudolf (1891–1966) professor of radiology in Zurich, S.'s friend. Hauff see S. to A. of 26 June 1946. "Little book", probably (Sigerist 1946a).

ACKERKNECHT to SIGERIST, New York, 22 July 1946

Dear Henry:

Thanks ever so much for the "University at the Crosroads" with the kind dedication which just arrived. I also owe you my thanks for a letter, the newspaper clipping on the Leipziger Messe, and the little pamphlet on medical conditions in Southern Germany, which I found <u>extremely</u> interesting. You will have more information in Switzerland. From my father's letter (Dr. Erwin Ackerknecht, Ludwigsburg, Stuttgarter Str. 85 – à tout fin utile) I gain the impression that the food situation is worse than ever. He never complained during the 9 months we have been in touch, but now he writes that the bread supply e. g. is just below minimum.

I very much hope that your plane business gets settled in time so that you stop working in time. It is on the other hand good that the hazardous planes got grounded before you left. I wish you a very pleasant time, and that Antaeus collects new forces in touching the Swiss earth.

I was very glad to hear that Illing and Plügge survived. I wonder what became of Scheunert, in my opinion the brightest of the little group.

I knew of Sprockhoff's death. Illing could now marry the widow which he admired so greatly. The trouble is that in the matter of passions, different from cabbage in this respect, "aufgewärmte" dishes don't taste so good in general. – I knew Baensch, of course, and hope he will succeed.

Lately I reread a great deal of Virchow, and was fascinated all over again. My thesis can give but a poor reflexion of his intellectual keenness and brilliancy. If I ever get a chance again to do what I like to do, I certainly will do a book on him as a politician, historian, pathologist and anthropologist. For the time being it looks as if Schuman and the end of the Opa [?] talked me into writing a quasi anthropologico-geographico-sociological goddamned popular book on the United Nations. It depresses me, but I can't help it.

Lucy and the children are fine, and send their love to the whole Sigerist tribe. Nora probably told you that she dropped in with her fiancé here. He makes an agreeable impression, and we spent a very pleasant half hour.

Kindest regards and best wishes

Yours as ever

Erwin

"University at the Crossroads" (Sigerist 1946a). "Leipziger Messe" = Leipzig Fair. Antaeus, a giant in the Greek mythology, who collected new forces on touching the earth. Illing, Plügge, Baensch see S. to A. of 18 July 1946. Gerhart Scheunert, one of A.'s Leipzig colleagues. "Aufgewärmte" = warmed-up dishes. The plan of a Virchow book materialized many years later.

ACKERKNECHT to SIGERIST, New York, 23 September 1946

Dear Henry:

If you got your plane on Sept. 20, you should be home by now. Welcome thus in "God's own country". We hoped that you might stop in New York on your way home – Stampar ought to be an attraction here for you now – we are extremely anxious to hear from you about Europe, ideas, people etc. – but with the hotel situation here, and your health you probably went straight home, and probably did the right thing.

I very much hope you will come here soon, and have some minutes for us. Otherwise I might have to go to Philadelphia, and would then try to make a jump to Balto for a few hours, in order to see you. I also have a long list of illustrations to look for, and I hate burdening Genevieve with it, if I can avoid it. The illustrations are for my Ciba series "Doctors as Statesmen and Politicians", which I wrote this summer, and which I intend also to use as a lecture this winter here. I am not dissatisfied with it; but I would still have prefered, to invest three more months in the subject and made it a real monograph. But nobody would pay me that, whereas...

I enclose the Leriche review. I have several bibliographical notes for you, but not at hand. They will follow later. Did you work on THE BOOK? I hope you had a good time, and profited physically as well as mentally and sentimentally from your vacation. We had some quiet weeks in the country, and still go there sometimes on weekends. The family is fine, and Sylvia, five now, goes Thursday for the first time to Kindergarten-School! I am measuring cadavers – it's the season again – and we try to introduce the Koenigswalds, who after five years of horror arrived with the most fascinating collection of Pithecanthropus material from Java last week, into the intricacies of shopping, appartment [sic] hunting, and other aspects of American civilisation.

We hope to hear soon from you.
    Kindest regards from all of us
        Yours as ever
            Erwin

Andrija Stampar (1888–1958) expert in social medicine and public health in former Yugoslavia, friend of S. Leriche see A. to S. of 5 December 1945. Gustav H. R. Koenigswald (1902–1982) German paleontologist and geologist.

ACKERKNECHT to SIGERIST, New York, 24 September 1946

Dear Henry:
    This is the Leriche review which I forgot to enclose into my letter yesterday. I apologize for my absentmindedness.
        Cordially
            Erwin

260

Dear Henry:

It looks as if I have to go to Philadelphia on Friday Oct. 4. I hope to be through in the morning, and to come to the Institute in the afternoon. Or to spend the night with the Blocks and to show up on Saturday morning. In case you are not available in Balto on Friday afternoon or on Saturday morning, please let me know before Friday.

Kindest regards
Yours as ever
Erwin

Block not identified.

Dear Henry:

The adress [sic] of Senator Wagner is 530 East 86 Str. Thanks in advance for your help. I am now all the more eager to settle this thing as quickly as possible, as I just found an invitation on my desk by Dean Middleton (do you know him? what kind of a fellow?) Madison, Wisc., to present myself as a candidate for an associate professor in the History of Medicine! I will be out there on Friday Oct. 11. I feel a little dizzy. It looks good. If we were more old fashioned, I would say: pray for me!

It was awfully nice to have met again. (though a little nostalgic for me, to hear of all these dear European places and attitudes) and I hope it was not too boring for you. I was so glad to see you physically in fine shape, and the "baby", THE BOOK, grown already so nicely. Thanks again for your wonderful hospitality.

Kindest regards from all of us
Yours as ever
Erwin

Robert F. Wagner (1877–1953) U.S. Senator. "Settle this thing": probably A.'s American citizenship. William S. Middleton (1890–1975) dean of the Medical School of the University of Wisconsin.

SIGERIST to ACKERKNECHT, Baltimore ?, 8 October 1946

Dear Erwin:

I am perfectly thrilled about Wisconsin. Good luck. Middleton is a very nice fellow, a Philadelphian, disciple of Riesman. He has taken a very active part in the life of the American Association of the History of Medicine and has written a number of historical papers that were published in the Annals. He is a good clinician and during the war was in charge of a large army hospital in England. I am sure you will find him very pleasant to deal with and I very much hope that he is going to write me so that I have a chance to recommend you.

You, of course, know William Snow Miller taught medical history and had a beautiful collection of books. I met him in 1931 and had a very pleasant evening with him. With Urdang, the new historians of science and medical history together a very good group could be developed, much broader than what we have here where Homewood is always afraid that it might be invaded by the Medical School. I will be most anxious to hear what you experienced.

Thanks for the address. I am writing right away and hope everything goes well. It was a great pleasure to have you here and you know that we always have a room for you.

Cordially as ever yours,

[Henry]

Middleton see A. to S. of 7 October 1946. David Riesman (1867–1940) medical historian. Annals of Medical History, a journal published from 1917 to 1942. William Snow Miller (1858–1939) professor of anatomy and history of medicine in Madison. Urdang see A. to S. of 23 March 1945. Homewood, the main campus of Johns Hopkins University on the North side of Baltimore, vs. the Medical School campus in the East.

ACKERKNECHT to SIGERIST, New York, 14 October 1946

Dear Henry:

I apologize for writing longhand, but this seems to be the only way to inform you quickly about the results of my Madison visit, from which I returned yesterday night.

The offer is a professorship for the History of Medicine at the medical school (collaboration with Urdang and the History of Science Department, but otherwise independence), $ 5000 a year going up to eventually 7500, clerical help, tenure, candidates for the doctorate (as the M.D.s write theses out there). Sounds all almost too good to be true. But I have no reason to doubt that Middleton's letter will differ from what he said. He makes a most pleasant impression (thanks a lot for your most valuable information), and I am glad that I will depend on him and not the Dean of the Arts and Sciences (Ingram). I am, of course, very excited and bursting with plans for lectures, papers, books etc. (The teaching lot is moderate) I would start at [sic] January 1, start teaching at February 1. Finding an appartment [sic] up there, selling the furniture here, moving the books etc. will, of course, be quite troublesome and costly, and for a while we probably will have to live in a hotel. But all that is not so important.

I think I got such a good offer for 2 reasons: I was very well recommended by my Malaria book, contacts, I had made, when out there for the book, and particularly Urdang, who has no money, but a tremendous authority up there, and refused (he was the 1. choice) with direct reference to me. Temkin was the 2. choice, but his infirmity [?] etc. spoke against him.

Furthermore they seem to feel that there will be more jobs of this kind open in the future, and they want to attract a competent person in time.

I am sorry to move away so far from you and other friends of the East Coast, but the offer is so very promising, and when I have more money, it's only 4 hours by plane from NY. Having been in a "marginal" position for so many years, I can not yet believe entirely in the good news. I am fully aware to what an extent I owe my luck to your help and feel deeply grateful for it.

I am a little tired, as I spent more than the half of four days and nights on the train, and was dragged around there a great deal, in order to produce the prescribed "good impression".

Thanks a lot too for the Wagner letter and the tablets! Awfully nice that you thought of the latter. Emmy should be back by now with Nora. Please give them our regards. I am very anxious to hear more of you – and the manuscript! I will have a very hectic time in winding up here, but I am so indescribably happy that I can drop now the silly Schuman book and all the other mercenary stuff. (Merck, translations, abstracts etc. – Ciba I hope to keep though Middleton is a little concerned about that)

Very best regards and wishes

Yours as ever

Erwin

Please give our love to Genevieve and show her the letter, as unfortunately I have no time to write her a separate one.

Urdang see A. to S. of 23 March 1945. Malaria book (Ackerknecht 1945). "1. Choice" = first choice. The first three departments of the history of medicine in the U. S. were Baltimore (1929), Madison (1947), and Yale (1951). Wagner see A. to S. of 7 October 1946. Genevieve Miller.

ACKERKNECHT to SIGERIST, New York, 16 October 1946

Dear Henry:

In the name of the whole Ackerknecht tribe I would like to thank you wholeheartedly for your thoughtful and cordial telegram. I have still a hard time to believe in the whole thing. But having it black on white now, there can't be any doubts about its reality.

May I ask you a favor at this occasion. I have been approached for co-editorship in a projected Journal for "Theoretical Anthropology" or something along these lines. But we will have to talk finances with a [...] foundation. Could you please let me have some data on what the Bulletin costs you at present? I trust you have them at hand in your report for the Association, which I have not yet seen in print. Thanks in advance.

Kindest regards and best wishes from all of us to all of you

Yours as ever

Erwin

Dear Erwin:

When I came to the office day before yesterday, your letter was on top of my mail and I was dying to read it since I well knew that its content would be important. But my office had been invaded by the Royal Dutch Army, the Surgeon General of the Medical Corps and the Colonel who heads the psychiatric services. They stayed here for hours and I had to wait until the afternoon before I could read your letter. All I could do at the moment was to send you a telegram.

This really is the best news I have had in a long time. You are a professor and not an anatomical preparator and although the time spent at the Museum was certainly not lost, your place is in a university and I am sure that you will be happy at Wisconsin. Madison is an enchanting place, a little cold in the winter but beautiful in the summer with a lake and the hills and to me this type represents the ideal community for a scholar. There is a university atmosphere as you would find it in a small town such as Göttingen or Heidelberg and you life [sic] infinitely better than in a city like New York. The University moreover attracts musicians and artists so that throughout the year you have very good concerts. I personally would much prefer to live in Madison or Ann Arbor or Ithaca than in Baltimore.

I had no idea that the Medical School was considering establishing a Chair of Medical History. All I had been told at the time was the Chair of the History of Science but I think it is perfectly splendid that a state university is going ahead in such a way and with the history of medicine, history of science and history of pharmacy combined you will be able to develop a very strong group. The endowed universities should feel ashamed that the state universities are taking the lead over them but shame is something that endowed universities never know. They are much too conceited.

I just heard that Emmy and Nora are not due before October 27 and I may be coming up to New York for that week-end. If plans materialize, I'll let you know. Emmy and Nora must be having an awful passage. They left Basel on September 27 and if all goes well will be in Hoboken on October 27. It seems unbelievable.

Well, there is a lot I would like to tell you but I must stop and get ready for my lecture. Once more, all good wishes for your future.

Yours as ever,
   [Henry]

P. S. Let me know when the news is official so that I can announce it in the Bulletin.

"The endowed universities' shame": S. thinks of Johns Hopkins which at that time supported McCarthyism under which S. suffered. "A lot I would like to tell you": probably S.'s plan to leave Johns Hopkins soon and settle in Switzerland.

ACKERKNECHT to SIGERIST, New York, 22 October 1946

Dear Henry:

Thank you very much for your kind letter of Oct 17, which was simultaneous with my letter, which you probably received meanwhile.

There is no possible doubt that the new job corresponds far better to my interests and abilities than the one here (which I have never regarded as anything but a fill gap) though, as you say, my time here was not lost. I have written 19 papers in 20 months, two or three of which are not too bad; I have learned a great deal through the Museum library and collections and a few people (Weidenreich, Hsu, Bidney); through the visitors and societies here I have made the acquaintance of a great many people, Americans and foreigners, whom I otherwise would never have met, and whom to know is useful. Eventually I have been able to form a first hand opinion on the shallowness, ephemerity and crookedness of New York's "spiritual life".

The news of Emmy and Nora are dreadful. This is almost as bad as our passages in 1941, in the midst of the war. What a "reconversion"! It would on the other hand be wonderful to have you here this weekend. I very much hope that your plan materialises. If you arrive after the Museum is closed (I am unlikely to go there on Saturdays) telephone messages can be send [sic] to us through our neighbors: Erich Schmidt Academy 2-3545.

Kindest regards and best wishes from all of us

    Yours as ever

    Erwin

19 papers are far more than given in the A. bibliography (Walser 1966). Weidenreich see A. to S. of 17 July 1945. Anthropologists Francis K. K. Hsu (1909–1999) and David Bidney.

Dear Erwin:

Thanks for your letter of October 18. I also had a very nice letter from Urdang who, in the whole matter, has really behaved admirably. The enclosed sheets will tell you what the cost of the <u>Bulletin</u> was during the year 1945. Please notice that the only overhead we have is the commission to the press. We still have a deficit of over $ 2,000 that had to be met by the Institute and since the cost of printing is rising steadily and our finances are deteriorating just as steadily, we have made plans to publish only one volume of 6 numbers next year. The <u>Bulletin</u>, in other words, will become a bi-monthly. This would also facilitate the editorial work that has to be simplified since we can no longer afford a secretary.

As long as the <u>Bulletin</u> was the only journal devoted to medical history in the whole English-speaking world, I felt that we should publish as much as we possibly could no matter what the cost might be. Now, that we have the <u>Journal</u> and that the Wellcome Medical Historical Museum in London is going to start another periodical, we can afford to cut down and to be more strict in selecting articles. Six numbers of about 150 pages each will still make a respectable volume for which $ 5.00 will not be too much.

Please let me have the name of the man who has been appointed Professor of the History of Science at the University of Wisconsin. Did I understand you correctly as saying that they plan to have two professors of the History of Science, one for the History of the biological and one for the history of the exact sciences? I would like to write a rather strongly worded note in the <u>Bulletin</u> to the effect that the University of Wisconsin has set an example that should put to shame the endowed universities that have been talking so much without ever doing anything. But I want the facts to be accurate.

With kind regards, I am
    Yours as ever
      [Henry]

Journal of the History of Medicine and Allied Sciences. A British counterpart (Medical History) was founded in 1957 only. A "strongly worded note" did not appear in the Bulletin of the History of Medicine of 1946 or 1947.

Dear Henry:

Thank you very much for your letter of Oct. 23, and the data on the Bulletin. I am answering immediately, (and therefore longhand, alas) in order to finish with this series of "crossing letters", though I do hope to see you, before you see this letter of mine.

The University of Wisconsin has created indeed 2 professorships in the History of Science: one in biology, which has been filled by a young man called Stauffer (good old Swiss name) a pupil of Sarton, who is supposed to have not published because he was in the service for 5 years. The other one: Physics-Mathematics was offered to Bernard Cohen, another pupil of Sarton who declined, and the job is still open. (I suggested Drabkin though I doubt whether he wants to leave New York). I have still to get the approval by the Regents, a formality; yet I would appreciate if nothing on my appointment is published before it is completed by this act. I will let you know immediately, once I have this approval. It seems that Prof. Reynolds of the History Department was very active in promoting the history of science idea. The great difficulty will, of course, be, when more such chairs are created, that almost no candidates to fill them have been trained, and they will have to have very young people of whom one does not know, how they will turn out and who also lack somewhat the authority to build up the new discipline in the school. But better doing something doubtful, than doing nothing.

I am somewhat grieved by the fact that Rosen seems a little "verschnupft" that he was not offered the chair, because personally he is one of the very few people I care for in this country. It is, of course, senseless that he should do public health instead of medical history. But as far as this Wisconsin job goes I feel perfectly innocent, because I was just as surprised by my nomination as anybody else (though he probably thinks I went to Balto in order to get your support). I also think that he would have refused anyhow as I am convinced that she [his wife] alone makes more money here than I will ever make in Madison. Neither of them could even get a license up there, as Wisconsin does not recognize foreign credentials. Well, I trust, being a nice character, he will overcome these feelings, and will eventually get a chair of medical history here or somewhere else in a big city which suits them better. Because anyhow besides Temkin he is the only possible candidate left, as I do not think that a medical school will easily hire a non-medical person for this kind of job.

I am winding up my collection here, doing other odd jobs, and have already started working on Virchow's anthropological writings of which we have a good collection here, having bought the books and reprints of his pupil von Luschan. We have all disagreeable colds, the children have been in bed for a few days. Otherwise things are all right. We hope very much to have you here for the weekend.

Kindest regards
Yours as ever
Erwin

Sarton see A. to S. of 23 March 1945. Bernard Cohen (1914–2003) became professor at Harvard. Drabkin see A. to S. of 13 February 1946. George Rosen and his wife Beate Caspari had German licenses to practise medicine. Only in 1969 did George Rosen get a chair at Yale. "Verschnupft" = offended. Temkin see A. to S. of 8 December 1937. Felix von Luschan (1854–1924) Austrian anthropologist.

ACKERKNECHT to SIGERIST, New York, 4 November 1946

Dear Henry:

I apologize for disturbing you. But we are getting kind of worried, what happened to Nora and Emmy? They were due last Sunday. One more week, and still no news of them. What happened? Could you please let us know?

Here nothing new. We are winding up our affairs, [xxxx]. Thanks a lot for the Hesse [?] newspaper clips with the little malaria item. Incidentally I knew the quoted Herrmann Rudy quite well, as I studied with him in Freiburg i. B. in 1924.

We very much hope that things have quieted down again, and you have been able to go back eventually to the BOOK.

Kindest regards and best wishes
As ever yours
Erwin

P.S. I just had a letter that the Board of Regents has appointed me professor of the history of medicine, beginning January 1, 1947. Thus the thing is definitely [?] official and publishable.

[xxxx] Half a sentence deleted as Chesney Archives' Protected Health Information.

SIGERIST to ACKERKNECHT, Baltimore ?, 4 November 1946

Dear Erwin:

I just received the enclosed letter which I think looks promising. If you do not hear from Senator Wagner's office "some time after election" you could always get in touch with his secretary.

Emmy and Nora arrived safely last Monday. Since I knew that they would not be in before Monday, I did not spend the weekend in New York but took a night train on Sunday. They sailed 28 days and had an awful time but they stood the hardship very well. It is a great relief for me to have them there. Nora is at Columbia and had the good luck to get a room at International House.

We had a visitor from Peru here for a few days, Professor Carlos Monge. He is a great expert on high altitude physiology and pathology. He came because he wanted to know something about the history of anoxia. He had heard vaguely of Paul Bert but had no idea that the book was full of historical references.

Yours as ever,

[Henry]

Wagner see A. to S. of 7 October 1946. Columbia University in New York. Carlos Monge (1884–1970). Anoxia: Lack of oxygen in the blood and tissues. Paul Bert see A. to S. of 2 August 1944.

ACKERKNECHT to SIGERIST, New York, 11 November 1946

Dear Henry:

Thanks a lot for your letter of Nov. 4, and the enclosed letter of Wagner's secretary. I hope that he is not too downtrodden after the results of the [?] election.

We were very glad to hear that Emmy and Nora arrived eventually.

Last Friday the Medical History Society had a very well attended meeting with Weinstein [?], the Health Commissioner. Rosen seems to have overcome his grudge.

I got a lot of French medico-historical geographical and anthropological books from the Embassy for review. Some might interest the Bulletin.

Guttentag contemplates spending his sabbatical at the Institute. I think that would be very good for all concerned. His other plan is to go to Germany as adviser for university reconstruction.

I hope that I will be able to read your manuscript before leaving for Madison.

I am ashamed of my longhand writing, knowing how little you like it, and close with my kindest regards

Yours as ever

Erwin

Wagner see A. to S. of 7 October 1946. New York (State) Health Commissioner, probably Michael Weinstein. Guttentag see A. to S. of 12 November 1945.

SIGERIST to ACKERKNECHT, Baltimore ?, 21 November 1946

Dear Erwin:

I wonder if you could publish the enclosed note in the Journal. I am sending it to you rather than George Rosen because it concerns a subject in your field. Lastres sent it for publication in the <u>Bulletin</u> but I have no time to translate it myself and have nobody else here who could do it. If the Journal cannot use the manuscript, please return it and I will see what I can do with it.

I hope to be able to send you the first part of my book next week and the second part one week later. I wish to read the typescript before I send it on and so far, I have not had a minute's time. I have not touched the book since July but I am making an effort to go back to it this week-end, and I hope it will succeed. For over 20 years I did all my research and writing at night but now I need part of the day for this kind of work and with the growing stream of visitors that we are having here, it is very difficult to squeeze out even a few hours.

I would also very much like you to help me in getting some illustration material from the Museum of Natural History, particularly for the sections on paleopathology and on primitive medicine. We will have to talk the matter over. I plan to be in New York December 21 to 23 for the annual meeting of the American-Soviet Medical Society and if you have no engagement for the 23rd and the Museum is still open, we could spend the whole day together. I even have a hotel room which means something these days.

Yours as ever,
   [Henry]

Lastres see S. to A. of 27 November 1946. "The book" (Sigerist 1951).

ACKERKNECHT to SIGERIST, New York, 25 November 1946

Dear Henry:

Thank you very much for your letter of Nov. 21. I have forwarded the "discovery" of Lastres to Rosen. Personally I feel it is not worthwhile to be published, neither by the Journal nor by the Bulletin. First because it is a carbon copy, and Lastres has therefore probably published it already in Peru (as he had his contribution to the Castiglioni volume). Second, because his contention that Pachacamac was an equivalent of Asclepius, is based on half a sentence of the adventurer Miguel de Estete. He does not even give those data on Pachacamac which can be looked up in every handbook, nor the source of his fancy pictures etc. If those fellows want to publish abroad, they should at least stick to certain minimum standards. But I might be too fussy.

I am very upset to hear that you still had no time for the book. I very much hope that you succeeded this weekend. But this situation is simply untenable that you play the Cooks Bureau for medical historians, instead of doing the essential thing, that is writing the book.

I am looking forward very much to your visit on December 23. Of course, I will be free. With illustrations we will have a hard time. Less on paleopathology, where we can have a few nice pieces fotografed [sic] here. But our picture collection offers little on primitive medicine, and we will have to choose such material rather from books and articles not tapped so far for this purpose.

We are pretty busy with the problems of liquidating and moving (seeing people for goodby [sic] included) Ellen coughs a lot at night, and Lucy gets thus little sleep. Otherwise the family is O.K. I was, of course, very pleased with Hesse's Nobel Price [sic]. Even financially it will be very helpful to him. I read several nice French medico-historical books (on

272

Dupuytren, Pasteur etc) If they are not original, they are at least well written. I am just reading the Contenau on Babylonian-Assyrian medicine, and very curious to hear how you liked it.

Kindest regards and best wishes
   Yours as ever
      Erwin

Lastres see also S. to A. of 27 November 1946; Castiglioni A. to S. of 3 April 1946. Pachacamac, ancient city in Peru. Miguel de Estete (born 1507) participated in Pizarro's conquest of Peru. Thomas Cook's, one of the first and best known travel agencies. Hesse, see A. to S. of 1 July 1946, was awarded the Nobel Prize for literature in 1946. Guillaume Dupuytren (1777–1835) French surgeon. Louis Pasteur (1822–1895) French bacteriologist. (Contenau 1938).

SIGERIST to ACKERKNECHT, Baltimore ?, 27 November 1946

Dear Erwin:

These South Americans are beginning to be a real pest. Their ignorance is abysmal and their conceit has no limit. There are, of course, exceptions but Lastres certainly does not belong to them.

Thanks for your many reprints. I am delighted to have them and this just reminds me that I have not sent you my recent reprints. You are going to get them in a few days. I have just reviewed our reprint list and we are going to send them out regularly again. Personally I have not much to send because I have not had the time for papers.

At long last I am writing again. I locked myself up for three days over the week-end and had only one interruption, namely an invitation to go to India for 6 weeks to attend their Science Congress as representative of the National Academy of Sciences and of the American Philosophical Society, with all expenses paid. It was not easy to refuse but I did it and now I am writing again a few pages every day. It is, however, a constant struggle to squeeze out a few hours for real work.

I am glad that you will be free on December 23. I will send you on Friday the first section of my book that contains the introductory chapters. You will find a few gaps, particularly in the footnotes. I am filling them in these days but I do not want to delay the manuscript. The second part on primitive medicine will follow next week. Keep both manuscripts until I come. We can then discuss them and also the question of illustrations. I, of course, have some picture material here but I would like to avoid reproducing those pictures that have been seen too many times. Well, we shall talk the whole matter over. I am finishing Egypt now and will then have Babylonia and what goes with it. I have not read Contenau's book yet. I read his book on Assyrian-Babylonian civilization and also his book on divination but I have not touched the medical book so far. The fact that he is a good Assyriologist and accidentally a doctor also does not necessarily make him a historian of medicine.

Friday I am having ten people who plan to found a journal of social medicine, Roemer, Terris, Falk and a number of others who seem to have money in sight for the purpose.

Last Monday we had an excellent meeting of the Medical History Club staged by Temkin in an admirable way. It was a joint meeting of the Club and the Society of Hygiene. It started with cocktails and a subscription dinner, had a capacity audience at the School of Hygiene and the discussion was excellent, very lively and very stimulating.

Looking forward to seeing you soon, I am

Yours as ever,

[Henry]

The manuscript of Lastres see S. to A. of 21 November 1946 was not published in the Bulletin or the "Journal" of 1947 or 1948. S. had been on a study tour in India in November and December of 1944. Contenau's book see A. to S. of 25 November 1946 (Contenau 1938). Instead of a Journal of Social Medicine an Institute on Social Medicine was founded in 1947 within the New York Academy of Medicine. Milton I. Roemer (1916–2001) health administrator, pupil and friend of Sigerist. Milton Terris (1915–2003) epidemiologist. Leslie A. Falk (born 1915) pupil of S.

ACKERKNECHT to SIGERIST, New York, 2 December 1946

Dear Henry:

Thanks ever so much for your letter of Nov. 27, and the manuscript, which arrived today. I am burning with impatience to read it; and I will start reading it tonight, and be it after midnight when I am through with all this darned technical stuff which chokes me ("business" letters, and letters for the appartment [sic] we never get etc.)

I am delighted to hear that eventually you started writing again. It is obvious that you can not write many papers during this period, and I think it is not too bad, as the book is more important, and anyhow you have written more papers in the past than most people would in three lifetimes.

I was rather pleased with Contenau's book. It is not very "deep", but well written, interesting, and sound, as far as I can see, except perhaps for his formulation of antecendents of Hippocratism in Babylonian medicine. He obviously does not know too much of the latter. Well, I hope we can talk over this and many other things very soon. Today I took out reservations for the 29th, and four weeks from today we should have arrived in Madison.

Kindest regards
　　Yours as ever
　　　　Erwin

(Contenau 1938).

ACKERKNECHT to SIGERIST, New York, 13 December 1946

Dear Henry:

Thanks ever so much for the second part of the manuscript which Emmi brought over. I read it, like its predecessor, with great pleasure, and will have very few critical remarks to make on details. I think the chapter on primitive medicine is just what is needed for such a book (and was never done), and I admire all through the manuscript your ability to develop difficult subjects with such an elegance (and without cheapening) so that they go down the readers [sic] throat very easily. I am all the more depressed by the idea that you encounter so many external obstacles in writing the book.

I had a very friendly letter of R. Redfield (who resigned as Dean of Social Sciences and kept only his job as professor of anthropology in order to remain able to do research) concerning my article in the Bulletin on "Natural Diseases and rational treatment". He rightly drew my attention to the fact that not only "effective methods are far from being always rational" as I emphasize heavily, but "rational methods are by no means always effective", a fact confirmed by the whole history of medicine.

It was awfully nice to have Emmi here. [xxxx].

You can imagine that we are terribly busy with saying goodby [sic], "initiating" my successor etc. But I still read some more Virchow. Admirable stuff. I am looking forward to have tonight "brühwarme" news from you through Otto Guttentag. Yesterday night I spoke in the New York Society of Medical History on "The Doctor as Physician and Statesman", a small crowd as usual, but a few nice students from New York University. The Koch letters are still here indeed, and it would be very good if you could take them with you.

I am looking forward to seeing you soon. Kindest regards and best wishes

> Yours as ever
> Erwin

Redfield and Virchow see A. to S. of 2 August 1944 and 27 April 1932, respectively. [xxxx] One sentence deleted as Chesney Archives' Protected Health Information. "Brühwarme" news = brand-new information. Guttentag, Koch see A. to S. of 12 November and 14 April 1945, respectively.

ACKERKNECHT to SIGERIST, Madison, WI, 3 January 1947

Dear Henry:

Thanks ever so much for the telegram which I found here yesterday morning at the Dean's office. We had a few extremely hectic last days in NY – Genevieve whom we saw the last evening can testify to it – arrived on Monday night after 28 hours of travelling, had two days rest in the hotel, where at the modest prize [sic] of $ 45 p. week we are allowed to stay for 3 weeks, and are now again in a complete topsy turvy condition, trying to get an apartment, to get settled professionally etc. Urdangs will arrive from NY to night. The fact that Lucy and the children are not yet "acclimatized" to the cold (and we had – 19 F the first day – and I had to rush them back to the hotel after ½ hour in the open and rub them for another half hour to bring them back to normal) also complicates things a little. Well, I trust it will all settle down after a while.

I had a very pleasant talk with Middleton yesterday. I will have to give a thirty hour introd. course for the second year students during the second semester (15 weeks) It will be rather hard sailing, as I have to get organized

276

simultaneously (my books are, of course, in the warehouse), and as 30 hours seems to me not an ideal time unit for an introductory course, I feel I cannot spend too much time for beginners on ancient medicine and have thus "too much time" for the 19th century, (22 hours would in my mind [be] the ideal time unit for an introductory course) But it is an experiment anyhow, and when they were generous with time, I did not want to refuse!

We hope you have had pleasant holidays and have been able to go back to the book. You will soon hear more from me.

Kindest regards and very best wishes from all of us to all of you
yours as ever
Erwin

My office, which will be in the library, is not yet ready because of lack of building material. Thus I have an office in the hospital for the time being. But send my mail to the indicated address please. I pick it up there every day. E

A.'s first letter from Madison. The letter-head: The Universtiy of Wisconsin. State of Wisconsin General Hospital. Madison 6.

Genevieve Miller. Urdang, and Middleton see A. to S. of 23 March 1945 and 7 October 1946, respectively.

Sigerist to Ackerknecht, Baltimore ?, 10 January 1947

Dear Erwin:

Thanks for your letter of January 3. Genevieve reported about the very pleasant visit she had with you and I can well imagine that you had a hectic time getting away. It must be quite a shock to be so close to the Arctic all of a sudden, and it will take the children some time to get acclimatized but you will enjoy the summer. The whole region is beautiful and you will find Winnebago Indians not so very far from the city. At least, I remember that we visited an Indian camp in 1940 when we drove through that region.

I was amazed and delighted to see in the last number of Science that the University of Wisconsin has purchased the Thordarson collection of books. It is a splendid collection, very important for the history of science, and I am sure that you will benefit by it too. It is simply astounding how state universities can go ahead and purchase such valuable collections while we have the greatest difficulties in buying cheap, new publications.

Some day when you have time, look up Professor Otto, the professor of philosophy at the University, and give him my kindest regards. He was born at Zwickau but came to this country at the tender age of five so that he probably never had the chance to cultivate a Saxon accent. He is familiar with the work of the Institute and has always be very kind to me. I think he is retiring this year.

Emmy has just spend [sic] a week in New Haven with the Kahns. I have spent most of the vacation working on the book.

I remember with pleasure the visit at the Museum and I am very grateful to you for all the trouble you have taken with the book and for the notes that you have very kindly sent me.

I can imagine that it will take you a lot of time to prepare a course of 30 hours, particularly in a new environment without familiar tools but you were very correct in accepting the time and not asking for a reduction because it is very difficult to obtain more hours while it will be easier in the future to cut down if you wish to do it or to divide the time between a lecture and a seminar course.

Well, I hope you will be acclimatized soon and wish that you will find an apartment. That's the most important at the moment. Please remember me to Lucy, the children, Urdangs and with all good wishes, I am

Yours as ever,

[Henry]

Genevieve Miller. Zwickau, a town in Saxony. The Kahns, possibly Louis Kahn of the Center for British Art, Yale University.

ACKERKNECHT to SIGERIST, Madison, 22 January 1947

Dear Henry:

Thank you very much for your letter of January 10. I do not know whether I wrote you already about our housing situation. This essential is at least, after many pains, settled for six months. We rented an old house at the city limits for six months. There is, of course, a lot of work to do around the house in general, and right now to make it look half way decent. But we were very lucky, and feel really very happy.

Professionally I also go slowly under way. I have now some secretarial help. This is one of my first experiments with that dreadful machine, the dictaphone. Friday I start teaching. First a kind of general introductory lecture, why Medical History should have a legitimate place in the Medical School. Mostly, of course, taken from your writings, and duly acknowledged. You are far better at these general things than anybody else. Then I go into paleo-pathology and paleo-medicine, as I have decided to baptize pre-historic medicine. And then up to the present. I devote about one third of the course to the 19th century. This might look horrible, but it is not as bad as Garrison, who spends 50% of his book on the modern period. I have done a lot of thinking about the division of my course, and I have the feeling that I am not entitled to burden these boys who, after all, are not to become medical historians, with too much historical stuff.

Tomorrow night I am also talking on some silly panel discussion. [xxxx], and our social life is also beginning. So you see we have quite a hectic time.

Yes, indeed, we bought the Thorardson collection. Unfortunately I had not the time to look at it. It is indeed very good. In general I am very delighted with Madison, professionally and personally. I enjoy tremendously the sight of the nature from my windows and sun coming in after two years in the New York darkness.

Emmy wrote about your resignation. Well, we have talked often enough about the subject. You know that as a medical historian I feel extremely sad about the fact, and it will bring a great deal of difficulties. But, as a personal friend, I feel that you have done the right thing.

Kindest regards from all of us to all of you,

> Yours as ever
> Erwin H. Ackerknecht

[xxxx] Half a sentence deleted as Chesney Archives' Protected Health Information. Thorardson collection see S. to A. of 10 January 1947. S.'s resignation: At the end of 1946 S. decided to resign from his post at The Johns Hopkins University and to retire to his native Switzerland. There were several reasons for such a step, the major one was to free himself to write the eight volumes of his *History of Medicine*. Only when he obtained a salaried professorship in absentia from Yale University was he able to resign. The official resignation took place in January 1947.

Dear Henry:

Could you please send me the Address of Artelt and your definite opinion of him. As you know, Howard Becker of this University is going soon to Europe in order to take care of the German University, and in talking with him about medical historians, I would like to know more about Artelt.

In working out my lecture on paleo-pathology, it occurred to me that there is one further method to get at the age of disease: that is, the epidemiological and immunological one. This is, of course, rather difficult, and needs a great amount of special knowledge. Unfortunately, I could not do much here about it, not having the books of Charles Nicolle here. But, you have them in Baltimore, and you might even like to add a footnote along these lines to your book.

Among other things, I went over Edelstein's old articles. I feel he over does a little bit the religious side of the hippocratic physician. Do you think that there is any point in publishing my first lecture which I have written up and which was about the value of medical history in medical education. The ideas are mostly yours. Formulation is a little different and I might have added the one or the other little traits. I have lately gone over a lot of papers for Schuman's Journal. Some of them were quite interesting and quite good. I think that nobody can mind that after my last experience with Schuman I have lost any interest in him and his enterprise. This fellow makes the naive and writes me letter after letter to squeeze me for information as he used to do. But this is over, and I also will try to pull out of his Journal as soon as possible without any dramatic side-effects. Perhaps the bulletin will have to have a larger editorial board after your departure, and that might give me an opportunity to change without any noise. I enclose a reference on a German book which I came across lately, and which might be interesting for the Institute. Well, soon it is you I hope who will send us the German language references, and you need no longer our assistance in this respect. We do hope that you are in good health, and getting along alright [sic].

Kindest regards and best wishes from all of us to all of you.

Yours as ever

Erwin

The letter-head now reads: The University of Wisconsln. Madison. The Medical School. Department of the History of Medicine.

Artelt see S. to A. of 14 May 1946. Howard Becker (1899–1960) professor of sociology at the University of Wisconsin. Charles Nicolle (1866–1936) French physician who wrote several books on infectious diseases. Edelstein see A. to S. of 2 August 1944. A. published his first Wisconsin lecture (Ackerknecht 1947a). Schuman's Journal: J. of the History of Medicine and Allied Sciences; A. was on the editorial board of the "journal" until 1952, however, he has never been on the editorial board of the "Bulletin". "Your departure": S.'s resignation and departure to Europe in summer 1947.

SIGERIST to ACKERKNECHT, Baltimore ?, 14 February 1947

Dear Erwin:

Walter Artelt's address is:

Frankfurt a.M.-Süd 10

Gartenstrasse 132

Edelstein, who knows him best, has written on his behalf to the American officer who is in charge of the University of Frankfurt. This was some time ago. I think there is no doubt that Artelt joined the Nazi party under great pressure during the war and that he did it primarily to prevent an SS man from taking over his Department. Edelstein says that Artelt behaved very well toward him and helped him to leave the country. I personally feel that of all the German medical historians, he is by far the most decent and I do not see why he should not be permitted to teach when opportunists like Diepgen and von Brunn have managed to keep their chairs.

I wish something could be done for Leo Norpoth whom you probably knew at Leipzig. He is still in French captivity and it seems that the University of Mainz is interested in him. He is a catholic and was discharged from Leipzig when Hitler came into power. Mainz, however, is French zone and I am afraid that your Professor Howard Becker could not do much in this case.

I had a long letter from Professor Thomas, the biochemist in Leipzig whom you certainly knew. He is dean of the Medical Faculty in Erlangen and is very much embittered. He is one of the very few Leipzig professors who, to the very end, refused to join the party. His Institute at Leipzig, at least the new part, was not destroyed, but when the American troops evacuated Saxony they took him and part of his staff along probably so that the Russians would not benefit by his work. He was then made dean at Erlangen and was given a dozen other administrative positions so that he cannot do any research any more.

The immunological approach to paleopathology has been tried in the past but not too successfully. I have made references to it in my book and Williams in his paper published in the <u>Archives of Pathology</u> summarized what has been done in the past. The method may yield results with Peruvian mumies [sic] rather than with those from Egypt. In Egypt the bodies were kept in a brine for a very long time which obviously affects the tissue reactions.

I quite agree with you about Edelstein's interpretation of Hippocratic medicine. He is a highly religious individual who finds religion everywhere. You were not here when we gave the Graduate week on the Renaissance. In a one-hour lecture, I discussed the primitive accumulation of capital toward the end of the Middle Ages, the increased demand for metals caused by the introduction of fire-arms, the demand for gold as a result of increased trade, the search for gold that started yoyages of discovery etc. etc. and then Edelstein spoke for an hour to prove that the Renaissance was a purely religious movement.

I would be delighted to publish your first lecture. I published the first lecture I gave at Zurich as well as the first I gave at Leipzig and such discussions of principles are always very fruitful.

What I would like to do with the Bulletin is, to make Genevieve managing editor and to give her an editorial board consisting of people with whom she could consult and who would advise her. You obviously should be on it and I might be on it myself as liaison man with Europe. However, I think that it is better to wait some time until plans have ripened for the future of the Institute. I had a one hour's talk with President Bowman who was very diplomatic, made profuse notes, but did not say anything. Your name obviously came up but I have no idea what his plans are. The good thing is that the issue of my successor cannot be postponed because the temporary grant of the Rockefeller Foundation which amounts to $ 15,000 a year and represents almost 50% of the total budget expires next year so that the University is forced to act soon and to evolve a program that will appeal to the foundations. One good thing is that George Corner is on the Committee that is looking for a successor. He is a very decent person and one of the few who has a judgment in the matter.

One change we are going to do immediately with the Bulletin is namely, that we are going to publish it bi-monthly, 6 numbers of about 130 to 150 pages. The cost of printing is increasing so tremendously that we are forced to cut down somewhat. People will still receive more than $ 5.00 worth but we cannot increase our annual deficit. Six numbers instead of ten will also relieve Genevieve.

Berghoff's book, the reference to which you sent me, is here but it is no good at all. Berghoff was one of the last students of Neuburger in Vienna who managed to escape to Yugoslavia in time and is now somewhere in Dalmatia. He is a dentist, if I remember correctly and may be a good tooth-puller but his historical work is superficial and unoriginal.

Next week I am going to Princeton for one of the bi-centennial conferences, 3 days on "The University in World Affairs." It promises to be quite interesting, few papers and mostly discussions and the whole group will stay together in the same hotel. Toynbee from England will be there and Rappard from Geneva besides Ulich, Flexner, Compton, Day, and a dozen or so other people.

With all good wishes, I am

Yours as ever,

[Henry]

Artelt see S. to A. of 14 May 1946. Edelstein and Diepgen see A. to S. of 2 August 1944 and 2 May 1945, respectively. Von Brunn see S. to A. of 14 May 1946. Becker see A. to S. of 7 February 1947. Erlangen, German town near Nuremberg. At the end of WWII American and Russian troops met in Saxony, however, the Americans had to withdraw according to the treaty of Yalta. The Graduate week on Renaissance medicine at S.'s Institute took place in 1939, i.e., years before A.'s arrival. Bowman see S. to A. of 6 December 1941. S.'s successor, Richard H. Shryock, was elected in 1949 only. Dalmatia, the coastal part of Croatia. Toynbee see A. to S. of 25 July 1945.

New names, in alphabetical order:

Berghoff, Emanuel, Austrian medical historian (Berghoff 1946)

Compton, Karl T. (1887–1954) president of MIT

Corner, George Washington (1889–1982) anatomist and medical historian. In the 1940s in Baltimore as director of the Department of Embryology of the Carnegie Institution

Day, probably George P., Treasurer at Yale

Flexner, Abraham (1866–1959) reformer of medical education in the early 20th century

Norpoth, Leo (born 1901) S.'s publisher in Leipzig

Neuburger, Max (1868–1955) professor of medical history in Vienna

Rappard, William E., professor at the University of Geneva, Switzerland

Thomas, Karl (1883–1969) professor of biochemistry in Leipzig

Ulich, Robert (1890–1977) professor of history and philosophy of education at Harvard
Williams, Herbert U., pathologist

ACKERKNECHT to SIGERIST, Madison, 21 February 1947

Dear Henry:

Thank you very much for Artelt's address. Would you please be so kind as to send me the address of Norpoth too. I will try my best to help him, which, unfortunately, consists only of writing a few letters to France, where I have, nevertheless, still some connections which might be useful. I knew Norpoth as a matter of fact already when I came to Leipzig. We had studied together in Freiburg and Vienna. I always found him to be a very learned and decent kind of chap.

I did not make myself very clear in the question of using immunity studies in paleopathology. I was not thinking of direct evidence which has given nothing. I rather thought of indirect evidence as for instance in the case of malaria, where the different reaction of the negro at least to the plasmodium vivax, the smaller size of his spleen tumor, the existance [sic] of a monkey plasmodium, which can be inocculated [sic] in man, and a few other facts speak in favor of a very long existance [sic] of malaria in, for instance, West Africa.

I enclose my introductory lecture, and appreciate very much that you intend to publish it.

What will become eventually of the Bulletin, depends of course on the general development of the Institute, and of the person of your successor. Otherwise I think your idea is very good, and I am glad that there is a hope for me to get rid of my Schuman connection without too much noise. I am really very curious whether they will give your chair to your "Wagner" which after all, they should do.

I trust you have had an interesting time in Princeton. I ordered the series of slides which Clay and Adams have brought out for Medical History. Even as they are, they are useful, but the series is composed with an appalling lack of imagination. 222 portraits, and nothing else. And in addition at least 10% of the portraits are those of rather unknown men. I have written them a letter, explaining that one needs more for the teaching of Medical History than portraits.

I wrote three popular articles for Merck last year on Primitive Medicine, Medieval Medicine, and the Dawn of Modern Medicine. They had so many requests for the first two articles, that they have reprinted the whole series under separate cover. I found this rather encouraging. We have had here our little worries on the general and a more private scale. That the Regents who are Republicans refused a professor of Political Science because he was a Democrat, was not too encouraging. And that we might have to move in July again because the house will be sold, is not too nice a perspective either. But, otherwise, everything is alright [sic], and we go on liking it here very much. I hope you find time for your book, and are physically alright [sic].

Kindest regards and best wishes.

Yours as ever,

Erwin

Artelt and Norpoth see S. to A. of 14 May 1946 and 14 February 1947, respectively. Plasmodium vivax is one kind of the malaria germ. "Wagner": The name here may refer to Faust's pupil in Goethes *Faust*; A. certainly means Temkin as S.'s pupil. Clay and Adams, probably the Company for Instruments, Visual Aid Materials etc. The three papers of the Merck series are (Ackerknecht 1946b,c, 1947b).

SIGERIST to ACKERKNECHT, Baltimore ?, 26 February 1947

Dear Erwin:

Thanks ever so much for your excellent lecture. I like it very much and will publish it as the opening paper of the March number. I think you have presented the principles of medical history in a very plastic and original way. I am sure that the students are much interested in your course.

I have more students than ever this semester because they know that these are my last courses. I had announced a seminar in the sociology and economics of medicine but so many and so different students came that I have to split the group. I have now an introductory lecture course on the sociology and economics of medicine, mostly for medical students and I have an advanced seminar for students of the School of Hygiene that is also attended by a number of Government employees from Washington. It's a lot of work but since these are my last courses, I want to make them as good as possible. The book is suffering, however, and all I can hope for is to finish Egypt. Babylonia I will have to write up in Europe.

The address of Norpoth is:

Stabsarzt Doz. Dr. Leo Norpoth
Prisoner No. 1098568
Depot P.G. 205
Baccarat
France

This at least is the last address I had. The trouble is that the French like the Belgians and the Russians need the German labor. Rene [sic] Sand told me some time ago that without German prisoners they could not operate the coal mines of Liege [sic].

Nothing has happened yet as to my successor but I would appreciate it if you could send me as soon as possible a brief curriculum vitae and the bibliography of your writings. This may be needed all of a sudden. Sidney Painter is chairman of the committee to recommend a successor and George Corner is on it too so that the matter is in good hands.

The Merck reprint looks very nice indeed and I am delighted to have a copy of it. So much for today. Best wishes from house to house.

Yours as ever,
   [Henry]

A.'s lecture (Ackerknecht 1947a). Norpoth and Sand see S. to A. of 14 February 1947 and 18 July 1946, respectively. Liège, city in Belgium. Sidney Painter (1902–1960) Johns Hopkins medievalist. Corner see S. to A. of 14 February 1947.

ACKERKNECHT to SIGERIST, Madison, 1 March 1947

Dear Henry:

I had just sent off a letter to you when I received yours. Thanks ever so much, especially for the address of Norpoth. [xxxx]. Therefore longhand and short. I enclose a vita and list of publications.

I understand fully that you want to take your fill in teaching before leaving. Though I do not regard it as my main purpose in life, I enjoy it very much myself, more than I thought I would. I am, of course, sorry that this puts another stop on THE BOOK.

Yesterday night we met (at the house of a German sociologist, H. H. Gerth) Rudolph Kolisch, a very nice chap, who wants to be remembered to you.

Kindest regards and best wishes
> Yours as ever
>> Erwin

Norpoth see S. to A. of 14 February 1947. [xxxx] One sentence deleted as Chesney Archives' Protected Health Information. Hans H. Gerth, German sociologist, coworker of Max Weber. Rudolph Kolisch, probably the violonist (1896–1978).

ACKERKNECHT to SIGERIST, Madison, 4 April 1947

Dear Henry:

I enclose an excerpt of a letter of Otto Guttentag on his work in Germany, as you also have sponsored in a way this work, and as he is a very bad letter writer, and I don't know whether he gave you any reports so far.

These days I had a rather fresh [?] rating experience. I found in an old lecture of V. Ziemssen mention of unpublished papers of Schoenlein, including a treaty [treatise?] on the influence of political history on the history of medicine! Imagine of what interest such a treaty [!] would be to all, a treaty [!] written by a friend of Herwegh and Eisenmann, and a treaty [!] written by a man who, I think, published never more than 120 lines during his lifetime! But where might these old papers be now? I think the only man who would have been able to answer this question would have been Erich Ebstein. But if I am not mistaken, he died even before Hitler, and did not leave any spiritual heir.

With all these centenaries around, the Wisconsin centenary 1848, the German centenary 1848, the Black Death centenary 1348, I take to the custom of thinking in centenaries. And therefore don't forget that in May it will be 100 years that Semmelweis applied his new method. (For exhibition).

I am going on as usual with courses, etc., and enjoy it. Did incidentally Klebs ever tell you, why after all his father, in spite of all his accomplishments, never got the fame, that minor men achieved?

I haven't heard from you for quite some time. I am certain you are most terribly busy. But I hope that at least you feel well. Kindest regards and best wishes from all of us to all of you.

Yours as ever,
Erwin

Guttentag see A. to S. of 12 November 1945.
   New names, in alphabetical order:
Ebstein, Erich (1880–1931) German physician and medical historian
Eisenmann, Johann G. (1795–1867) German revolutionary
Herwegh, Georg (1817–1875) German revolutionary
Klebs, Edwin (1834–1913) German pathologist and bacteriologist
Klebs, Arnold C. (1870–1943) son of Edwin, physician and medical historian in the
   U.S. and Switzerland
Schoenlein, Johann L. (1793–1864) German professor of medicine
Semmelweis, Ignaz Philipp (1818–1865) obstetrician in Vienna
Ziemssen, probably Hugo von (1829–1902) German pathologist

SIGERIST to ACKERKNECHT, Baltimore ?, 15 April 1947

Dear Erwin:

Thanks for the letter of Guttentag that I read with great interest. It is very interesting and I can well imagine that his recommendations meet with some difficulties because the limitation of the number of students admitted to the medical school runs against the basic concept of the European university that is meant to be open to all people who have successfully completed gymnasium. But I suppose the time has come to make new departures and to recognize the medical faculty as what it is, a professional school like engineering or agricultural schools. The Russians went the whole way by separating the medical schools from the universities altogether.

Yes, a manuscript of Schoenlein on the influence of political history on the history of medicine would indeed be a most interesting document. Where could it be? Würzburg, Berlin, Zurich? Who knows. At any rate, I am making a note and will keep the matter in mind when I am in Switzerland although I am not too hopeful.

We have not forgotten the Semmelweis centenary and we have even anticipated it by publishing a bibliography in the December number.

I think that one of the chief reasons why old Klebs never was given the credit that is due to him was the result of his unbearable character. He antagonized everybody wherever he went. In Zurich where he was professor of pathology, he was thrown out of the Medical School because in the middle of the academic year he would spend entire weeks sailing on the Lake without even notifying his staff so that nobody knew where he was. He had a complete disregard for every convention and finally came to Chicago because no institution in Europe wanted him.

I think the case is by no means unique. John Billings deserves a great deal of credit that is usually given to Welch, Osler and other Hopkins men, but Billings had a very austere personality and no sense of humor at all in a world that appreciated jokes, and expected them from a great man.

There is not much to report from here. I am still very busy with the two-hour Seminar and the one-hour Lecture course and trying to finish a few things. Time is getting short. Emmy may have written Lucy that we, in all probability, have a house about 10 miles from Lugano. My mother is buying it for us. It is not quite definite yet but I could not wish for anything more. It is removed from the tourist traffic yet connected with Lugano by a small electric railway and it stands in the midst of vineyards. The place is Pura and the name of the house is Casa Serena. If nomina sunt omnia [sic] there could not be a better name for the kind of house I am trying to find.

>With kind regards, I am
>>Yours very cordially,
>>>[Henry]

Guttentag see A. to S. of 12 November 1945. Schoenlein, Semmelweis, Edwin Klebs see A. to S. of 4 April 1947. John S. Billings (1839–1913) medical historian and bibliographer. William H. Welch (1850–1934) pathologist, hygienist, medical historian. Osler see A. to S. of 12 April 1946. The Casa Serena in Pura became indeed S.'s refuge for the final ten years of his life.

ACKERKNECHT to SIGERIST, Madison, 26 April 1947

Dear Henry:

Thanks ever so much for your letter of April 15th. I wish I could be present at your speech concerning the future of medical history in this country. I hope it will be printed. Personally I am not too optimistic about the future. We are now in a decisive period for the establishment of our discipline in this country. If we succeed in having two or three more chairs during the next two or three years, I think we will be established. Otherwise our discipline may die a lingering death together with other humanities. In order to have established these chairs we need a united effort and leadership. Now that you leave us, where will we find such leadership? I am extremely skeptical that your successor, even if it is a competent man, which seems to me to be not certain at all, will have the same authority, the same dynamic spirit, and the same ability to unite the very different tendencies in our ranks.

In a time when you probably have hardly the leisure to read your letters, not to speak of answering, I am somewhat ashamed to write you long epistles. But I like to talk to you as long as possible and I also have a few practical points to puzzle. First of all, could it be possible that you could have sent to me twenty more copies of my malaria monograph? I am out of stock. You have always been very liberal in this respect, but I doubt very much whether your successor will be.

There is another problem connected with your return to Switzerland. As you know, I have still some debts over there, which I was unable to repay because of the regulations. My librarian creditor has now suggested, whether you might be able to take a smaller sum, let's say $ 100 with you and pay it out to her at the normal exchange rate. Eventually in arranging your books if you find such which you do not want to take with you, and which are in the Welch library, they will always be most welcome out here. Do not forget, please, that I am kind of a medico-historical Beaumont, and that every book is a treasure to me out here.

I am now very near completion of my collection of essays on primitive medicine. As you know, I don't want to deal any longer with Schuman. Which publishers would you recommend to me to approach in this case?

The reference of Ziemssen to the Schoenlein paper is to be found in his 26th and 27th Klinische Vorträge, Leipzig, 1900, p. 14. The papers were at that time in possession of Schoenlein's grandson, Graf Puckler. Ziemssen then had a certain Dr. Kerschensteiner – I wonder whether this is the later educator – working on them. Thus at that time they should have been in Munich.

Thank you very much for your very interesting information on Klebs and Billing [sic]. Eventually I am not going to read a paper in Cleveland, thanks to Dittrick. He never sent me an invitation, and the first I saw about the meeting was the program. When I wrote him, all he had to offer me was to read a paper by title, which I refused as being too silly. Nevertheless, the light preparation which I made for the paper, "Social Thought in French Medicine Around 1830", has paid. I think I have struck a mine. I found an enormous literature on public health, published in France between 1818 and 1848, and now obviously forgotten by everybody, even the French. What I will do with this material is, of course, another question, as it is mostly in Washington.

I have also started a little research on German "48'ers" in American medicine, and discovered to my very great surprise, that there were some very outstanding men, but that the bulk of those who achieved fame in American medicine, came over in the late 50's. These are mostly the specialists. Rosen in his doctor's thesis, deals already with the foreigner as a specialist in this country. By the way, in re-reading Rosen's thesis, I found it even more excellent than at the first time. It is a great pity that this study of his, which is undoubtedly the best thing he has ever done, has been published in such a form that it remains practically unknown. I re-read simultaneously Stern's "Society and Medical Progress", and I must say that this one loses just as much at a second reading as Rosen's wins. It is really terribly superficial.

I sent you the Guttentag letter without comment. But I would like you to know that I do not at all identify myself with his opinions. The measures they are taking over there I can regard only as dictated by dire necessity. Otherwise, in view of the amazing ignorance which I have observed in so many cases here, I would not feel so very superior in educational matters. All this talk about greater social obligations (the necessity of continuously begging for funds?) is sheer bunk. I feel that taking out medicine from the university and making it a professional school would be the end of humanistic medicine.

Yes, we heard from Emmy the wonderful news about Casa Serena. We congratulate you wholeheartedly. The whole thing really sounds as beautiful as a fairy tale. Kindest regards and very best wishes.

Yours as ever,
Erwin

Malaria monograph (Ackerknecht 1945). William Beaumont (1785–1953) physician and physiologist; he had a patient with a gastric fistula whom he used to investigate the gastric juice. Ziemssen, Schoenlein, Billings, Klebs see A. to S. of 4 April 1947. Georg M. Kerschensteiner (1854–1932) German educator. At the end of May the annual meeting of the American Association for the History of Medicine was held in Cleveland. Howard Dittrick (1877–1954) physician, medical historian, and collector for a museum of medical history. "48'ers": German revolutionaries of 1848. Rosen's thesis was published in book form (Rosen 1944). (Stern 1941). Guttentag see A. to S. of 12 November 1945. Casa Serena see S. to A. of 15 April 1947.

Sigerist to Ackerknecht, Baltimore ?, 2 May 1947

Dear Erwin:

Your paper [stationery] is getting fancier with every letter which shows that your Department is being established more and more firmly. Before I forget: you may receive a letter from a Dr. A. J. F. Zieglschmid who is professor of German at the University of Oregon. He has published a very interesting "Chronik der Hutterischen Brüder", a sect that was quite widespread in Central Europe in the 16th and 17th centuries and a number of its members settled in America, particularly South Dakota. The professor wants to publish a number of other documents and manuscripts concerning the sect among which there is an Arzneibuch of 1635. I hear that the book is based to a large extent on Paracelsus and the professor asked me if I could help him and advise him in the preparation of his edition or if I could recommend somebody. I gave him your name and address because I thought that you might be interested in the matter. I should think that the book must contain many elements of popular medicine. At any rate if Professor Zieglschmid writes you, you will know what it is all about.

My lecture on medical history in the USA is still in its embryonic stage. I wish to take advantage of the opportunity to say a few things that I have at heart and the address, of course, will be published as soon as I have the time to write it. I am not too optimistic myself and I am sure that a great deal will depend on what happens in Baltimore in the next few months. Genevieve showed me your letter and I only hope that your prognosis will not materialize although it very well may.

I am, of course, very glad to let you have 20 more copies of your malaria monograph. The book belongs to the Institute and I feel free to dispose of it in any way I please. You will receive the books from the Hopkins press directly.

There should be no difficulty at all in my taking a hundred dollars along for your creditor in Switzerland. I will continue to have a bank account in America since I will be receiving foundation money and I will transfer some money every month or every few months. A certain amount can be exchanged every month at the high exchange rates.

I was glad to hear that your collection of essays on primitive medicine is almost completed and I can imagine that you would prefer to have another publisher rather than Schuman. You will not be astonished to hear what happened to me. Schuman was to publish the new edition of my book on Soviet medicine and had made a contract about it with the American-Soviet Medical Society that I had presented with the copyright of the book. Schuman promised to have the book on the market early this spring and received the manuscript ready for the press last August. A few weeks ago, he notified the American-Soviet Medical Society that he was unable to publish the book as he had so many other financial committments, and so after nine months we had to look for another publisher. The Citadel Press will now undertake to bring out the book and a week after they had taken over the contract, the manuscript was already being set into type.

It is very difficult to advise you as to a publisher as you probably know better who handles anthropological literature. Under normal circumstances I would not have hesitated to bring it out in one of our Hopkins series but now that I am leaving, I cannot mortgage the future. Why not try Paul Hoeber (69 East 33rd Street, New York City)? He is still interested in medical history, is backed by Harper and I would be delighted to recommend the book. I will probably see him in New York next week and he will undoubtedly also come to Cleveland.

Kerschensteiner was the editor of the Münchener Medizinische Wochenschrift. As far as I remember, he was the son or brother of the famous educator. He died in the 1930's.

I feel as you do about the program of the Cleveland meeting and I told Shryock just a few days ago that I considered it very poor policy to have the entire program on invitation.

Time is getting short now, and yesterday at the Hamilton Street Club I started the series of farewell dinners and addresses. I hope that my stomach will survive.

We had an excellent Seminar on Chinese medicine. Hume had the good idea not to give the course himself but to bring a Chinese scholar along, Dr. P.C. Hou, who is not only a distinguished pathologist but a real scholar who knows the history of Chinese medicine. I am including a copy of the program.

So much for today and my warm wishes to Lucy and you.

Yours

[Henry]

Head of the mentioned sect was Leonhard Hutter (1563–1616), an orthodox Lutheran. Arzneibuch = pharmacopoeia. S.'s lecture on medical history in the U.S. was published (Sigerist 1948). Kerschensteiner compare with A. to S. of 26 April 1947. Shryock see A. to S. of 23 March 1945. Hamilton Street Club, a Club of Hopkins professors. Edward H. Hume (1876–1957) staff member of S.'s Institute.

ACKERKNECHT to SIGERIST, Madison, 7 May 1947

Dear Henry,

I was just reading over Deutsch on the great world citizen, and looking into the mirror, and wondering whether I should reduce a little bit my pilosities in order to become a better historian, when your letter arrived. Thanks ever so much for everything, the malaria reprints, the offer to transfer, the tips for publishers, etc. I'm looking forward to a letter from Dr. Zieglschmid. – I most sincerely regret that I could not assist at the Hou seminary [sic]. Will the lectures be published? It certainly would be worthwhile. I have a little material on all three problems, but I would welcome more most wholeheartedly. – What day are you leaving Baltimore? Fejos just wrote me that they will pay me a trip to New York, and thus I will go to Washington and look up my French public health literature and drop in at Baltimore on June 9th. – I wrote already to Genevieve about my teaching experiences, and wouldn't repeat it here therefore, all the more as these problems are now no longer so important to you. By the way, did you read B. Allen's "Medical Education and the Changing Order"? I thought it not bad and though he doesn't mention you, the influences are unmistakable.

As far as the successor problem goes, at second thought I feel that the story of the young man who shall develop, is perhaps only a piece of politics, and is to soften up people for accepting Larkey as the minor evil. I personally, since the time of Bruening, have always been opposed to all evils, minor and major. I feel that Larkey would be a first-class burial for the institute at which, it is true, a lot of alcoholic beverages would be consumed.

The primitive medicine manuscript is ready, and may, [sic] I ask you formally to give me the permission to re-publish the articles from the bulletin?

Looking forward to seeing you soon,

Yours as ever,

Erwin

Deutsch see A. to S. of 23 March 1945. Pilosity: hair growth. Zieglschmid and Hou see S. to A. of 2 May 1947. Fejos see A. to S. of 17 July 1945. Raymond Bernard Allen's book (Allen 1946). Larkey see S. to A. of 8 May 1945. Heinrich Bruening (1885–1970) conservative German chancellor 1930–1932.

ACKERKNECHT to SIGERIST, Madison, 3 June 1947

Dear Henry:

I enclose a manuscript which might be suitable for publication in the Bulletin. I was not so sure, but Urdang urges me to submit it. If you can't use it, you know there will never be hard feelings. I also enclose a little book review. I can proudly announce to you that I am now the only man in the United States who possesses the Buschan. My father got it for me after a two year's search. It's a well written compilation, and I was very satisfied to see that his bibliography is not better nor more extensive than mine though he had forty more years' time to collect it.

The dinner in Cleveland was an agreeable surprise to me. I had a wonderful day with Herskowits and Hallowell in Chicago. The children are still running slight temperatures, but up again, as they don't exhibit any other symptoms. Everything else by word of mouth next week.

Kindest regards to all of you.

Yours as ever,

Erwin

Urdang see A. to S. of 23 March 1945. Georg Buschan see A. to S. of 15 April 1946, (Buschan 1941). Melville Herskowits (1895–1963) and Alfred I. Hallowell (1892–1974) anthropologists.

Ackerknecht to Sigerist, Madison, 16 June 1947

Dear Henry:

This is my bibliography on Primitive Medicine as it stands now (without Buschan). I came back yesterday afternoon, finding everything o.k. (Lucy and children delighted with Emmy's gifts) As this was my first morning in the office, and a terrible mountain of mail, I might have overlooked some typing errors in the bibliography, for which omissions I apologize.

I got through my odd 60 books in W., but it was a terrific experience in view of the heat and the moisture. Villermé comes out of my studies as far more than just the describer of factory conditions, and strong influence on his contemporaries.

Thanks again for the delightful evening. Good luck to all of you
Yours
Erwin

Buschan see A. to S. of 15 April 1946. "W.": Washington, DC. Louis René Villermé (1782–1863) French physician and sociologist.

Sigerist to Ackerknecht, Baltimore ?, 19 June 1947

Dear Erwin:

When you were here the other day I mentioned the possibility that Yale University might appoint me Harvey Cushing Fellow in the History of Medicine. This was not correct and please do not mention it to anybody because I do not want rumors to develop. Actually I will get my fellowship money through Yale University but Cushing's name will not be involved.

It was a very great pleasure to have a glimpse of you. The packing week was quite strenuous and when the two lift vans were full, 80 boxes of books were left over that will have to be shipped extra. The storage company misestimated everything.

We are all set for the trip and only hope that the weather will be a little better than what we have now.

With all good wishes to you all, I am
Yours very cordially,
[Henry]

296

This is S.'s last letter from the U.S. before he moved into the Casa Serena in Pura, Switzerland.

SIGERIST to ACKERKNECHT, Pura, Switzerland, 6 August 1947

My dear Erwin,

Just a few lines to tell you that Europe is still a good continent and Switzerland a beautiful country. What I like particularly here is the lack of hysteria. Russia is obviously not popular, and the Neue Zürcher Zeitung writes regularly articles to denounce Russian wickedness. They are all written by Waldemar Jollos, who has written the same articles for the same paper ever since February 1917. The Labour Government in England is probably even more unpopular to the Neue Zürcher Zeitung because it is so much closer to home, and the English method of socialization seems much more dangerous to the conservative forces here than the Russian one. But Switzerland is very prosperous at the moment, having a regular economic boom, and so there is not much tension. The atomic bomb of which so much fuss is being made in America appears here like some kind of fairy tale.

We are delighted with the house. It is a little small, particularly for the many books, but we have all we need, and the location on the slope of a hill is simply beautiful with an overwhelming view on the lake and the mountains. I had to turn my desk around so that I would not have the full view that I find too distracting when I work. Now I look on a vineyard, have a visteria and a figtree right in front and a charming village, Neggio, with a hill in the background.

Pura is an interesting community of about 500 people. Most men are craftsmen in the building trade, masons, carpenters, cabinet makers, painters, decorators, stucco workers, who before World War I used to go to France every spring, work there during the building season and then came home in the early winter with their pockets full of money. They all have a bit of land with vines and corn that is usually attended to by the women, who in true Mediterranean tradition do all the heavy work.

I hope to be ready to resume my work on THE BOOK by September 1. By that time my library should be in working order, at least more or less. In the meantime I am writing book reviews and articles that you will find in the Bulletin. I am Writing 500 words a day as I used to do in the past, and from August 15 on I will gradually "raise production" to 1000 words a day. That should be my routine from September 1 on.

I remembered how you helped me moving the books on Cloverhill Road and how simple this was compared to what we have now, where I have not only all the books that I kept at the Institute, in addition, but also 27 boxes of books that I had stored in Basel for 15 years. But what a joy to open these boxes and to find many old friends that I had missed all these years.

I hope that you and the family are well, and I am anxious to have news from you.

> With all good wishes I am yours very cordially,
> Henry E. Sigerist

"Lack of hysteria": S. had suffered under McCarthyism in the U.S... Neue Zürcher Zeitung: the leading conservative newspaper in Switzerland. Waldemar Jolles wrote novels, books on Russian history, and translations of Russian books. "Delighted with the house": Casa Serena in Pura in the Italian-speaking South of Switzerland, near the Lake of Lugano. "Many books": About 10.000. THE BOOK: S.'s planned 8-volume *History of Medicine*. "1000 words per day": S. liked to plan his work in quantitative terms which often had to be revised or proved outright unrealistic (Bickel 1997). Cloverhill Road: S.'s address in Baltimore. "Basel": At S.'s mother's.

ACKERKNECHT to SIGERIST, Madison, Wisconsin, 14 August 1947

Dear Henry:

It's already two months since we met last, and meanwhile you have put an ocean between us. We have'nt [sic] heard directly from you, and we sincerely hope you have arrived safely and you can adjust yourself, as they say here, without too many difficulties.

I have just sent off my article on "French Hygiene 1815–1848" to the acting editor, but I am still so used to submitting every new child of my typewriter to you that I enclose a copy of it. This will show you what I have been doing during the last two months, and that I have been rather busy. I hope that you find time to have a look at the manuscript, particularly p. 23 ff. but I am obliged to warn you before hand that it's dull. It is not much more than an extended bibliography, although I hope that it contains some data and ideas that make the reading worth while. If I would have really developed the different parts of the article, I would have had to write a book, for which I have neither the inclination, nor the time, nor the appropriate material available here. Together with the hygiene stuff, I read a good deal of Saint-Simon, Condorcet and other French writers of the period, and enjoyed it very much. Now I have to turn into local history, and I cannot pretend that it is particularly pleasant.

For the time being, my health is, unfortunately, such that I cannot do much. We have all had our fifth infection, about three weeks ago. I had it last, and combined it with a nasty flare-up of an old sinus. Never mind! We have had a few hot days, but on the whole, the summer is far more benign than on the east coast. I could never have written this article in the same lapse of time down there during this season.

Besides working, not much has happened. People seem to be for the most part on vacation, and thus one gets little mail. Tant mieux! Perhaps you'll come across a Frenchman over there who would be interested in this French hygiene business, to follow it up and to develop it. It is, after all, a little paradoxical, after my experiences there, that I, of all men, should be advertising their accomplishments.

I very much hope that you are feeling good, that you have been able to start work on the book again, and that I hear from you soon.

Kindest regards and very best wishes from all of us to all of you.

Yours as ever,

Erwin

French Hygiene (Ackerknecht 1948a). "Acting editor" of the Bulletin of the History of Medicine after S.'s departure was Genevieve Miller, followed in 1948 by Owsei Temkin. Claude-Henri Saint-Simon (1760–1825) French social philosopher. Antoine-Nicolas Condorcet (1743–1794) French philosopher and politician. Tant mieux = all the better.

ACKERKNECHT to SIGERIST, Madison, 17 August 1947

Dear Henry:

"You beat me to it" I had just sent out a more detailed letter to you (with a carbon of my last opus) French Hygiene 1815–1848) when your letter of Aug. 6 arrived. Thanks a lot. That was the first authentic news we had from the Sigerist family from Europe, and we were very glad (though not surprised) to hear that you are happy. It made me a little more nostalgic than I am anyhow. How I would like to see Paris again and hear French instead of the native noises! Will it ever come true?

We pass now through the most disagreable period of the year in this country: summerheat, and the eternal diseases and housing insecurity become more annoying in proportion to the increase in moisture and temperature.

I was glad that you have resumed writing, and am looking forward to the results. I am also doing a lot of bookreviewing right now, unfortunately nothing very good. An "essay" of Leonardo on medicine and philosophy unbelievably bad.

Yesterday night we were at Urdangs at one of the here customary parties where there are so many people that you can't talk to any. Something transpired which I think is fairly typical: when the president wanted to submit Claget's [sic] appointment to the regents they found out that they had hired him without having any data on him (there won't be any except birth and graduation anyhow), this contrasts vividly with the fuss they raised when the problem was to get a foreigner who had a reputation anyhow. And with human material so carefully chosen we will build that great center of history of science research that you so generously advertised in your valedictory (as I was told by visitors: Janet Koudelka, and one of Edelstein's students, Cole)! And as I am bilious, a story which you might like to tell to those who want to become professors here. A Southerner was invited with Booker Washington in Boston. When he came home they asked him how he handled the delicate situation. "Well, I could'n call him nigger, I didn'want to call him mister, thus I called him professor." – You see its [sic] really hot here from the stuff I write. It's night, but still around 80.

Did you have a chance to give my regards to Dr. Gertrud von Waldkirch? I hope you will find more sensible things in my other letter.

Kindest regards and best wishes from all of us to all of you
Yours as ever
Erwin

"Carbon": Carbon copy. *French Hygiene* (Ackerknecht 1948a). Urdang see A. to S. of 23 March 1945. Marshall Clagett, historian of science. Janet B. Koudelka, librarian at the Hopkins Institute of the History of Medicine in Baltimore. Edelstein see A. to S. of 2 August 1944. Booker Washington (1856–1915) educator and activist. Gertrud von Waldkirch, probably a coworker of A.'s father at the Deutsches Literaturarchiv in Marbach, Germany.

Dear Erwin,

Many thanks for your letter of August 17 and also for that of August 14 which I just received. I am awfully glad that you reminded me of Dr. v. Waldkirch. When I arrived in Switzerland I planned to bring her the money personally, but then I was only a few hours in Zürich and had no time for the library. Afterwards, I forgot the matter, but as soon as I received your letter I sent the $ 100.– to Dr. von Waldkirch, who wrote me a very nice letter in which she spoke very warmly of your father. I assume that you have heard from her meanwhile.

Your paper is extraordinarily interesting, a real contribution that advances our knowledge of the history of hygiene quite considerably. I knew several of Villermé's books and had also browsed in Fodéré's big book. Clendening had a copy of it, and I remember spending a whole day once reading this book in the beautiful historical reading room of the University of Kansas. I wonder if anybody uses that collection now. Your paper mentions dozens of names that I had never heard before. I suspect very much that there was a similar movement in other countries, perhaps Italy, and it would be worthwhile to go into the matter. In Italy malaria was a constant challenge, and the drainage of the Pontinian Marshes was a much better job than that of Mussolini, who drained the land so much that nothing grew on it afterwards. In Italy, too, the Roman aqueducts, the Cloaca maxima, and similar ancient monuments were a constant reminder of what public health had once been. I also liked your very pertinent remark that the Swedes had once been the terror of Europe.

I am just reviewing a very delightful book on <u>Mexico en la cultura médica</u> by Ignacio Chavez, one of the few truly great clinicians of Mexico. It strikes me how different the Spanish colonization policy was from that of the French in Canada. You once wrote that the Canadian hospitals were nothing but "soul traps". Not so in Mexico, where there was no compromise and no wooing of the natives. Traps were not necessary. Either the natives became Christians right away or they were slaughtered without further ado. But once they were Christians, Spain gave all it had to give, – hospitals, foundling asylums, convalescent homes, schools, a university, printing presses, etc.

Things are going well here, except that my mother fell and broke a leg, and that I will have to go to Basel for a few days just when I was resuming work on my book. The fracture is fortunately not a complicated one, but at 82 this is not a joke.

The season is perfectly beautiful now; the heat is over; the weather is perfect still, and the grapes are ripe.

By the way, have you read Carlo Levi, <u>Christ stopped at Eboli.</u> I have just read it in Italian, and I am most enthusiastic about the book. Levi was a physician who became a painter and writer and was confined by Mussolini to a small place in Calabria. The book in which he pictures the people is a superb anthropological monograph besides being good literature. An English translation came out last spring and you will undoubtedly find it in the Library.

I hope that you have all recovered by now, – you better do before the winter sets in – and with kindest regards I am

Yours as ever

[Henry]

Von Waldkirch see A. to S. of 17 August 1947. Louis René Villermé (1782–1863) French hygienist. (Fodéré 1822–24). Clendening History of Medicine Library at the University of Kansas Medical Center. (Chavez 1947). (Levi 1945).

ACKERKNECHT to SIGERIST, Madison, 2 October 1947

Dear Henry,

Thanks ever so much for your letter of September 9, and for having settled the Waldkirch business. Thanks also for your appreciation of my paper – I was so very glad to have it. I myself have the feeling that at least it offered valuable material, but in my isolation I very much like to hear it from somebody else who knows better. The paper is, of course, primarily descriptive, but I have tried also to refer at least to the influence of philosophical tradition and the relations with social theory. I also feel that the parallels with clinical development and the influence of military surgeons are quite striking. The few allusions to the relations between Cabanis, Gall, and Broussais that I made in the manuscript rendered poor Temkin quite jittery. He sent me immediately page-proofs of his (by the way, excellent) Gall article to show me that he had not gotten the "inspiration" concerning these relations out of my manuscript. He definitely is a strange fellow.

302

In my bibliographical studies for this paper I did not come across any Italian material, but this, of course, does not mean that there does not exist some. Still, the Italians who had indeed the excellent traditions of papal physicians like Lancisi, lacked a few of the important stimuli for this movement in France; the industrialization, the experience of the Napoleonic Wars, and its condensation by military physicians. As always, the war had trapped a number of very good men in military medical service. Military medicine is very largely rather negative medicine, the chasing of goldbricks; thus there was only one way of positive medicine open to them, as it still is to the professional military medical men, <u>Prevention.</u> I think this is the reason for the great accomplishment of an otherwise not too brilliant branch of our profession in preventive medicine.

I trust that Clendening's books will still be used, as long as Major is around down there. Waters, who was lately down there and browsing in that library, told me that Mrs. Clendening, the poor, poor woman, has still not yet given the books to the library, as she hopes to sell them to them. They are somewhat reluctant to buy, as Mrs. Clendening, holding large lumber interests in this state, is not exactly needy.

Thanks for the tip to the Chavez and Carlo Levi books. I very much hope that your mother is better now, and the whole thing had not too much of a disturbing effect on your work. Here, too, now the weather is very fine. You know how lovely autumn is in this country, the best, if not the only, good season of the year. I'm glad to report that we have had no disease lately. We were out for a short vacation in August, and I took it easy also for two weeks afterwards, read French novels and went to the movies. We saw a very interesting Irish movie, "Odd Man Out". We had the National Student Conference here, at which occasion Lewis Corey gave a talk, rather disappointing generalities. We also had a big symposium on the use of isotopes in medicine.

Our greatest trouble for the time being is to find housing before November. I got a 15% raise, but, as you probably have seen from the newspapers, increase in prices continues to be so rapid that the effect is, unfortunately, not very great. I also have my first candidate for a doctor's degree. He wants to write on Greek and Latin terminology in medicine. Of course Edelstein would be a better sponsor there, but I think I will manage it, all the more as our classical philologist of the campus, Agard, is interested in the problem and also has written a little book on it. I'm preparing courses now and writing a little on the history of this school.

In October I go to a meeting of the History of Science and History of Medicine Committee to New Haven. Genevieve probably wrote you already about that, and about the Conant meeting in Princeton in December. I wonder what will come out of all their talking. Shryock has developed lately so many tender intentions for me that I almost suspect him of being inclined to take over your job in Baltimore.

We very much hope that everything is all right with you and the work is progressing.

Kindest regards and best wishes from all of us.

Yours as ever,

Erwin

Waldkirch see A. to S. of 17 August 1947. Pierre-Jean-Georges Cabanis (1757–1808) French physician and philosopher. Franz Joseph Gall (1758–1828) German brain anatomist. François Joseph Victor Broussais (1772–1838) French physician and physiologist. Temkin see A. to S. of 8 December 1937, was S.'s coworker in Baltimore. Giovanni Maria Lancisi (1654–1720) Italian physician and epidemiologist. Clendening (Library) see S. to A. of 9 September 1947. Major see A. to S. of 10 May 1945. Ralph Waters, AAHM member at Madison. Lewis Corey not identified. Chavez, Levi see S. to A. of 9 September 1947. Edelstein and Genevieve Miller see A. to S. of 2 August 1944 and 28 February 1945, respectively. Conant meeting not identified. Shryock see A. to S. of 23 March 1945.

ACKERKNECHT to SIGERIST, Madison, 26 November 1947

Dear Henry,

I haven't heard from you for quite a while. You will have heard from other quarters about some of the more external aspects of our existence as moving, diseases, and the committee meeting in New Haven. As far as the bunch assembled there is concerned, Guerlac was undoubtedly the most interesting. Personally he seemed rather ambitious. In technical matters he seems just as unreliable as the rest of them, Dean Stimson excepted.

During the last weeks I have been working rather steadily on my Virchow. Among other things, I have been going over 170 volumes of the Archives. And, in view of the fact that the old man produced more than 2000 papers and books, this is only the beginning. It is a lot of glutaeus work; still I like it very much. What I miss is the opportunity to discuss things with other medical historians. Paradoxically enough, I have now splendid opportunities to discuss anthropology, or general history, or sociology. Our contacts in this respect are really most gratifying, visits of my Chinese friend Hsu (anthropologist) from Chicago included. But of our group here, Urdang is too much concentrated on his darned pharmacy, (What a pity that such a good man picked such a rather secondary subject), and the two boys don't know enough details. Same holds good for the medical people here. Temkin is, as you know; my relations with Rosen are still rather ambivalent, although his accomplishments in public health should by now have bolstered his ego a little bit. So my best bet remains, for the time being, one of my students, a rather gifted and intelligent boy.

By the way, in reading a great number of contemporary material to Virchow, I have become rather certain of the fact that those Schoenlein papers I wrote to you about this summer must have been in the Leipzig Institute. I got this clue from Ebstein's "Aerztereden". Thus, if you ever hear of the Leipzig material turning up somewhere in Russia, please let me know. I would like very much to have a photo copy of that Schoenlein manuscript on medical history and politics. I am a little mad at myself that I could sit for years practically on these papers, without ever realizing their presence or value for my work. This background reading, by the way, is most depressing. In their speeches and autobiographies all these great scientists come out to be such terrible philistines and bootlickers of the "princes", that one can hardly believe it. Fortunately, Virchow makes an exception; and Waldeyer is a little bit better than the rest.

Nine third year students have signed up for my seminar (texts on contagion from Fracastoro to Koch). Unfortunately, I continue to be a popular lecturer, and "meetingitis" being one of the outstanding culture traits of this country, as you know, this takes up quite some time.

There is, of course little time left for non-professional reading. Still, I had time to enjoy Jacques Barzan's [sic] "Teacher in America". I found the man much better than his reputation. I like very much the new novel of Camus, "La peste". I just saw the catalogue of medical books of Huber, Bern, and was very much impressed. No American medical publisher could show a similar catalogue. Intellectual life in Switzerland must be quite active at present.

By the way, do you know the name and the approximate address of a medical man in Kansas collecting Virchow? Henry Schuman once told me of this man (he sold to him, among other things, the Virchow portrait by Lieberman). I am, of course, very anxious to get in touch with this man, and, on the other hand, I am no longer on speaking terms with Mr. Schuman as far as I am concerned. We very much hope that everything is going all right with you and the family. Kindest regards and best wishes from all of us to all of you.

Yours as ever,

Erwin

Guerlac, Henry E. (1910–1982) professor of history of science at Cornell University. Dean Stimson not identified. "Archives": Virchows Archiv für pathologische Anatomie und Physiologie und für klinische Medizin, founded 1847. (Ebstein 1926). Wilhelm von Waldeyer (1836–1921) German anatomist. Girolamo Fracastoro (1478–1553) Italian physician, anatomist, poet. (Barzun 1954). (Camus 1947). Huber, publisher in Switzerland. Lieberman: Possibly Max Liebermann (1847–1935) German painter.

Names mentioned before;

Hsu	see	A. to S. of 22 October 1946
Koch	"	A. to S. of 14 April 1945
Rosen	"	S. to A. of 27 March 1945
Schoenlein	"	A. to S. of 4 April 1947
Schuman	"	S. to A. of 27 March 1945
Temkin	"	A. to S. of 2 October 1947
Urdang	"	A. to S. of 23 March 1945
Virchow	"	S. to A. of 27 April 1932

SIGERIST to ACKERKNECHT, Pura, 22 December 1947

My dear Erwin,

I have not written for a very long time but now I want to wish you and yours a very happy New Year and hope that will find a permanent abode, at least so far as there is any permanency in this changing world.

I heard from you occasionally through Genevieve who met you in New Haven and now again at Princeton. You heard that she is leaving the Institute also, so that Temkin and Larkey will soon be the only leftovers of the ancien régime and will be able to do their business without being disturbed. If it continues like this, and the University cannot make up its mind, the Institute will soon become a completely sterile place, and this at a time when the chances are better than ever. When I first came in 1931, the general interest in the history of science was extremely small, while now everybody is talking about it, so that the chances of building up something are infinitely better. I know that there are still very few people who do serious work, but universities are paying attention to the subject, conferences are being held, the Cornell Press is launching a series of classics in science, and it would really be tragic if the Baltimore Institute with its splendid collections would go to pieces instead of doubling its activities.

Here in Europe and particularly in England the interest in the history of science including of course history of medicine is growing also. You probably read that a British society of the history of science has just been founded with Charles Singer as president. You probably also received or will receive soon the Archives internationales d'histoire des Sciences, which is a revival of Archeion subsidized by UNESCO. UNESCO furthermore is paying travelling expenses of all delegates (including American) who attend international conferences in the history of science. Efforts are made to revive the International Society of the History of Medicine, and Gomoiu plans to call an international meeting in Switzerland in the autumn of 1948. If we could get rid of the dead wood such as Laignel-Lavastine, Tricot-Royer and Gomoiu himself, some serious work could be done and some real projects could be launched.

One very tangible difference that I foresee in all such international work is the decided animosity of European scholars towards American scholars. I have seen so many symptoms of it recently that it struck me very forcefully. You know yourself how the French used to feel towards America, and when the Marshall plan comes through, which it undoubtedly will, to prevent an economic crisis in America, the Western European countries will not be grateful to America, but will hate her for having been humiliated. Seen from the European perspective the problem does not at all appear as one of West versus East, but much rather as one of Europe versus America.

I had an interesting visitor here some time ago who spent three afternoons with me, Paul Wandel, the Minister of Education of the Soviet Zone of Germany. You may have known him in the early days because he must be about your age. He was seriously ill and the government sent him to Switzerland for recovery, where he spent some time in a village close to ours. From him I learned a lot about the German universities, and the difficulties they had with the reorganisation. The professors who are still in their chairs are mostly old catholics or Deutsch-Nationale à la Diepgen, Hueck, etc. who either were too old to be pressed into the party or stayed out because they did not consider the Nazis "salonfähig". This is poor material to reorganize a university with, and a trained young generation is non-existent. At the University of Berlin 25 % of the student body is now of working class origin. Following the Russian example, they founded a German Academy of Science with full-time jobs and institutes. They did it by taking over what was left of the Kaiser-Wilhelm-Gesellschaft and the Prussian Academy. The other academies, such as the Saxon Academy, are now branches of the German Academy. You can imagine the opposition that was brought against all these new measures, but they are going on steadily. In Leipzig Hueck was dean of the medical school for a while, but was discharged as such because th [sic] opposed the government on every measure. On the other hand, they do not hesitate to re-instate former Nazis if they need them. Thus Schede, the Leipzig orthopedist, was re-instated recently because they had nobody to replace him.

It will amuse you, by the way, to hear that within a few weeks I was offered the chair of the history of Medicine and Science at the University of Berlin, Diepgen's chair, and the Chair of the History of Medicine at the University of Jena, the one that Meyer-Steineg formerly held. This was all before I had met Wandel and I would like to know who has been pulling wires behind the scene.

Here things are going their normal way. My mother made an astonishing recovery from a bad pneumonia and is at home now after four months in the hospital. We shall all be in Basel for Christmas.

This letter is so unduly long that I will write you about my work in the next letter. Volume I of the <u>History</u> is not quite finished, but should be soon.

Once more all good wishes to all of you.

    Yours as ever,

      [Henry]

Genevieve Miller (see A. to S. of 28 February 1945) left the Baltimore Institute to study history at Cornell University. Larkey see S. to A. of 8 May 1945. "The University cannot make up its mind": Hopkins did not fill S.'s vacated chair until 1949. Charles Singer (1876–1960) English medical historian. P. M. Maxime Laignel-Lavastine (1875–1953) French medical historian. Gomoiu and J. P. Tricot-Royer (1875–1951) were presidents of the International Society of the History of Medicine. Marshall Plan: U.S. plan for the rebuilding of war-ravaged Europe. Paul Wandel (1905–1995), a German communist who spent the Nazi period in Soviet Russia. Diepgen see A. to S. of 2 May 1945. Werner Hueck (1882–1962) pathologist; Franz Schede (1882–1976) orthopedist, both at Leipzig University. "Salonfähig" = fit for society. Theodor Meyer-Steineg (1873–1936) German medical historian. S. declined the offers for chairs in Berlin and Jena, then part of the Soviet zone of Germany. Volume 1 of S.'s A History of Medicine took years to be finished and eventually appeared in 1951.

Dear Henry,

Thanks ever so much for your letter of December 22. I was particularly interested in your news concerning international efforts in the history of science, that had not yet percolated to my backwoods. The understandable animosity of Europeans against Americans granted, I still hope that there might be some possibility of "harmony" in the history of science field. Eventually it will, of course, depend upon the attitude of Americans. Anyhow, it might provide us with a possibility of traveling. By the way, what about the rumor that you are coming over here this spring?

My "news" is of a far more homely character. I had to waste a week in December in reviewing the "great" new Mettler book for our State Journal. In enclose, for the sake of simplicity, a carbon of my review, which is as mild as I could possibly make it. I also reviewed the autobiography of Dr. Plesch, "Janos", for the Bulletin. A most disagreeable character. Princeton ended, as was to be forseen, without any results, and was a terrible and most tiring mess. The only good part of it was that I had a chance to read Jacob Burckhardt on the train.

I have finally finished writing the history of this school, which I had to do for our centennial year. The dullest thing I have ever turned out. Difficult to do anything else in writing the history of people with whom one has lunch every day. Still, the thing had one advantage in that I came into rather close personal contact with several members of the history department (Curti, Carstensen, Jensen) and through them I am now trying to persuade the historians to do something more relevant in this centennial year, that is, to make a symposium of 1848, not only on this country but on England, France, Germany, etc. I feel that a book of this kind might be quite interesting. I will have to take up the German "48"ers for my Virchow anyhow. Personally, I am also doing a little reading on two other '48 centennials which interest me even more than this one: the 1348 and the 1648.

Have you seen the blast on "Changing Medical Care in our Changing National Life" with which Edward A. Park, the retired pediatrician of Hopkins, came out in the December number of the Journal of Pediatrics? It is rather interesting in view of the fact that I remember having very violent discussions with the gentleman on the streetcar back in Baltimore concerning your attitude toward the problem. Now he has become almost a Paulus.

I remember vaguely a newspaper man called Wandel. This is probably the one you mentioned. By the way, did you know that George Sacke, the historian from Leipzig, whom you probably knew too, perished a few days before the end of the "1000 years" in a concentration camp? Another Leipzig historian friend of mine, (Schuerer,) wrote the sad news to me from London.

May I bother you with two technical details? All my attempts to sell my essays to commercial publishers (Macmillan, Hoeber, Charles Thomas) have failed. But I have now a chance to get a grant for it and to bring it out with the University of Wisconsin press. For that I need a statement of yours as the editor of the Bulletin that you authorize reprint of the articles. Would you please send it to me?

In my last letter of November 26th, I also asked you for the name of the Virchow collector in Kansas. Can you by any chance remember his name?

I am very much interested in the news about the progress of your work and hope very much that the first volume will soon be finished. Your house looks wonderful on the New Year card (for which we thank you very much) and it must be a delight not to have to shovel snow every morning in order to get out of the door. We still seem unable to get rid of the continued infection, which is all the more annoying as Lucy is now greatly absorbed by her teaching and studying. Very best regards to all of you from all of us.

Yours as ever,

Erwin

"Coming over here": During his ten years in Pura S. has never returned to the U.S. (Mettler 1947). (Plesch (1947). Princeton: A meeting. Jacob Burckhardt (1818–1897) Swiss historian. "History of this school": University of Wisconsin School of Medicine. Virchow see S. to A. of 27 April 1932. 1348 begin of the "black death" plague epidemics. 1648 treaties of Westphalia at the end of the 30 years war. (Park 1947). Wandel see S. to A. of 22 December 1947. George Sacke and Schuerer not identified, see also S. to A. of 23 February 1948. "1000 years": The Nazi leaders boasted their empire would last 1000 years; it collapsed after 13 years.

Sigerist to Ackerknecht, Pura, 23 February 1948

My dear Erwin,

Thank you very much for your two letters of November 26 and January 19. First of all, I would like to state emphatically that there is absolutely nothing to the rumor that I might come over this spring. I could not possibly interrupt my work at this moment and besides I do not plan to show up in America before I have at least 2 or 3 volumes of the History finished. Quite apart from the fact that travelling makes me very tired. When I can live peacefully here in Casa Serena I feel perfect and work every day until midnight without any effort. But travelling wears me out. I was a week in Zürich in January, where I had to give three lectures at the University. I could not refuse an invitation of my old alma mater. But once I was there I had to give five lectures instead of three, had to attend every day a lunch and a dinner, and it took me a week to recover from the strain. The weather, moreover, was disgusting. I do not think that any city in Europe has a worse climate than Zürich. First a Föhn that split your head, then rain and slush and you never see the sun in that city. I caught an awful cold on the second day, and gave all my lectures tuffed with drugs and trying to appear normal. So you see why I stay in Pura whenever I can. We had a delightful winter, unusually mild, and the sun shines almost every day. The local paper wrote that January had been a very bad month because the sun did not shine on 9 days.

I do not know who the Virchow collector in Kansas is. Why don't you write to Ralph Major who must know of him.

I wonder whether the Schoenlein papers were really at the Leipzig Institute. If they had been there, Sudhoff who never missed an opportunity to write a paper, would in all probability have written something about them or Ebstein would have published them. I hesitate to write v. Brunn because I have not yet resumed diplomatic relations with the Leipzig Institute except with Richter, the old Institutsdiener, to whom I am sending a food parcel every month. Did you hear that Diepgen has left Berlin and now has a chair at the University of Mainz. Schlau muss der Mensch sein! You see a good many Germans in Switzerland. I met the son of v. Brunn in Zürich; he had tuberculosis and managed to stay in Davos throughout the war. A few days ago we had the visit of the son of Hansen, who was formerly at Heidelberg with Weizsäcker and Krehl and is now in Lübeck as

Director of the Hospital. Yes, I did know Georg Sacke and I was sorry to hear that he perished in the last minute. I knew his brother the physician who wrote a dissertation on Zemstvo medicine, but the faculty refused him because he was a Communist. I once heard from him from Prague and heard that he had gone to Russia.

Congratulations upon the completion of your history of the Wisconsin school. I know what a nuisance this kind of work may be but I am glad to know that you are working on your Virchow. It must be an interesting experience to go through the 170 volumes of Virchow's Archives. After all, the entire history of pathology is reflected in them. Your review of the Mettler book is very tactful indeed; I received a copy of the book from the publisher's, but fortunately not for review, and all I had to do was to write them a polite letter. It is a terrible book, and I cannot understand how a husband can expose the abysmal ignorance of his dead wife in such a way.

I am glad to hear that you liked the book of Camus La Peste. I have half a dozen new books on plague here, and I will say a few things about Camus in this connection, because it is interesting to see that the subject still attracts good writers, and this is one of the best existentialist experiments I have seen so far.

There is little news here. I had hoped to be through with volume 1 by now, but am not and will still need a few more months. The first volume is the slowest. When I was about through with Egypt I heard that the Belgian Egyptologist Jonckheere had just published a 3-volume book on the subject. I ordered it immediately, but getting books in Europe takes many weeks. He probably did the work that Grapow planned to do. While the Germans [sic] scholars were busy with the war, those of the occupied countries were thrown out of their jobs, and had the leisure to do work of such magnitude. I want to compare his results with mine, and of course I am anxious to see whether he has some new material. This may force me to revise some chapters. If the book had come out 6 months ago, it would have saved me a lot of time, but I am glad that it came out now and not 6 months later.

I would very much like you to read my sections on Egypt and Babylonia when they are ready, because they fall to a large extent into your field. I have emphasized the magicreligious side much more strongly than my predecessors, in Egypt also. I disagree with Breasted in a great many points, and find him sometimes incredibly naive. Luckhardt was a poor adviser.

312

You are probably still buried in snow, but spring is not too far off, and I only hope that the family is well.

With all good wishes from house to house I am

Yours as ever

[Henry]

The enclosure to this letter is an authorization to reprint articles from the Bulletin of the History of Medicine. Föhn: Swiss name of a southerly wind. Ralph Major see A. to S. of 10 May 1945. Schoenlein and Ebstein see A. to S. of 4 April 1947. Walter von Brunn see S. to A. of 14 May 1946. Robert Richter: Servant of the Leipzig Institute. Food parcels: The post-war food supply in Germany was still poor. Diepgen see A. to S. of 2 May 1945. "Schlau muss der Mensch sein": Better be smart. Walter A. L. von Brunn Jr. (born 1914) medical historian, son of Walter von Brunn. Hansen not identified. Ludolf Krehl, German pathologist. Weizsäcker see S. to A. of 18 July 1946. Sacke see A. to S. of 19 January 1948. "Wisconsin School" of Medicine. Virchow's Archives see A. to S. of 26 November 1947. (Mettler 1947) was edited by her husband after the author's death. (Camus 1947). Frans Jonckheere (1903–1956). James Henry Breasted (1865–1935) archeologist and historian. Hermann Grapow, German egyptologist. Arno B. Luckhardt, physiologist and medical historian.

ACKERKNECHT to SIGERIST, Madison, 12 March 1948

Dear Henry,

Thanks ever so much for your letter of February 23rd. I was very sorry to hear that your coming here was only a rumor. One more reason not to go to this year's meeting in Philadelphia, where to go would be very difficult for me anyhow as I am still teaching at that time.

My suspicions that the Schoenlein papers were in Leipzig stems from the fact that Ebstein did publish a piece out of the lot (a speech of Schoenlein's in his "Aerztereden"). While I enjoyed hearing from Urdang that Artelt has been rehabilitated, I was rather nauseated by the idea that Diepgen got a chair in Mainz. But that is the way it works everywhere at all times. I am looking forward very much to the Egypt and Babylonia chapters of your book. These are undoubtedly some of the most difficult, but also some of the most fascinating chapters in the history of medicine and civilization. I never miss going to the collections either, in the University of Chicago campus or in the Field Museum when I pass through Chicago.

Right now I am very much absorbed by teaching. I give my introductory course, and my seminar on classic texts on contagion. As I have a nice group of seven intelligent students, I enjoy the latter very much in spite of the heavy preparatory work that it involves for me. I think we even bring out a few aspects in the history of the doctrine of the contagium animatum that had not been dealt with in the literature. Anti-contagionism seems to have been stronger than contagionism in the first half of the 19th century (partly for economic reasons), and it seems that Henle's fight looked to his contemporaries as a rear guard rather than as a vanguard action. Pasteur's successes brought a surprising change in the whole picture, that has often been projected into the past by later historians. I hope I will be able to write up some of this material, although I doubt it. Besides teaching there is still this lecturing for clubs, and a rather active social life. I have to prepare, between the two academic years, a report on 1848 in Germany (I "sold" my idea of a symposium on "1848 in Europe and America", but have to pay with making one of the speeches). At the same time, I have to write a Ciba number on the history of legal medicine for miserable money's sake. I will start out the next academic year with a new course on the history of diseases that will take up quite some time for preparation. I also have a second candidate for the M. D. thesis. This one wants to write on Wisconsin medical history. I am looking forward very much to the day when one will show up that wants to write on what I want him to write.

Have you seen the new book by Shryock on medical research? It is rather good; in spite of some repetition of book number one, not simply a rehash. I also very highly appreciate the absence of chauvinism in his books, so rare with most historians.

For amusement we read a book of E. E. Kisch on his youth in Prague that a friend sent us from Berlin. Kisch wrote it in Mexico. Provoked through an occasional remark on the otherwise miserable Berghoff, I read a biography of Campanella of whom I did not know much. A strange man, and a great poet.

Yesterday I had a visit by the "Chinese" Hume. He is writing a horrible book on medical missionaries, and has been squeezing me for about a year in letters. Now he came to do it in person. For 72 and a pernicious anemia he is doing very well physically. I guess that his intellectual limitations are no result of his age. They must always have been with him. His naive enjoyment of this world somewhat consoles me with his less lovable traits.

314

It is funny to listen to him over the phone, where he barks exactly like a Chinese.

Our bad luck in matters of health has been faithful to us. Sylvia has been out of school since Christmas. A continued low fever and increased sedimentation rate of unknown origin. They didn't even want to take her tonsils out; but those finally came out last Saturday, and now we are hoping for the best. All through the month of February my stomach was atrocious, and I had a hard time keeping up my teaching. Lucy fortunately keeps going in spite of her extraordinary, and for the rest of the family somewhat disturbing, activity as a teacher and student. We are celebrating our "spring" month of March with temperatures around -20. Really, why should you want to come over here? I very much hope I didn't write too much nonsense, and that you are in good health and the work on the book is progressing satisfactorily. Very kindest regards.

Yours as ever,
Erwin

Ebstein see A. to S. of 4 April 1947. *Aerztereden* see (Ebstein 1926). Urdang see A. to S. of 23 March 1945, Artelt S. to A. of 14 May 1946, Diepgen A. to S. of 2 May 1945. Contagium animatum: living contagious agent, see also (Ackerknecht 1948b). "Ciba": Ciba Symposia, a medical journal. Shryock see A. to S. of 23 March 1945 and (Shryock 1947a). Eugen E. Kisch (born 1885), his book on his youth in Prague not found in major libraries. Berghoff see S. to A. of 14 February 1947. Tommaso Campanella (1568–1639) Italian philosopher and poet. Hume see S. to A. of 2 May 1947, his book on medical missonaries has probably not appeared.

ACKERKNECHT to SIGERIST, Madison, 20 May 1948

Dear Henry,

I am taking the liberty of enclosing another brain child of mine. Two months ago the Fielding H. Garrison lecture was thrust upon me, and the only thing I could work up in such a short time were my studies on anticontagionism, of which I told you in my last letter. I hope the paper will meet with your approval. Besides teaching I have had no time during the last two months for anything else but this paper, and I am now trying frantically to work up what has been left undone. We also moved for the fourth time, and the children have been sick. Right now they seem all right. I'll write more after the Philadelphia meeting. Kindest regards and very best wishes to all of you.

Yours as ever

Erwin

Anticontagionism see A. to S. of 12 March 1948 and (Ackerknecht 1948b).

ACKERKNECHT to SIGERIST, Madison, 3 June 1948

Dear Henry,

I have just returned from Philadelphia. Let me give you a few impressions on the meeting. I proceed chronologically and assume that you have a program at hand. I came too late to hear the first three lectures (Jarchow [sic], Trent, and Bell), but have heard that they were competent. In the afternoon I delivered my own lecture, the text of which you have already received. I think it went off all right, although the audience is nor particularly inspiring.

The evening meeting on history in medical education was a good idea. Rosen's paper was solid, although a little dull. Leake's and Jacobs' discussion remarks lacked content. Leake made a much better intervention later on in the discussion. Heaton was rather refreshing in telling them a few frank words about so-called useful and so-called useless subjects in medical school, and that the solution of the trouble is in hiring full-time teachers and paying them a living wage. Shryock made a very good intervention. I have forgotten the rest. They had invited the five deans of the five Philadelphia medical schools, and two of the gentlemen (Jefferson and Temple) went on record in saying that only the "Oslerian method" could be practiced in their schools. This is, of course, sheer hypocrisy. They don't want to have any medical history taught, but can't admit it openly. I came out very strongly against this hide-and-seek game, and probably antagonized most people in being too outspoken, too young for this august assembly, too much of an outsider, foreigner, professional, etc., and in touching at the Osler taboo. Never mind. Somebody has to tell the truth.

The main result of the business meeting is Viets as President, Major as Vice-President, (both poor choices because of their inactivity). Spector as

Secretary is, I feel, an excellent choice. Forman as Treasurer is probably as good as any, and Temkin as editor will probably go nuts with his fussiness, but he will bring out the Bulletin all right.

Leake and Fulton were far more active in the organizational matters than I had ever seen them before. I have a sneaking suspicion that you had written them some "pep" letters. I think this was a most excellent idea, because the Association is not in a very good way at all and needs the active cooperation of all able bodied men very badly. I hope you keep them going, and I also hope that Shryock doesn't loose interest in the Association. These three are probably the key men in the Association right now. Norton and Spector are very reliable for technical jobs, but do not carry enough weight for more. Rosen, Temkin, and I seem not to be destined to play much of a role in the Association for many years to come. You should perhaps consider whether you couldn't interest a few more men in a more active participation in the Association's affairs. For instance, Emerson Kelly who I am sure would be very susceptible to a letter of yours, is a good man and as a prosperous surgeon more acceptable to the crowd than the above mentioned German trained trio. I also wonder whether some use couldn't be made of Galdston. Not very sympathetic as a person, but influential. I suppose that not much can be done about G. Corner; Trent really seems not bright enough and too much under the control of Henry Schuman, who, by the way, was absent. I have used my presence in the old nominating committee to obtain at least such a new nominating committee, and such additions to the executive committee that should not make it too difficult to carry out positive plans if you ever have such in the future.

I am afraid that you will have to have an eye on this child of yours in the future. The meeting was rather sad; it now was fully realized how much your absence and the paralysis of the Institute meant to the Association. A lot of resignations and no new members is a very bad sign. They have an entirely unjustified defeatism as to the Bulletin. The honors that the meeting bestowed upon you this time (honorary membership, toasts, etc.) were far more spontaneous than those of last year (when it was to many a formal affair), and really resulted from a general feeling of profound loss. I do hope that they help keep up your interest in the Association.

I cannot tell you about the afternoon paper, because I preferred to go to the art gallery and to read them in the transactions. In the evening the dinner speaker had let us down, but Chauncy Leake gave a technically excellent, improvised talk on medical ethics (of course nothing new to those who knew his writings.) Personally, I had a good time at the meeting, mostly with Rosen, Temkin, and Spector, but as said above, the impression of the meeting as a whole was rather disquieting. Kindest regards and best wishes from all of us to all of you.

Yours as ever,

Erwin

P.S. A suggestion of Middleton's to obtain either a new edition or a supplement of the Kelly-Burrage Dictionary was dumped into the lap of a committee with me as chairman. If I succeed in getting it, I really do not want to do the editing. Wouldn't that be something for Genevieve, or Bell, or who else? — The Army Medical Museum (Dr. Sloan) looks for a physician-historian (starts at 7,000, goes up to 10,000). Neither I nor Rosen nor Temkin are interested. Of whom would you think? I will suggest Fritz Lieben or Walter Riese. It is a vicious circle. Either there are no jobs or there are no candidates.

E.H.A.

Between dictating and signing the letter I almost kicked the bucket: intestinal obstruction, never mind, after 8 hours of hell my guts [...]. Unkraut vergeht nicht.

Meeting in Philadelphia of the American Association for the History of Medicine (AAHM). Garrison Lecture of the AAHM see A. to S. of 20 May 1948. Jefferson and Temple: Philadelphia universities. (Kelly-Burrage 1928). "Unkraut vergeht nicht": Ill weeds don't die.
New names:
Forman, Jonathan, member of the AAHM
Jacobs, Maurice, member of the AAHM
Jarcho, Saul (1906–2000) medical historian
Kelly, Emerson C. (1899–1977) surgeon, member of the AAHM
Lieben Fritz (1890–1966) author of a history of biochemistry,
Norton, not identified
Spector, Benjamin (born 1893) member of the AAHM
Trent, Josiah Charles (1914–1948) member of the AAHM
Viets, Henry R.(1890–1969) medical historian
Names mentioned before:
Bell S. to A. of 20 December 1945
Corner S. to A. of 14 February 1945
Fulton S. to A. of 26 February 1945
Galdston A. to S. of 2 August 1944

Heaton A. to S. of 23 March 1945
Leake A. to S. of 14 April 1945
Major A. to S. of 10 May 1945
Middleton A. to S. of 7 October 1946
Riese A. to S. of 27 November 1938
Rosen S. to A. of 27 March 1945
Schuman A. to S. of 2 April 1945
Shryock A. to S. of 23 March 1945

SIGERIST to ACKERKNECHT, Pura, 16 June 1948

Dear Erwin,

I can hardly believe it that I have not written you for several months, but this seems to be true and it just shows how time flies. I was terribly upset when I read your P. S. and saw that you had had an intestinal obstruction. It must have been an awful shock and of course very painful. With the guts you have, you must never get too far away from a medical center, which is rather sad for an anthropologist.

I was very glad to have your report about the Philadelphia meeting, and I wish to congratulate you most sincerely upon having been invited to give the Garrison lecture. I read your manuscript last night with very great pleasure and found it an excellent paper. One really has quite forgotten that the anticontagionists had a very good case indeed. I was particularly interested in the point you make that commercial interests had a stake in the matter. It had never occurred to me, but is is [sic] very true. Some time ago I was rereading some volumes of Casanova's memoirs and it struck me not only what a terrible nuisance quarantine was, but also that there were a number of loopholes. Venice was very strict as far as maritime quarantine was concerned, but if you disembarked further south, where there was no quarantine and entered the republic by land as Casanova did several times, you could escape quarantine, I suppose these were the corrective mechanisms that growing commerce developed as early as the 18th century. I am glad that your paper will be published in the <u>Bulletin</u>, which I hope will be continued. Chesney-Temkin Inc. bungled the whole affair badly or rather one should say Chesney did, because Temkin is probably too scared to do anything in the matter anyway. He is, moreover, in a very difficult position.

John Fulton, Chauncy Leake, and Shryock, I am quite sure, have the Association very much at heart, and I of course count on you, Rosen and the younger generation to play an increasingly active part in it. Spector was an excellent choice for Secretary, because he is interested in the matter, is conscientious and has time. He wrote me a long letter, saying how honore [sic] he felt about having been elected. Galdston is interested in the Association also, but you never know how much he is going to do. The symposium on social medicine we gave at the Academy more than a year ago and for which we had to rush in the manuscripts by special delivery has not even come out yet. Of course, I am pleased to hear that I am still remembered and it was very nice of you to elect me an Honorary Member. I sincerely hope that the Association will continue to be an active centre. A country the size of the U.S. with such an enormous number of physicians should really be able to have at least as many active members as Sweden or Holland.

The only meeting I will attend this year will be that of the Italian Society of the History of Medicine. They are having their convention in October in Milan, and Castiglioni is President, so that I could hardly refuse to join them. But it is a great nuisance because they expect me to read a paper in Italian and to write it so that it may be published afterwards, and at the moment I just have not the time for such extras. I suppose I shall speak on some problems of Egyptian medicine, translating a few pages from my book. There are some very good local studies that could be made here. My village has death registers since 1685 so that one could make a good study on mortality of a small circumscribed community. The history of the three epidemics of plague that ravaged the Ticino from 1525 to 1630 also remains to be written, but I will not touch any such thing until I have at least two volumes of the book written.

Volume one is nearing completion at long last, although it will be August until I am entirely through. I discussed Egypt in great detail because it was the first civilization that I tackled, and also because there is so much to be said about it. I devote much less space to Mesopotamia emphasizing particularly what is different from Egypt. I find the four Contenau books very useful. While I am finishing volume one I am preparing the outline of volume two, which I hope to be able to write in much less time because I have my method now well established.

Otherwise there is not much to report about us except that the season is perfectly beautiful and that Nora and her husband are with us for the whole summer, on their way to Rome. You probably heard that they are going to spend two years at the American Academy in Rome because Jack was awarded the American Prix de Rome. Sarton and his wife were here the other day. He has a new volume out, and we expect the Singers who both have volumes in the press and also Shryock who had two very good books out this year. What an activity! Genevieve and her mother will come at the end of August. Do not burden Genevieve with a new edition or supplement of the Kelly-Burrage dictionary. Since she has decided to get her PhD at Cornell I think she should concentrate on that and should not accept any special assignments. The project of course is a very good one. Why not make it a joint project of you and your students and Shryock and his students, Bell, Phyllis Allen, etc.

Switzerland is as peaceful as ever, and if one did not read the papers one would not know that anything is wrong with the world.

My love to you all.

 Yours as ever,
  [Henry]

P. S. I was interested to hear that the Army Medical Museum has a job available with such a good salary and that nobody is interested in it, but I really could not encourage anybody to consider a government job under the present circumstances. If you do you can be sure to have the FBI after you all the time unless you are an outspoken fascist. They would probably even suspect Temkin of being a Bolshevik because he was born in Russia.

(Casanova 1930). Alan M. Chesney (1888–1964) professor and dean at Johns Hopkins School of Medicine. For names mentioned before see A. to S. of 3 June 1948. "Association" AAHM, see A. to S. of 3 June 1948. "Academy": New York Academy of Medicine. Arturo Castiglioni see A. to S. of 3 April 1946. The Milan paper has not been published. S.'s A History of Medicine: Once more his gross miscalculation as to completion of volume I. Georges Contenau, see A. to S. of 25 November 1946, published on Assyria and Babylonia, see S. to A. of 10 July 1948. S.'s daughter Nora married the composer Jack Beeson. (Sarton 1948). Charles Singer (1876–1960) English medical historian; his wife Dorothea. (Singer/Rabin 1946). (Shryock 1947a,b). (Kelly-Burrage 1928). Phyllis Allen, medical historian. The P. S. shows S.'s disgust with McCarthyism of the late 1940s.

Dear Erwin,

I remember that you once told me that the American Geographic Society was preparing an atlas of diseases. I would greatly appreciate it if you could give me any details about it, because I would like to mention it in my book.

Cordially as ever
     Yours
          [Henry]

SIGERIST to ACKERKNECHT, Pura, 10 July 1948

Dear Erwin,

Yesterday I received the March/April number of the Bulletin and today your reprints came, and I wish to tell you how deeply I appreciated it that you dedicated your splendid paper on Hygiene in France to me with such warm words and in a language that is dear to both our hearts.

I also received your review of my article on Brunschwig. It is really nothing new, but I am glad to know that you got a copy because I had only very few.

At present I am deep in Babylonia and find Contenau's four books very useful. You probably saw his most recent opus La magie chez les Assyriens et Babyloniens, Paris, Payot, 1947. I quite agree with you that his book on medicine is a very good piece of work, and to me it is also a kind of insurance that I am not going to miss any important new literature.

I am also reading with much pleasure The Intellectual adventure of ancient man, published a couple of years ago by members of the Oriental Institute of the U. of Chicago (Frankfort, Wilson, Jacobson, Irwin). I like particularly the perfectly beautiful versions of Babylonic poems by Mrs. Frankfort.

I just bought The heathens; primitive man and his religions by William Howells, Doubleday, 1948, but have not had a chance to read it yet. He is one of your Wisconsin men. What do you think of the book?

Dr. Reucker, the editor of the Ciba journals in Basel, was here yesterday. He knows a lot about medical history and his first suggestion was that somebody should make a new Bartels, whereupon I told him that you were going to write THE book on the subject. He has a staff of 60 people and from his office he conducts Ciba publications in half a dozen different languages. They finance Gesnerus and the Swiss Academy of Medical Sciences because they and the other chemical factories make so much money that they hardly know what to do with it.

Shryock and his wife are in Lausanne and I expect them in the near future although it is not quite sure that they will come, because the American military government wants him to lecture in Germany. Next week I expect an Ethiopian doctor, who just graduated at the U. of Zurich. I think there are only 2 or 3 Western-trained Ethiopian physicians at the moment. Victor von Weizsäcker, the Heidelberg clinician is coming Sunday, so that we actually have a lot of what is going on in the world. But the more I know the more I bless my village.

Cordially as ever yours,
[Henry]

Hygiene in France (Ackerknecht1948a); his dedication: "A Henry E. Sigerist qui a guidé mes débuts dans l'histoire de la médecine en témoignage de mon affection et de ma reconnaissance". S.'s Brunschwig article (Sigerist 1946d). (Contenau 1947). (Frankfort et al.1949). (Howells 1948). Karl Reucker (1890–1961). (Bartels 1893). Gesnerus: Swiss Journal of the History of Medicine and Sciences, founded in 1943. Weizsäcker, Victor von see S. to A. of 18 July 1946. S.'s numerous visitors in Pura provided a connection to the outside world but also contributed to the slow progress of his opus magnum.

ACKERKNECHT to SIGERIST, Madison, 15 July 1948

Dear Henry:

Thanks ever so much for your letter of June 16 and your line of June 25. I apologize for answering only so late. But I have been sick practically ever since June 2nd; after the intestinal accident, it became obvious that my bladder is about as rotten as my GI-tract, I had to undergo an operation on June 22nd, and have started working again only yesterday. It wasn't too funny, and I cursed especially the loss of time.

In a conference held on May 20, 1944, in which participated about 20 medical men and geographers, the American Geographical Society decided to bring out an Atlas of Diseases, dealing with cholera, the typhoid group, malaria, yellow fever, goiter, plague, beri beri and pellagra, filiarasis [sic], encephalitis, and schistosomiasis. The Atlas is destined to be primarily a tool of research. The driving spirit is Richard U. Light, a neurosurgeon from Kalamazoo, Michigan, ignorant, but wealthy and dynamic. A short report on the conference and the plan for the atlas are given in an anonymous article: "A Proposed Atlas of Diseases", Geographical Review 34: 642–652, 1944. In later numbers of the Geographical Review, which unfortunately were available to me today, because they were with the binder, there were signs that work on the atlas had actually started. The conference adopted a rather lukewarm attitude toward the incorporation of historical maps. The maps are to deal primarily with the relation between environment and disease.

Because of my sickness I have not been able to do much since I wrote you last, although I have started working on a series on the history of legal medicine for Ciba, and I hope to be able to travel to Baltimore and Washington at the end of the month in order to look up the literature which we do not have here. In bed I read lots of books, but unfortunately it was all bunk except for the Whitehead "Science and the Modern World", that has now come out as a Pelican book and that contains some fine historical insights. I read also a very good German biography of Georg Buechner by a certain Hans Meyer.

Thanks for your comment on my Anticontagionism. It is not difficult to see the economic motive in the first half of the nineteenth century, because people had still a good conscience, and were very outspoken about it. The hypocrisy in this field starts only later, when self confidence is shaken. As far as your comments on the Association go, I am afraid that your appreciation of Iago Galdston is correct.

Lately I ran into a discovery of Pasteur (in his work on fermentations) on the bacteriostatic effect of onion juice, which might amuse you as completing and somehow explaining Paré's empiric observation.

Lucy and the girls go for a swim – one of the lakes is only fifteen minutes from our home – every morning, and look wonderful. In the evening Lucy goes to the library. We very much hope that you all have a good time with your visitors, and that on the other hand interference with your work doesn't make you too unhappy. I hope you received my reprints meanwhile. Kindest regards and very best wishes to all of you from all of us.

Yours as ever,

Erwin

(Whitehead 1947). (Meyer 1946). Georg Buechner (1813–1837) German poet, revolutionary, and physician. Galdston and Pasteur see A. to S. of 2 August 1944 and 25 November 1946, respectively. Ambroise Paré (ca. 1510–1590) French surgeon.

SIGERIST to ACKERKNECHT, Pura, 2 August 1948

My dear Erwin,

Thanks ever so much for your letter of July 15. I was terribly sorry to hear that you had an operation. What a family you are! I do not think that I have had one letter which did not report of somebody's illness. At any rate I am glad to know that you have recovered, and I sincerely hope that the end of the summer will be better than ist beginning.

Thanks very much for the information about the Atlas of Diseases. This is just what I needed. Of course, I was most excited to hear that Pasteur already found that onion juice has a bacteriostatic effect.

I expected Shryock and his wife, but he suddenly got scared about the Berlin situation and thought that war would break out at any moment. So he sailed back to America on the first opportunity. I had a long telephone call with him, and I suspect that the American embassy frightened him. He was caught by the last war, und gebrannte Kinder scheuen das Feuer. In my opinion, there is no chance in the world of having a war at this time, because nobody could possibly afford one, certainly not Russia.

Nils Bohr recently said to a friend of mine that 50 atom bombs dropped anywhere on the globe would be enough to sterilize the whole of mankind. One bomb dropped at Bikini was sufficient to increase radioactivity so that it could be measured at Copenhagen. Generals usually are idiots, but there are limitations even among idiots and I am quite sure that nobody is foolish enough to start a war now.

Genevieve will be sailing soon, and I expect her and her mother here around the 20th of August. It will be a very great pleasure to see her and get through her the latest news from the States.

I sincerely hope that your guts will behave in the future, and with all good wishes to yourself and the family

I am yours as ever

[Henry]

Pasteur see A. to S. of 25 November 1946. "Berlin situation": Although located in the Soviet zone of post-war Germany, Berlin, like Germany as a whole, was divided into four sectors; in June 1948, the Soviet Union attempted to control all of Berlin by cutting surface traffic to and from West Berlin. The Truman administration reacted with a continual daily airlift.

"Gebrannte Kinder scheuen das Feuer": Burnt children shun the fire. Nils Bohr (1885–1962) Danish physicist. Bikini: A Pacific atoll where the first American H-bomb had been tested in 1948.

Ackerknecht to Sigerist, Madison, 10 August 1948

Dear Henry:

Thanks ever so much for your letter of July 20. I have just returned from a week's expedition to the libraries of Baltimore and Washington. I was extremely lucky insofar as it was unusually cool, and I was rather satisfied with the amount of material I collected. Otherwise the Institute is really an incredibly sad sight to see. It reminds one of the abandoned mining towns in the West, or a dead village in France. Temkin is as usual, or even worse. It is to be hoped that this state of affairs will now soon be finished, and as they have a new president for January 1, Detlef Bronk (neurophysiologist from Pennsylvania), who has a reputation of being a good and intelligent man. Streeter died recently at 75; and so did George Corner's daughter, a Yale student, within a few days from acute leukemia. I was again fascinated with the Hopkins collection. It is really a pleasure to work there, and people who have it at their disposal don't know how much time and trouble they are saved. Although you are probably better off than I am so far as books go, you probably are having a similar experience now. The Army Medical Library in Washington is just as inefficient as ever.

Karl Pelzer, whom you might remember from Hopkins (the geographer who was kicked out by Bowman because his wife worked with the National Association for the Advancement of Colored People) was here for a few days, and gave a few very good lectures. He is now at Yale.

I have heard a lot about the "Intellectual Adventure of Ancient Man", but unfortunately didn't yet get around to reading it. The "Heathens" by Howells seems to me a well written compilation without any ideas of his own. It is a rehash of Howells' Harvard teacher Toller [?], just as his book

326

on physical anthropology is a rehash of his Harvard teacher Hooton. Howells is a competent physical anthropologist from a very old and wealthy New England family, deaf, and not much else to say about him.

We hope that the book and everything else is going all right. Kindest regards and best wishes from all of us to all of you

Yours as ever

Erwin

A. is referring to S.'s letter of July 10, not July 20. Detlev Bronk (1897–1975) President of Johns Hopkins University. Edward C. Streeter (1874–1947) medical historian. Corner see S. to A. of 14 February 1947. Bowman see S. to A. of 6 December 1941. *Intellectual Adventure* ... (Howells 1948). Hooton see A. to S. of 6 August 1945.

ACKERKNECHT to SIGERIST, Madison, 17 September 1948

Dear Henry;

Thanks ever so much for your letter of August 2nd, which arrived just when I had written you. Meanwhile I have finished my series on the history of legal medicine, and been busy with the German revolution of 1848. It is painful, but interesting. Many things have happened since I studied the problem in 1930 which give me another outlook; quite some books have also appeared, especially the great standard work by Veit Valentin (two volumes). It is a rather good book (Valentin also brought out a quite readable one-volume German history in English before he died as an (Aryan) refugee in this country last year). Of course, he was a German liberal professor with all that is implied by this status, and I personally prefer a more masculine author like Ricarda Huch. Valentine is still forceful compared to Lamprecht and the other professors who are just as exasperating as their 1848 ancestors in their queer mixture of talent and servility. In this whole 1848 literature, contemporary and later on, Marx and Engels with whom I disagree on a great many points in the 1848 question, nevertheless are of a rare maleness and consistency. In working on 1848 I have discovered, by the way, that my beloved Levy-Bruhl who had gone into anthropology only in his fifties (he died in his eighties) has written a very fine little book on the development of national consciousness in Germany between Leibnitz and 1848. (He has also written fine books on Comte and Gall besides his purely philosophical books.)

I took at least one week off in August, swimming, doing water colors, going with the children to the drugstore for ice cream sodas, and reading nothing but French and nonprofessional books (I am a Simenon addict, and like Fr. Mauriac very much, although I don't know why; so far nobody has been able to discover a trace of Catholicism in me). I remain also fascinated by the Utopian St. Simon.

It is not difficult to spend a fine vacation in Madison, if one only takes the time off. You might have seen that Life in one of its last numbers has declared Madison the best spot to live in the United States. Which, as much as I like Madison, is not exactly complimentary to the rest of American cities. LeCorbeiller, a Harvard physics professor, former "polytech-nicien" who visited us recently driving home from California, has the interesting theory that in order to enjoy travelling in this country, one should not stick to the European pattern of looking for an (inexisting) history crystallized in buildings, but rather observe geology, in order to get the same emotions out of this country. One of our students died from polio (thirty, two small children), though we have had so far only three cases in town; but they are plentiful in Milwaukee, California, etc.

I do not believe either in the immediate danger of war, because the Russians are too weak to start one at the moment, and I do not feel that this country will start one. But of course in a situation like in Berlin accidents can happen, and it is really difficult, and not very popular either, to keep one's mind cool, within the periodical outbursts of war hysteria that we have been witnessing here during the last few months.

Have you seen the last book of Bernard I. Cohen? It is interesting, but, I am afraid, not as good as it should be in view of the author. Cohen is really among the very few interesting people I know in the history of science, a fine scholar and a most delightful person.

In spite of all we have had a good summer (I have still some trouble with my reflux into the right kidney, but am otherwise all right). Now unfortunately the old winter routine starts again: "preaching" with little time for research, children going to school and being infected with the native manners and bugs, Lucy teaching and studying, etc., etc. We hope you are all doing well.

Kindest regards and very best wishes from all of us to all of you.

Yours as ever,

Erwin

328

A.'s history of legal medicine was published in 1951 only (Ackerknecht 1951a). 1930: (Ackerknecht 1931). (Valentin 1930–31). (Levy-Bruhl 1890). Gall and Saint Simon see A. to S. of 2 October 1947 and 14 August 1947, respectively. LIFE magazine. Cohen see A. to S. of 24 October 1946. (Cohen 1948),

New names:
Comte, Auguste (1798–1857) French philosopher and sociologist
Engels, Friedrich (1820–1895) German social economist and politician
Huch, Ricarda (1864–1947) German poet and historian
Lamprecht, Karl, German revolutionary leader in 1848
Le Corbeiller, Philippe (1891–1980) Harvard physicist
Leibniz, Gottfried W. (1646–1716) German philosopher and mathematicien
Marx, Karl (1818–1883) German social economist
Mauriac, François (1885–1970) French writer
Simenon, Georges (1903–1989) Belgian writer

SIGERIST to ACKERKNECHT, Pura, 18 September 1948

Dear Erwin,

I just notice that I have not answered your letter of August 10, but there was not very much to report recently. We had a lot of American visitors including a number of old Hopkins students. There seems to be a stream of American students going to Prague and Eastern Europe, you can imagine what brand, and the way apparently is via Pura. Horsley Gantt was here also last week, an old crony of the Hamilton Street Club, and Genevieve and her mother spent several weeks in the neighborhood, so that I feel very up-to-date with the latest American gossip.

Genevieve must have had a very hard time at the Institute during the past year. Our friend O. T. seems to be more difficult than ever, and I am very much afraid that he will get the job after all. This would be very much in the Hopkins tradition. First you do nothing for a year or two, then you ask a few people who refuse and finally you appoint the local man at the lowest possible salary. This is what happened in medicine, pediatrics, pathology, ophthalmology, etc. You undoubtedly know that the Institute was offered to Shryock and that the University approached the Rockefeller Foundation for an annual grant of $ 50,000. There is a chance that they may get 30,000 a year, but no decision is expected before January and Shryock therefore has not given any answer yet. With 30,000 from the Foundation and close to 20,000 from endowment the Institute would have almost twice as much as I ever had, and with such a budget a great deal could be done. However, I am not sure that Shryock will accept, because he is deeply rooted in Philadelphia, where he has all he wants. Hopkins offered him $ 12,000 a year, 2000 more than I had, but this is not much more than his present salary. And if Shryock does not accept, the Rockefeller money will not come forth, and Temkin will then be the automatic choice. (This, of course, is all very confidential.) Shryock has inhibitions also because he is not a medical man, but I am sure that the AMA would much rather swallow a PhD than a member of the fraternity. In these days of nationalism and narrow parochialism it might be quite good for the Institute to have a native-born American who has no foreign accent, who is a good administrator, could raise funds and make friends. With a budget of 50,000 moreover, he could appoint a staff of competent people who could carry out the research. I was astonished to hear that Chesney is very much against Temkin, while Corner is very much for him. Well, we shall see what happens.

Hopkins should be congratulated that the trustees appointed neither a general nor an admiral as president, and Bronk is probably a brilliant man. Still, I deplore that universities seem to think that a president must be a scientist and if ever possible a physicist. The sciences are well taken care of anyway, and I would much rather see a humanist or social scientist at the head of an important university.

I am still not quite through with Babylonia, and I curse the fact that Campbell Thompson never collected his papers in one book. The whole literature, as you know, is scattered in dozens of short articles in a variety of journals, and I always hesitate to put on the finishing touches before I have all the material in hand.

From Germany I hear a lot; Diepgen, v. Brunn and whoever is left of the old guard are writing long letters. Of course, nobody has ever been a Nazi in Germany, as you well know, and they all have always been my very dear friends (although they kicked me out of the German society) and they all hope that I will send them foodparcels.

I think I wrote you that Verlag Werden und Wirken in Weimar, the Thuringian State Publishing Company, wanted to publish German editions of four of my books, a new edition of <u>Grosse Aerzte</u>, <u>Civilization and Disease</u>, <u>Medicine and Health in the Soviet Union</u>, and a collection from the papers that I published in America during the last 15 years. The first was to be the new edition of <u>Grosse Aerzte</u>. All of a sudden, they had a new director who came from a training school of the Sozialistische Einheitspartei, and altough he had never seen my book because they have no copy of it he nevertheless decided that a book that had once been published by Lehmann in Munich could not possibly be any good, whereupon I told them to go to hell. In the meantime, the Hippokrates-Verlag in Stuttgart wants to publish <u>Medicine and Human Welfare</u> and has also applied for the German rights for the <u>History of Medicine.</u>

Hoping that you had a good summer, not too hot and with no illness in the family and with all good wishes I am

Yours as ever,

[Henry]

P. S. You may be interested in the publication mentioned on the enclosed card.

HES

Horsley Gantt (1892–1980) physiologist, student of Pavlov, later at Johns Hopkins. "That he will get the job" as S.'s successor. AMA: American Medical Association. Chesney and Corner see S. to A. of 16 June 1948 and 14 February 1947, respectively. Bronk see A. to S. of 10 August 1948. Campbell Thompson (1876–1941) British archeologist and assyriologist. Diepgen see A. to S. of 2 May 1945. Von Brunn see S. to A. of 14 May 1946. "German society" of the History of Medicine and Sciences. S.'s books mentioned are (Sigerist 1932,1941a, 1943, 1947).

ACKERKNECHT to SIGERIST, Madison, 14 October 1948

Dear Henry:

Thanks ever so much for your letter of September 18th. I sure enough wrote you on the same day. Thanks for the dope on the Institute situation. I am not so sure that Temkin will get it even when Shryock turns it down. God knows what new tricks they will cook up. In any case it is a pity to see the place wrecked this way.

It would certainly be better to take non-scientists for University presidents, but as we have already reached the level of generals and unsuccessful politicians, one has to be grateful if it is at least a scientist. Diepgen and Co. are really nauseating. I quite accidentally acquired here recently a little pamphlet of 1937, Introduction into the Study of Medicine, and sure enough it contained the usual thing about the blessings of national socialism written by – Diepgen.

I am not too much surprised by your adventures with the Thuringian State Publishing Company. The stupidity and cowardice of bureacrats [sic] and dogmatists prevails usually independent of their official color. Reprinting especially of The Great Doctors would have been very much worthwhile. It is good to hear that at least Medicine and Human Welfare will come out. I just reread it for some lectures, and found it an extremely rich and stimulating little book again. Thanks for the tip on the German book on primitive mentality.

Teaching has started again, and the first weeks were quite busy with my leading off other people's courses with historical introductions, a method I approve of in principle, but I dislike in practice. Fortunately it's over and I can now concentrate on my course and studies on the history of diseases. (I fortunately finished my paper on 1848.) Right now I am trying to catch up with the newer plague literature. I will also give a lecture on the historical role of diseases for The Viking Fund at New York on December 3rd. From several suggestions for a seminar next semester, my students have to my surprise not picked the clinical, but the philosophical subjects. Thus we will read Hippocrates' On Ancient Medicine; Paracelsus' The Defensiones; Cabanis On Certitude; Blane's and Oesterlen's Medical logic; Bartlett's Philosophy of Medicine; we will spend a great deal of time on Bernard's Introduction to Experimental Medicine, and we shall close with Charcot's general chapter in his Senile Diseases, and Albutt's [sic] short introduction to his Systems of Clinical Medicine. In this whole seminar business as I am practising it one is of course greatly handicapped by the paucity of translations available. You might enjoy Evelyn Waugh's The Loved One, a quite amusing satirical little novel on the undertaker racket in the U.S.

We very much hope that the whole Sigerist family is doing fine. Kindest regards and best wishes

Yours as ever,

Erwin

This letter is largely based on S.'s last one. Diepgen see A. to S. of 2 May 1945. Apparently A.'s paper on 1848 has not been published. Books mentioned: (Hippocrates 2004?), (Paracelsus 1941), (Cabanis 1823), (Blane 1822), (Oesterlen 1853), (Bartlett 2005), (Bernard 1927), (Charcot 1881), (Allbutt 1896). (Waugh 1967).

Dear Erwin,

It really is amusing how we are writing letters to one another the same day. Thanks for yours of October 14. Some time ago I sent you some German journals that a student brought me. Do not return them because I have read them. Perhaps that Urdang might care to see them. The German publishers are extraordinarily enterprising. Georg Thieme just published a German translation of the Welch biography by the Flexners. Venezianisches Credo, poems by Richard [sic] Hagelstange, was issued by the Insel-Verlag in 20,000 copies on excellent paper, and they would probably have printed and sold twice as many copies if they had had the paper.

I just had the visit of Dr. Siegfried Behrsing, whom you may have known in Leipzig. He is a Sinologist and Sanskrit scholar and was assistant in the Indological Institute when we were in Leipzig. His sister-in-law was Margarete Blank, my last Leipzig "Doktorand", who was beheaded by the Nazis a few weeks before liberation. At the moment he is in charge of the Berlin museums in the city administration and he had many interesting reports. Like myself, he does not believe in the imminence of war, although he is in the center of the danger area.

Actually I think that France is a much greater dangerspot, because the polarization of society is about complete there, so that the possibility of a civil war must be considered very seriously. De Gaulle is a fool, but he has a good braintrust. Did you know that Pasteur Vallery-Radot is with him and is preparing to be Minister of the Interior. André Malraux will be the French Goebbels. De Gaulle has learned a lot from Hitler's experience; he will not persecute the Jews, but will have them finance his venture.

There are several new books on the plague, and I have been preparing a comprehensive review for a long time, but unfortunately never was able to finish it. One new book is A. Francesco Da Cava, La Peste di San Carlo visto da un medico, Milan, Hoepli, 1944, a very good and thorough monograph on the epidemic of 1576–77, one that almost wiped out the population of the Ticino. The Italians also reprinted the monograph of Giuseppe Ripamontik [sic] La Peste di Milano del 1630, Milano, Muggiani (1945). This is the epidemic that was described by Manzoni in the Promessi Sposi; it was particularly interesting for the psychological reactions. A number of people were executed as unctores, as it was believed that they were spreading the plague by anointing places with the virus.

My first volume should be finished soon now because I have all the materials in hand, but the Babylonian medical literature is frightfully sterile. Dozens and dozens of texts all saying the same. Egypt was much more pleasant.

Now that Genevieve is in Ithaca, I hear very little from Baltimore. I forgot to say in my last letter what I think is obvious, that if Shryock does not accept the chair and if the university is willing to take a foreign-born, you of course would be the best choice. I do not see why Temkin does not accept the job at Stanford University. He would probably fare much better in a new environment.

There are rumors that you may be coming over next year, and if you do I count on your including Pura in your itinerary.

It is autumn now and the trees are changing color very rapidly. We made 60 quarts of wine last week and I will save a few bottles for when you come.

With best regards from house to house

[Henry]

Urdang see A. to S. of 23 March 1945. Rudolf Hagelstange (1912–1984) German writer. Blank see S. to A. of 18 December 1945. Charles De Gaulle (1890–1970) general, head of the French government after WWII. Louis Pasteur Vallery-Radot (1886–1970) Pasteur's son. André Malraux (1901–1976) French author and statesman. Goebbels: Hitler's propaganda minister. Books mentioned: (Da Cava 1944), (Flexner/Flexner 1941), (Hagelstange 1946), (Manzoni 1913), (Ripamonti 1630).

ACKERKNECHT to SIGERIST, Madison, 28 October 1948

Dear Henry:

Thanks ever so much for your letter of October 23rd, and for the German journals that arrived a few days ago and came in very handy as I am working on the second part of the 1848–1948 speech. I will actually write very little, but I would like to base my assertions as largely as possible on facts. To write on present day Germany is a rather depressing job. In the course of these studies I came across a fascinating little book, written by a disappointed Hitler youth, Dietrich Meichsner: "Versuchts noch mal mit uns".

The situation in France indeed looks pretty grim. Pasteur Valléry-Radot has been a Fascist for a long time. De Gaulle is probably more intelligent and more honest than any of the modern dictators since Napoleon III, which will probably make his adventure not any better, but rather worse. He will be a product of despair, like our late bum from Austria. I spoke with a young Socialist who is by definition anti-De Gaulle and travelled this summer in France (he grew up in Belgium and therefore knows the language well), but after being in France for two weeks he also felt feelings creeping up in him, like: Why not De Gaulle? It can't become worse. We know that song.

It is good that the Milan plague of 1575 has been taken up again, unfortunately in Italian, which makes it not very accessible. I have always felt that it is fundamentally far more interesting than the one of 1630 which probably due to Mazzini [?] (and also to Robert Fletcher in this country) has received undue emphasis. After all[,] there have been scapegoats in almost every major epidemic, not only of plague, but just the same for instance of Cholera, even in the 19th century (see Heinrich Heine's Franzoesische Zustaende). It would probably be a far more worthwhile adventure to write a comparative study on the scapegoats in epidemics, instead of sticking always to the old Milan story.

I was particularly interested in the last pandemic of plague (1895, etc.) and in the economic consequences of the black death. Among the more recent writings on the latter subject I like best the article of H. Robbin in the Journal of Political Economics, 34 (1928). A relatively good overall piece on the history of plague is the introduction to W. J. Simpson, Treatise on Plagues, (1905) which is rarely mentioned. Even on the black death there is no good monograph. Cardinal Gasquet was too much interested in clergymen, and his anticlergymen counterparts like Coulton are equally silly. Thorndike's 1927 article on the black death is pitiful (American Hist. Rev.). Well, we will see him out here at our Symposium in January, together with the Chicago Dean (some Mac), Nagel, Black, Lecorbeiller, Lark-Horowitz, Temkin, and Ogburn.

A propos Temkin, he couldn't possibly accept the chair at Stanford, as this chair does not exist. Just like a number of other jobs with which this joker – Dean Faust – is peddling around. Stanford is now the third of these phantom chairs about which people get unduly excited (the other ones are Yale and New York University) and of which I hope that I will be able to fill the one or the other at best some ten years from now with my future pupils, your scientific grandchildren. Urdang probably wrote you that he has obtained money to train a young man, G. Sonnedecker, as his successor, which is all for the better, as the young man makes an agreeable and serious impression. Urdang is still in pretty good shape, but he is 65, will be automatically retired in five years, and anyhow nobody ever knows, as the sad sudden death of Ruth Benedict four weeks ago showed.

The question of our European trip next year is still entirely in the embryonic stage, and depends on a lot of variables like money, time, and transportation facilities. We will, of course, do our level best to come and admire the spiritual and natural beauties of Pura. Not much has happened here since my last letter. I have now passed from plague to cholera on which I had fortunately already analyzed the bulk of the material for my Garrison lecture. Some of our students have manifested their discontent with our football team at their last game. Thus the president had to apologize to these heroes (the footballers), the press was full of the incident for many days all over the country, and we were unpleasantly reminded of the fact that for a great many people this whole scholarly stuff in Universities is only an obnoxious appendix to the gladiators. This feature we were at least spared at Hopkins. By the way did you ever meet the late George Crile, and what were your impressions of him? I have to review his autobiography, written in that spirit of brazen self-advertisement to which we are used here by now. I cannot make up my mind whether he was a genius or a fake. Probably a little bit of both.

We too have an unusually beautiful and mild autumn here. Lucy is going on with her studies, and everybody seems to be healthy for a change. We hope that at Pura too everybody is healthy and happy, and I hope that you will be through soon with the Babylonian drudgery, after having passed through the Egyptian captivity. Kindest regards and very best wishes from all of us to all of you.

Yours as ever,

Erwin

(Meichsner 1948). Valléry-Radot see S. to A. of 23 October 1948. "Late bum from Austria": Hitler. "Mazzini": A. probably means Manzoni, see S. to A. of 23 October 1948. (Simpson 1905). Le Corbeiller and Benedict see A. to S. of 17 September 1948 and 2 August 1944, respectively. (Crile 1947).

New names:

Black, Max, historian of science
Coulton, George G. (1858–1947) wrote on plague
Crile, George W. (1864–1943) surgeon
Fletcher, Robert, H., medical historian
Gasquet, Francis (1846–1929), wrote on plague

Heine, Heinrich (1797–1856) German writer
Lark-Horowitz, Karl, historian of science
Nagel, Ernest, historian of science
Ogburn, William F., historian of science
Sonnedecker, Glenn A. (born 1917) Urdang's successor as head of the American Institute for the History of Pharmacy
Thorndike, Lynn. (1882–1965) historian of science

SIGERIST to ACKERKNECHT, Pura, 11 January 1949

My dear Erwin,

I have not written you for a long time but before I forget it I would like you to check two references for me. The American Journal of Physical Anthropology must be easily available to you. I have two references that are not complete and of which one at least must be wrong. If you could complete the references on the enclosed sheet I would be ever so grateful. A week ago I sent most of the manuscript of volume 1 of the History to the Oxford Press. I would have liked you to read the sections on Egypt and Babylonia first but the publisher seems to be in a terrific hurry as publishers always are – which does not mean that he is going to print the book soon. I will see to it, however, that you get galley proofs when the time comes because I am anxious to have your opinion. The end of the volume is still being typed and I am working on appendices, illustrations, etc., looking forward to volume 2. The Greeks will be a real relief after the evil spirits of Babylonia.

I saw in Science the program of your symposium on the History of Science but I am not sure if this is the beginning or the end of your centenary celebrations. You must be glad when it is all over.

I just had a long letter from Genevieve who attended the annual meeting of the HSS in New York but she does not mention you and I assume that you have not been there.

We are buried in snow. On New Years [sic] day we had a terrific snowfall and the electricity and telephone went out of order. The mail could not reach the village for two days. This is very unusual here and I wonder how long we are going to keep the snow.

At the end of November I gave a lecture at the University of Berne. I postponed it for a couple of years but then I enjoyed giving it more than

I had expected. The University would like me to come once every week to give a regular lecture course and a seminar but this is obviously out of the question.

Your Xmas card was charming. The girls have changed so much that we hardly recognized them.

With all good wishes I am
    Yours as ever,
      [Henry]

HSS = History of Science Society. The offer of the University of Bern tempted Sigerist, as can be seen in his correspondence with Hintzsche, the university's anatomist and medical historian (Bickel 2008). Eventually, Sigerist turned the offer down as he did with offers from other Swiss and German universities.

ACKERKNECHT to SIGERIST, Madison, 20 January 1949

Dear Henry:

Thanks ever so much for your letter of January 11. I enclose the references for the Candela article. I was extremely glad to hear that volume 1 is now with the Oxford Press. I am looking forward very much to the galley proofs and am sending you my very best wishes for number II.

Meanwhile we had the 1848 symposium. It was a success, but printing of the essays was just as successfully sabotaged by the Chairman of the Department of History who could not overcome his grudge, that the idea had not been one of his, and that two of the lectures had been given by non-members of his department, one even an M.D.! Good old academic politics.

I have also finished my first round on the History and Geography of Diseases, dealing after malaria, plague and cholera with yellow fever and cancer. I have also worked up already typhus. I enjoy the thing tremendously and hope, after having dealt with a dozen more diseases, to come out with a book in some three or four years. I also hope to have two pupils of mine running this year for the Garrison medal with detail studies out of the field, one on the history of leprosy, the other on the history of cholera.

Urdang flew in December to a Pan-American Sandwich Architects (pharmacists) Congress in Cuba, and had a good time. But he probably wrote you already himself about his triumphs.

We also had our Symposium on Science and Civilization last week. Although only the papers of McKeon and Temkin were really good (by the way Temkin is getting deafer and deafer) it was much better than I had thought it would be, thanks mostly to the panel discussion speakers who were all very excellent. I am including a short report that I wrote for the Archives Internationales d'Histoire des Sciences. The centennial celebrations of the University started last May and will go on till next May, but as far as we are concerned, fortunately we are through.

Guttentag became on Christmas Eve at the tender age of at least fifty the father of his first daughter (in case he did not announce it to you). He had divorced his sterile and energetic wife, and married a girl he met in Germany. But you know all that from Genevieve.

Genevieve just wrote me the first letter since she went to Cornell. She seems to have had a very hard time in adjusting to the new situation, but I think she is doing much better than she thinks herself. Guerlac [?] was full of praise for her.

I have of course read and reviewed a lot of books, but I can't remember any one as worthy of mention except for the new edition (practically a new book) of Kroeber's twentyfive-year-old textbook of anthropology. (It does not contain anything on primitive medicine.) He uses at least as much ancient history, as anthropology, in order to make his point. At seventy-two the old boy still has more to say than all the younger men.

Saunders just offered me to bring out a revised edition of the Garrison. I told them that neither did I want to make the revision (I want to do my own creative work, and I hope to have during the next months again some time to work on Virchow besides my philosophy seminar) nor do I think that there is much point in bringing out a "revised" edition in view of your forthcoming book. The first two hundred pages would have to be rewritten entirely, and yet they would never live up to your books. I told them that in case they want to make just a reprint (perhaps in having references checked by a more or less professional bibliographer like Proskauer) I would be glad to write an introduction, and to add a chapter on trends since 1929. We will see how they react. If nothing comes out of the whole thing, I won't shed a tear. I am surprised that they are trying to do anything. In general[,] publishers here are now at the lowest level of their free enterprise. Contacts with them on occasion of that new edition of the Kelly-Burrage dictionary that we tried to stimulate have shown that clearly to me.

I was not at the New York meeting as I couldn't afford it financially or physically. My stomach was again very disagreeable in November and December, and I had been in New York anyhow in order to give a lecture on the influence of disease on the growth and decline of societies for the anthropologists. Of the medico-historical people, I saw only Rosen who probably wrote you that he has become now a bigshot in the New York Health Department. You also probably heard about the death of Trent from malignant tumor. Hania Wislicka's husband, apparently a very nice and quiet chap, has accepted a job out here, so they will come out here in the summer.

We were surprised to hear about your snow. This year all rules seem reversed. We have had so far an extremely mild winter, but now with -15 we eventually live up to true form. We were very glad to see you all happy and healthy on your Christmas card, and hope you go on being so in your paradise.

Kindest regards and very best wishes.

  Yours as ever,
   Erwin

A.'s book on the history and geography of diseases appered much later in German (Ackerknecht 1963), followed by an English translation. McKeon, professor of philosophy at the University of Chicago. Kroeber's book is possibly (Kroeber 1922). Fielding H. Garrison (1870–1935) medical historian; his classical textbook of the history of medicine (Garrison 1913) was published by Saunders and went through several editions.

 Names mentioned before:

Guerlac	A. to S. of 26 November 1947
Guttentag	A. to S. of 12 November 1945
Kroeber	A. to S. of 25 July 1945
Proskauer	A. to S. of 31 August 1945
Rosen	S. to A. of 27 March 1945
Trent	A. to S. of 3 June 1948
Wislicka	A. to S. of 12 November 1941

SIGERIST to ACKERKNECHT, Pura, 28 April 1949

My dear Erwin,

Again I have not written for a very long time but I have not forgotten you, and I was very glad to receive the reprint of your Anticontagionism paper with that excellent picture of yours. If only the reproduction were better, but I see that cuts in the <u>Bulletin</u> are as bad now as they were in my time.

The manuscript of my first volume has been with the publisher for some time. He wanted to rush it through the press so as to have the book out in the fall, but I succeeded in dissuading him from doing it because I very strongly feel that such a book should not be printed in a hurry. I wish to check my references and quotations carefully, and the fact that there is an ocean between us does not accelerate matters. I finally agreed with the press to have the first volume published in the spring of 1950. This will give us a whole years [sic] time and thereafter I hope to have a volume out every spring.

I sent the manuscript of the section on Egypt to Dr. Temkin and asked him to pass it on to you whenever he was through with it. The section on Mesopotamia will follow in a couple of weeks. I would greatly appreciate it if you would read these sections and let me have your comments and criticism. I postponed Jewish medicine to a later volume where it will appear as a link between the Ancient Orient and the world of the Middle Ages.

At the moment I am deeply involved in volume II, which I think will be very unorthodox because I plan to give India almost as much space as Greece. I found that medicine in both civilizations ran a parallel course throughout Antiquity and long thereafter, and that ancient Indian medicine was at least as effective as that of Greece. The turning point in the West came with the Renaissance and it looks to me as if India has its Renaissance now.

I am also preparing volume III in which Arabic medicine will take the central part. The Arabs, after all, were the immediate successors to the Greeks and were the link between East and West.

When are you coming to Europe? We very much hope to see you. I saw Gregory Zilboorg in Zurich a few days ago and found him quite unchanged. In a few days we expect to see Hamilton Owens and his wife, the editor of the <u>Baltimore Sun</u>, whom you probably met in Baltimore. Thus we are not quite cut off from the world.

I probably told you that Erica left me in January to take a job with the World Health Organization of the United Nations in Geneva. Nora is still in Rome for one more year, and at the moment she and her husband are in Sicily exploring the island and attending the annual meeting of the International Society of Contemporary Music.

Pura is beautiful at this time of the year, but you must come soon and see it for yourself.

With kind regards from house to house, I am

Yours as ever,

[Henry]

Volume I of *A History of Medicine* appeared in 1951, volume II posthumous and incomplete in 1961. Zilboorg see A. to S. of 5 August 1941. S.'s daughter Erica as her father's secretary in Pura in 1947 and 1948; her successor was the American Claire Bacher. Daughter Nora and her husband see S. to A. of 16 June 1948.

ACKERKNECHT to SIGERIST, Madison, 5 May 1949

Dear Henry:

Thanks ever so much for your letter of April 28th. I was very glad to hear that the book is now settling down to some kind of routine, and I am anxiously looking forward to receiving the galley proofs from Temkin. I was also very interested to hear concerning your plans for Volume II. I hope we will be able to discuss the India-Greece problem viva voce. You should run there into quite some trouble with dating, and differences in underlying philosophy. The Renaissance problem also seems rather knotty, as we had no medicine to import in our Renaissance, while the Indians do.

We have got so far two essentials for our trip to Europe: the money, and the airplane reservation. We are still fighting for the permit of the military government to enter Germany, but I hope we will get it. We have airplane reservations from New York to Paris on June 19th. We will stay for a week in Paris. <u>By the way, could you be so kind as to drop me a line by airmail, if you are able to recommend to us a hotel (preferably not too big, no bed bugs, and as few American tourists as possible)</u>. If you should be unexpectedly in Paris during this week I can always be reached through Mr. J. Hundert, 99 Rue du Temple, Paris 3rd. From Paris we will proceed to Ludwigsburg (my address there will be Dr. Erwin Ackerknecht, Stuttgarter Strasse 85, Ludwigsburg, Wuerttemberg, Germany, U.S. Zone). The main purpose is, of course, to see my parents again after 17 years, and to show them Lucy and the children. Lucy has also her mother and sister in Stuttgart, unless the mother gets meanwhile the American visa, which is promised, and comes here, and the sister and her husband go either to

England or Switzerland (he is offered a job in St. Gallen). I will be able to stay with my parents for only a week, because then I will have to work for the grant with which we finance the whole thing. This implies travelling all over the Western Zone, and making a survey in the different universities on German anthropology (research, teaching, personnel). Lucy intends to do some research on the German-Jewish mixed marriages in the Stuttgart region. When this research trip of mine is over, that is in the second half of August, I hope there will still be enough time and money left to visit Pura. We hope so very much to make it, but we are not yet sure of it. Switzerland seems also very expensive for Americans.

By the way, do you know of any French medical historian who is worthwhile to be looked up? I am in a somewhat odd situation, working continuously with French problems, and yet having no personal medico-historical relations with France. Do they do any work besides Valléry-Radot's hospital histories? There should be a man about my age who has similar interests.

I have spent the better part of the last months on two papers on "medical philosophy" which are just being typed. I will send you the carbons next week. The shorter one is for the Scientific Monthly. The second one will go first to the Bulletin, but Temkin may have "no space", feeling offended by my trespassing into his philosphy domain. I will then place it in the Archives Internationales or the Journal probably. Besides there is the usual teaching, and speeching, and book reviewing, and the blasted "social life", and now that it is spring (on Easter we still had snow, but since a few days temperatures above 80) there are also quite a number of things to do around the house and garden, and the preparations for the trip certainly take up a lot of time. I am getting continuously more "respectable". Now I became also a member of Phi Beta Kappa.

The review books are all without much interest. Your old friend Kagan has written another Garrison where he tries to fill in the gaps to which you pointed in your review. That is a laudable endeavor, but he's just too plain dumb to write a book. There is an interesting little novel of a 19-year-old Negro student, William Gardner Smith on his experiences as an occupational soldier in Germany ("Last of the Conquerors"). Urdang has just celebrated the 40th anniversary of his marriage and one of the young historians of science, Stauffer, has married the widow of the anthropologist Mekeel, no less than ten years his senior, but an agreeable person. As he was anyhow so far, well, a personal friend of Joachim Wach, whom you probably remember, this is perhaps an appropriate transition.

If you read American newspapers, you can guess what a tremendous amount of rotten nonsense concerning so-called socialized medicine we are obliged to listen to, not the least in this school. (The Hopkins people, by the way, adopted an attitude far superior to the average of the profession, see the "manifesto" in the J. A. M. A.) One of the saddest experiences in this direction was a speech of the old physiologist Carlson from Chicago here on no less than "Science, Society, and the Future of Mankind", where he gave besides other nonsense, of course, also his expert judgment on socialized medicine. It is rather funny to se these beneficiaries of socialized education bark at "socialized medicine".

We very much hope that you and the family are all right and that we will see you in a couple of months. Kindest regards and very best wishes.

Yours as ever,

Erwin

Western Zone: The British, U.S., and French zones of occupation of postwar Germany. Vallery-Radot see S. to A. of 23 October 1948. "Journal" of the History of Medicine and Allied Sciences. Phi Beta Kappa, a national academic honorary society. Garrison see A. to S. of 20 January 1949. S. R. Kagan wrote a biography of Garrison (Kagan 1938) which was criticized by S. (Sigerist 1939). The second Garrison biography is (Kagan 1948). (Smith 1948). Stauffer see A. to S. of 24 October 1946. Joachim Wach, possibly the historian of religions (1898–1955); he taught at Leipzig in the 1920s and immigrated into the U.S. J. A. M. A., Journal of the American Medical Association. Anton J. Carlson (1875–1956).

SIGERIST to ACKERKNECHT, Pura, 11 May 1949

Dear Erwin,

Thanks ever so much for your letter. Look here, you must plan to come to Pura in August or whenever it suits you best. Switzerland is not more expensive than any other European country, and here in Pura you, of course, would stay with us or I would put you up in the village as our guests, so that you would not have any expenses at all. I am most anxious to have you here, at least for a few days, so as to have a chance to discuss our various problems.

As far as hotels in Paris are concerned, I can recommend Hotel des Saints Pères, Paris-6e, several of my friends have been there recently and are very satisfied. It is on the left bank, has hot and cold water in every room and no bedbugs, and the rate for a single room is Fr. 600, which is equivalent to $ 1.50. Breakfast is Fr. 100, which is about 25 cents. There may be some Americans in the place, but not enough to make it unpleasant.

Much more difficult is the question of medical historians, and I do not know of any younger man active in the field. The subject is still monopolized by the old guard, Laignel-Lavastine and Co. I heard that Gaston Baissette, who wrote that silly Hippocrates book, is at the moment writing a history of medicine in many volumes similar to mine, but I have no contacts with him. I would, however, advise you to call on Dr. Genty, who is librarian of the Academy of Medicine, and editor of France médicale. He knows everyone in French medicine, and Erica and his daughter are working together in Geneva.

I am anxious to see your paper on medical philosophy because I have a half a dozen books on the subject here for review, mostly German and Italian. When the people have no money for experimental research, they write philosophical or historical books because this can be done with a pencil and paper, but the result is sometimes rather sad.

Yes, I do read American papers and magazines, and I thank heaven that I do not have to listen to all that asinine talk on socialized medicine. Fifteen years of it was enough. I am sorry that old Carlson is making a fool of himself. It just shows that at a certain age people should shut up.

If there is anything I can do in Europe for you, just let me know. I do not plan to be in Paris as I hardly ever leave my village, but I count on your visit.

With all good wishes from house to house, I am

    Yours as ever,

      [Henry]

Maxime Laignel-Lavastine (1875–1953) French medical historian. Gaston Baissette (1901–1977) wrote on medical history, but did not publish a (multi-volume) history of medicine. Carlson see A. to S. of 5 May 1949.

Dear Henry:

Thanks ever so much for your prompt answer of May 11. I have just returned from the Association meeting in Lexington, Kentucky; so let me first give you a short report on that. Because of the cockeyed location, attendance was very poor. Many of the familiar faces like Galdston, Krumbhaar, Leake, Long, Larkey, McDaniel were absent; Fulton because of diabetes, and Heaton because of a coronary. The meeting was run mostly by Viets and Spector. Some role was also played by Dittrick, Shryock (you certainly know that Shryock has accepted the Hopkins chair), Temkin and Rosen. Major and Norwood were present but not heard of. The only result of the business meeting that I can remember, was that the William H. Welch Medal was eventually instituted, and that Viets got a little sum for defraying his expense (like the signing of Chesney's lovely contract concerning the Bulletin). The poor boy apparently needs money. This was probably also the reason why he gave the Garrison lecture which after all carries $100. The Osler meeting, quite apart from the subject, was even more lousy than it looks on the program, as only two papers, those of Davis and Spector were actually delivered. The other papers next day were mediocre. The last one was a heavy onslaught on me by a friend of the grandson of Sappington, who had to defend the Sappington family honor. I had a chance to talk and I think I got even with the family interests. The Garrison lecture was considerably better than I had been afraid it would be, as V. had done some original research.

I can't tell you anything about the dinner, and the third day, as I was so disgusted with this Southern city (you have to be used to these inbred, sour faces of the white, the special buses and special drinking fountains and special waiting rooms for the "colored", and the whole mouldy air of past glory in order to take it) that I pulled out on the evening of the second day like many others (Rosen, Shryock etc.). The organisational side of the thing was also poor, the proverbial "Southern hospitality" so inexistent, that I was even afraid the next day's program which involved an automobile trip would not materialize properly. Next year we will go to Boston, and I trust it will be a better meeting, as on the other hand there are still sufficient people in the Association who are interested enough to carry on.

I then spent two days with Herskowits in Evanston to prepare my trip for Germany. I went over thousands of cards of anthropologists all over the world (H. prepares an international directory), picking the German ones. It is, by the way, lovely to see how these panders of death have re-built their reputation. Racist Hans F. K. Guenther, for instance, writes under special interests: "rural sociology, religion".

Thanks for your prompt information concerning hotels and Dr. Genty. We will surely try our best to come and see you, but we just can't promise, and forsee exactly. There are too many variables in the whole equation. We had for instance just to postpone our departure for ten days. We supposedly leave now by June 28th, as Lucy's mother is arriving in New York on June 18th, and we have first to initiate her into the American way of life.

You will have received meanwhile my two papers. I am afraid they will help you little in reviewing the German and Italian philosophical books, as they are really rather historical than philosophical. You are undoubt-edly right on the sources of this increased interest in medical philosophy in Europe. Nevertheless one or the other of these books may turn out to be good. I reviewed for instance the "Philos, Grundlagen der wissenschaft-lichen Erkenntnis" by Anton Fischer from Budapest not so long ago, and found it a rather good book. I could not say the same for the Posthumous Essays of Maurice Cohen, which are disappointing.

Kindest regards and best wishes from all of us to all of you.

Yours as ever,

Erwin

"Association": American Association for the History of Medicine (AAHM). (Fischer 1947). Maurice Cohen's book not identified.

New names:

Davis, member of AAHM (there were four of this name at the time)

Guenther, Hans F. K. (1891–1968) German anthropologist

Herskowits, Melville J. (1895–1963) anthropologist

Edward B. Krumbhaar (1882–1966) pathologist in Philadelphia and founder of the American Association of the History of Medicine in 1929.

Long, Esmond R. (1890–1979) pathologist and medical historian

McDaniel, Walton B. (1897–1975) medical historian

Norwood, William F., member of AAHM

Sappington or Sapington, not identified

Names mentioned before:

Chesney	S. to A. of 16 June 1948
Dittrick	A. to S. of 26 April 1947
Fulton	S. to A. of 26 February 1945
Galdston	A. to S. of 2 August 1944
Genty	S. to A. of 11 May 1949
Heaton	A. to S. of 23 March 1945

SIGERIST to ACKERKNECHT, Pura, 8 June 1949

Dear Erwin,

Many thanks for your letter of May 30. I had several reports of the Association meeting. Henry Viets thought it was perfectly splendid. He would since he is the president and gave the Garrison lecture. Genevieve liked the atmosphere, but I fully sympathize with your reaction because I always felt very much like you do about the South. I suppose the Yankees are glorifying the South from an old guilt complex, and maybe also because they sometimes wished they could be as lazy as their southern brethern. You certainly are going to hear "all about Osler" this year. The Hopkins club had to devote a meeting to him, and I suppose there are going to be many more.

The chief reason why I am writing now is that Temkin just wrote me that he had mailed you the section of my book on Egypt. It will probably reach you at a most inconvenient time when you are getting ready to leave. The section on Mesopotamia is on its way to Temkin, but will not be sent to you. If you come in the summer there will always be time to discuss a few points.

If you have the time to read the chapters on Egypt, let me know what you think of them and whether you have found any mistakes, and be good enough to forward the manuscript to the Oxford University Press, (Attention Mr. Philip Vaudrin), 114 Fifth Avenue, New York 11, N.Y.*

Your papers have not come yet because mail is frightfully slow, but I am looking forward to seeing them.

Bon voyage, I will be anxious to hear how you will find old Europe.

    Cordially as ever yours,

      [Henry]

* They have had a copy since Jan. but want a second one. Do not bother about typographical and similar errors.

Viets see A. to S. of 3 June 1948.

Dear Henry:

Thank you ever so much for your lines of June 8th. I have already sent back the Egypt manuscript to Temkin, as I was anxious not to get it stuck here, and I will advise him now to send it on to the Oxford University Press. I read the chapters on Egypt with extreme pleasure and profit, and I am sure it will be a great success. I haven't found any gaps or mistakes. Minor detail: you might like to mention in a footnote that the Smith Papyrus is now in the New York Academy of Medicine.

The Smith Papyrus brings up of course the problem of symptoms in general. Laennec in his doctor's thesis realized very clearly that there are actually two sets of symptoms, and it depends entirely on your approach, which one you emphasize: the "prognostic" ones, general and unspecific, and that were mostly studied by Hippocrates, and the diagnostic ones, specific, but physiologically often irrelevant, which, Laennec felt, came now to the foreground for the first time. I wonder whether you care to bring up this question already at this very early stage. A realization of the difference between these sets of symptoms is of course much older. I remember having run into it not only in Pinel, but also in Sydenham, and passages in Celsus could probably be interpreted in the same way, although I have never found the point made with such clarity as in Laennec.

I don't know whether I wrote you already that we have to postpone our departure till June 28th, as Lucy's mother is arriving in New York on June 18, and Lucy has to pick her up there. Thus, in spite of the postponement of our departure, we are under no less pressure. Also my secretary is leaving tomorrow, and I therefore better close for today. You will hear more from me on the other side. (Dr. Ackerknecht, Stuttgarter Str. 85, Ludwigsburg, Wuerttemberg, Germany, U.S. Zone)[.]

Kindest regards and very best wishes from all of us to all of you.

Yours as ever,

Erwin

René Théophile Hyacynthe Laennec (1781–1826) French professor of medicine. Pinel see A. to S. of 14 June 1945. Thomas Sydenham (1624–1689) influential English physician. Aulus Cornelius Celsus (1st century AD) Roman author, wrote on medicine.

ACKERKNECHT to SIGERIST, Cologne, 3 August 1949 (Postcard)

Dear Henry:

While working up my way north I would like to send you all at least […] cordial greetings as time for letter so far lacking. […] a good deal of the Artelts in F. (Good […]) and with my own eyes Diepgen's reprint of his last book where dedication "den med. stud. des 3. Reichs" is now changed into "m. l. Freund und Schüler Lammel […]"!

Very Cordially yours as ever

Erwin

Diepgen see A. to S. of 2 May 1945, his former dedication: "To the medical students of the Third Reich", changed into "To my dear friend and pupil Lammel". Hans-Uwe Lammel: German medical historian.

ACKERKNECHT to SIGERIST, Madison ?, 22 September 1949

Dear Henry:

We came back last Saturday night, after a rather disagreable last week in Paris, Lucy running 103 (tonsillitis) and being transportable only with high doses of penicillin. She still is not very well, and I am now fighting with the same bug. This together with a course and seminar to do, 2 reports and 1 paper to write, and lots of business mail makes it still impossible to write the "real" letter I owe you. But I thought I run off to you this little piece of information that might interest you. I have been all over Western Germany (Tübingen, Stuttgart, Frankfurt, Mainz, Köln, Münster, Hamburg, Göttingen, München), found things better than I expected them to be, but still bad and especially strange ("fremd") enough to leave without tears. I couldn't say the same for Paris, beautiful, unchanged (except for the silly baby mass production). Too bad that we couldn't come to Pura. But I was afraid it would work out this way. We hope you had a good summer.

Kindest regards and best wishes from all of us to you all

Yours as ever

Erwin

By 1949 post-war conditions had considerably improved in Germany. At the same time France, frightened by a decreasing birth rate, subsidized births. A. sent S. the copy of a letter to Shryock, dated 22 September, describing his experiences in Germany and France.

SIGERIST to ACKERKNECHT, Pura, 3 November 1949

Dear Erwin,

Of course I was disappointed that you could not come to Pura last summer, but I know from my own experience how things go on such a trip, particularly when you have the family along. Well, there may be a chance next summer. UNESCO will probably pay the way of a number of Americans who attend the Amsterdam congress and I hope you will be one of them.

Your letter to Shryock was very interesting and gave a good account of conditions of medical history in Germany. Artelt really seems to be the best man in the field today. I find his book extraordinarily useful and on account of it, was able to reduce the appendices of my first volume to a minimum. I have very little contact with Germany and do not care to have any. Dr. Buess, who teaches medical history at Basel, just spent a couple of months as visiting lecturer at the "Free University" of Berlin and found it rotten with bureaucracy and as traditionalistic as could be. The founding of a new university would be such an opportunity to create an institution of a totally new type with new curricula.

We had a good summer with glorious weather all the time. We had some very welcome visitors, such as the Guerlacs, the Fultons, the Stevensons, Zilboorg, Adolph Schultz, Hamilton Owens, of the Baltimore sun and his wife, and a few others. I attended two meetings, the one of the Swiss Society of the History of Medicine at Lausanne and the one of the Italian Society that was held early in October at Milan. Castiglioni was president and primarily for his sake some of us from abroad had to attend the meeting. But I enjoyed seeing Italy again. On the surface things look fine; there are no ration cards, meals are as good as before the war and not more expensive than in Switzerland. Reconstruction is going on at a tremendous pace. Under the surface, of course, things are very different. The agrarian problem has not even been touched and the recent, very serious strike, of the farm laborers revealed how bad conditions were even in the north. There is much activity in medical history, chiefly I suspect, because the country is too poor to offer opportunities for experimental research. The work done is not very profound, but there are some good people, and Pazzini in Rome is using his clerical connections to build up an institute that will undoubtedly become the chief Italian centre of medical-historical activities.

351

My own work is progressing slowly but steadily. Volume I is scheduled for publication in the early spring, and I expect galley proofs any time. I am writing Volume II and greatly enjoy spending a year with Greek and Hindu civilizations.

So much for today. There is, of course, more that I have to tell you but we shall have to get our correspondence going gradually.

With warm wishes to you and your family, I am

Yours as ever,

[Henry]

Amsterdam would be the site of the first post-war congress of the International Society of the History of Medicine in 1950. A.'s letter to Shryock see A. to S. of 22 September 1949. (Artelt 1949). Heinrich Buess (1911–1984) Swiss medical historian. Stevenson, possibly Lloyd G. (born 1918) medical historian. 1949 was the first post-war year that allowed normal travel between European countries. Certain food staples were still rationed in some European countries in 1949, such as Britain. Adalberto Pazzini (1898–1975) Italian medical historian.

Names mentioned before:

Artelt	S. to A. of 14 May 1946
Castiglioni	A. to S. of 3 April 1946
Fulton	S. to A. of 26 February 1945
Guerlac	A. to S. of 26 November 1947
Owens	S. to A. of 28 April 1949
Schultz	A. to S. of 16 May 1946
Zilboorg	A. to S. of 5 August 1941

ACKERKNECHT to SIGERIST, Madison, 10 November 1949

Dear Henry,

Thanks eversomuch [sic] for your letter of November 3rd. We too regretted that we could not come to Pura, but you were really lucky that we did not. During that last week of our European stay Lucy came down (it was now Paris) with a rather bad tonsillitis, which with the children, and the hotel etc. was not so pleasant. Only with high doses of penicillin did we get her on the plane, and God knows how we would have succeeded in less metropolitan surroundings.

I didn't look up any of the German medical historians except Artelt and his wife of whom I am rather fond. As far as professors go the German

Universities are just as stuffy as ever. Much better were my experiences, at least in the field of ethnology, as far as the younger generation, privatdozenten and students are concerned. They are no longer militaristic and authoritharian at all — the six years they spent in uniform were too much of a lesson. They are very different from what their brethren of 1919 used to be, and would be promising, if not the whole situation in Germany would be so terribly narrow and hopeless. We achieved our main goal, seeing my family, and had many pleasant and interesting impressions but we were very glad to pull out again.

Paris was delightful as ever, and expensive as it is in general, second hand books – especially if one is rather attached to the beginning of the 19th century – are still cheap and I made a few nice buys in spite of the fact that I had not much money to spend.

After returning here I was of course hard pressed with all the accumulated work of the summer: correspondence, my candidates for their M. D., lousy little papers and lectures one cannot avoid giving etc. that I have not come to myself entirely.

I am mostly absorbed by the history of diseases. I am giving my course again this semester. This year with another set of diseases: typhus, leprosy, influenza, polio, encephalitis, goiter, syphilis, avitaminoses. I am also participating in the official bacteriology course, where in eight lectures on the "big" diseases like influenza, Plague, small pox, etc. I am giving half an hour of history-epidemiology. This seems to be a better form of integration than the one hour leadoff I usually give to many courses, and I rather like it, except for the fact that these fellows teach at 7:45 in the morning.

My seminar in the second semester will be this time about texts in pathological anatomy (Celsus, Morgagni, Bichat, Laennec, Bright, Virchow, Rotitansky [sic], Welch). You see I am trying to get back this way to my other main subject: Virchow. I'm very much frustrated that I haven't been able to do so yet, as I had planned. But with all the other obligations waiting for me I failed to do so.

I was very much interested in what you wrote about Italy. Maybe the same conditions will also make for a new flowering of medical history in Germany, and they will do a more conscientious job probably then [sic] the Italians. Here of course there is less attention than ever in medical historical work, now that a new wonder drug ACTH (a pituitary hormone) is around the corner. It will be years until they will really know what it is and until they will be able to produce sufficient quantities; but if 1/10th of the expectations is realized, it will be an indeed great progress (rhumatic fever, nephritis, all allergic conditions etc.)

We are looking very much forward to Volume I. Very best wishes for the progress of Volume II.

Kindest regards from all of us to you all,

Yours as ever,
Erwin

Artelt see S. to A. of 14 May 1946; his wife, Edith Heischkel (1906–1987) is likely to be the first professional woman in medical history. Celsus see A. to S. of 14 June 1949. Giovanni Battista Morgagni (1682–1771) Italian pathologist. Marie François Xavier Bichat (1771–1802) French anatomist and physiologist. Laennec see A. to S. of 14 June 1949. Richard Bright (1789–1858) British physician and pathologist. Karl Rokitansky (1804–1878) Austrian pathologist. Welch see S. to A. of 15 April 1947. ACTH = adreno-corticotropic hormone (corticotropin).

Sigerist to Ackerknecht, Pura, 22 February 1950

Dear Erwin,

I just notice that I have not answered your letter of November 10. What you wrote about Germany and Paris, of course, interested me very much. I have not been in Paris since 1946, but I read the "Nouvelles Littéraires" and a few other journals so that I am not quite out of touch. I have completely lost my urge to travel, however, and hate to leave the place. As a matter of fact, I spend twenty hours a day in the same room, which is bedroom and study combined. Nevertheless, I accepted to give a few lectures in England in June and may spend a week in Rome as long as Nora and Jack are still there, chiefly with the purpose to get illustrations for Volume II. It is much easier to secure them from museums and photographers when you are on the spot then [sic] if you have to do everything by correspondence. About half the illustrations for Volume I I had from the Wellcome Museum, thanks to Underwood who was extremely co-operative. Dr. Reucker of Ciba was also very helpful. They have an enormous collection of photos.

The history of disease is a fascinating study and so much remains to be done in that field. I sent you the announcement of Pazzini's book, but

I have not seen it yet. It is probably pretty superficial but shows that there is a need for such a book.

We had a very quiet winter. The children came from Rome and Geneva for Christmas. Nora obtained a Fulbright fellowship and is studying at the University of Rome, where they have some good professors for Slavic languages and literatures. The University, however, is closed half of the time, either on account of strikes or because a professor has died or for some other reason. Spring is beginning now; the spring flowers are all in bloom, while you probably still have snow, or at any rate winter.

At the end of March a small group of Swiss medical historians will hold a two-day conference in Pura, with seven papers on the program and plenty of time for discussion. The official meetings in the fall are always so rushed that we decided to come together informally in the spring, and I expect much more from such a gathering than from the large conventions. This is also the chief reason why I am not going to Amsterdam; I can do very well without Laignel-Lavastine and other similar soap-box historians. Genevieve is arranging for an Anglo-American meeting in Pura in the week preceding Amsterdam, and I only wish you could come also. We had an old "Pension" near-by, which has been completely rebuilt and is now a very delightful and inexpensive hotel.

I hope your family has not had too much illness this winter and with warm regards from house to house, I am

Yours as ever,

[Henry]

The Wellcome Library and Museum in London is the center of medico-historical activities in Britain. E. Ashworth Underwood (1879–1980). Reucker see S. to A. of 10 July 1948. (Pazzini 1947) and S. to A. of 3 November 1949. 1950 saw the first annual Pura Conference of the active Swiss medical historians. Laignel-Lavastine see S. to A. of 11 May 1949. Amsterdam meeting see S. to A. of 3 November 1949.

ACKERKNECHT to SIGERIST, Madison, 28 February 1950

Dear Henry:

Thanks eversomuch [sic] for your letter of February 22nd. I had wondered already what had happened. Many thanks also for sending me the announcement of the Pazzini book. It was the first news I had of it, and

I ordered it immediately. It hasn't arrived yet. Even if it is a hasty Italian salad, as it might well be, I will have to look into it. I feel that the man probably tried to do too much. There is no point of attempting a repetition of the Hirsch. One individual just can't handle any longer the history and geography of all existing diseases.

You are unfortunately right that we are still in the snow and ice stage (although for a change we had a thunderstorm last night) and will be probably for one or two more months. I sure envy your Swiss professors for the lovely spring meeting they will have with you. I am sorry that I will not be able to participate in the Anglo-American meeting in August, as I am not going next summer to Europe (Genevieve wrote you probably already). The main reason is that I want to work this summer, and when we go to Europe there wouldn't be much work done. I also am by no means keen for this congress. You know how little I feel attached to the country of my birth which after all "vomited" me, but on the other hand I would feel it incongruous to go to a Congress from which people are excluded not for what they have done, but for where they are born, when I happened to be born on the same spot. When the Nazis did such things it was called "racialism". Urdang will go. As long as my parents are alive we have on the other hand to go from time to time to Europe, and we hope to find money to work the summer of 1951 in Paris (as frustrating as that might be to live two months in Paris and then have to leave again) and have the children stay with their grandparents and pay there a short visit. I will go to Boston this spring although I have little hope that much inspiration will come out of it.

I started writng the Virchow book around Christmas, and am progressing slowly. I have so far done about sixty pages. (one fifth?) A short biographical sketch, and a chapter on Virchow's general ideas. I am now involved in a detailed discussion of his medical work, pathological and public health. A lengthy discussion of his political work, and of his anthropological work will follow. In spite of my many preparatory studies it is still a terrific amount of work because of his prolific writing. If I'm lucky I will be through next spring. The main problem, is of course, to keep writing in spite of all the distractions by teaching and other things, and this is not easy, as you know. I am not very satisfied with what I have done, having discovered that writing a biography is not the best way of writing history. The method I used before: to write the history of movements, seems to me to come far closer to reality. But it is too late now. The cake has been cut and has to be eaten. In rereading old Leipzig publications (yours, Hirschfeld's, Pagel's, Temkin's and mine) I realize that at that time the whole Institute group was somewhat puzzled by the Virchow problem, and I feel quite nostalgic for these days of intellectual and physical youth.

You probably realize that Hanja, now Ris has been a resident of Madison for about half a year. Through some queer accident her name is in everybody's mouth, she is mentioned every second day in the newspapers, and has become a "cause célèbre". She applied for admission to the license examination and the Board that has refused here every foreign graduate since 1937, refused her because the Board could not judge whether the University of Zurich from which she graduated was "on the same high level as Wisconsin Medical Schools". As there had been some hard feelings about the practices of the licensing Board for a long time, in the general public, and this seemed to be a particularly nonsensical argument, the political opposition has taken up her case, and brought the licensing Board into a rather unpleasant situation, although it sticks to ist guns. Hanja is definitely not happy about having become a test case, but she will get her license this way and also quite a number of patients. Her husband is very agreeable, quiet, a typical natural scientist, and the baby is a very nice little boy too. It so happens that just during these fights Karl F. Meyer of California whom you probably know too, was here to give a lecture on international public health and showed slides of new Swiss University Hospital and Medical School buildings that were really overwhelming, and far superior to anything I have seen here. It is sad to think that the whole of Europe could look this way without these stupid wars.

Lucy has been working very hard in teaching languages, and studying anthropology. She published her first small two papers, and hopes to take her Masters [sic] degree in spring. She is also taking driving lessons. Her mother is a great help, as she practically has taken over the household, and a most agreeable companion. From diseases – I knock wood – we have fortunately been free since our return. Only Lucy was laid up for a week with a sore knee after a fall around Christmas which was all for the better as it forced her to relax a little. We very much hope that you are all doing well.

Kindest regards and very best wishes,
 Yours as ever,
 Erwin

(Pazzini 1949). (Hirsch 1893), "Keen for this congress": Amsterdam, see S. to A. of 3 November 1949. Boston: AAHM congress. Hirschfeld see A. to S. of 11 April 1939. Walter Pagel (1898–1983) German medical historian in England. Hanja Wislicka Ris see A. to S. of 12 November 1941. Karl F. Meyer (1884–1974) pathologist at UCLA.

ACKERKNECHT to SIGERIST, Madison, 26 May 1950

Dear Henry:

This is just to give you a short report on the Association meeting in Boston from which I returned yesterday. You most probably have the program. As Genevieve unfortunately couldn't be present on account of her exams, you might like to have a few comments.

In the business meeting nothing of importance happened. As far as I can remember the list of officers looks like follows: Ralph Major, President; John Fulton, Vice-president; Iago Galdston, Secretary; Emerson Kelly, Treasurer; Owsei Temkin, Editor. I have forgotten who besides Shryock was elected into the Executive Committee.

Under report of constituent societies, Shryock developed shortly his program for the Institute that you probably know already. He tries to make it an institute for the History of Medicine and Science, somehow in the vein of the late Berlin Institute. For us medical historians this might be regrettable in a certain way, but it is the logical consequence from the fact that he is a historian, that medical history will and should always be largely a medical discipline, while history of science, at least in this country, is far more history than science. There is in addition a total vacuum in the history of science here in spite of all the opportunities this field has. Sarton, I. B. Cohen, Guerlac, our boys here are complete flops from the administrative point of view, Shryock might therefore be successful along these lines, and fill a real need. I hope that everything will work out all right.

The Welch celebration was far better than the Osler orgie of last year, due to the quality of the papers (especially Temkin's) as well as to the subject of the performance. The papers of the Monday morning session were not breath taking but decent, Rosen's paper being of more than average interest, Hyman Goldstein was unvolontarily comical as usual. Monday afternoon you were awarded the William H. Welch medal as you probably know. The Garrison lecture was a fine performance of ecclesiastic rhetory [sic]. The visit of historical places was charming. Sarton's dinner address fine as long as he stuck to Boyle. But when he used the whole thing as a background to a violent emotional attack on "modern art" (which I do not happen to like either) rather illogical and philistine. The papers of the Tuesday morning session were dull, but they had the good sense to put at the end of the session a man who was a very good speaker. As a whole the meeting was very well organized, probably due to Spector, and left pleasant memories, far more so than the last two meetings in Philadelphia and Lexington. Viets performed a veritable marathon race of little speeches here and there.

Everyone [sic] of my spare moments during the last months has been, of course, devoted to the Virchow book. It has by now grown to seven chapters (out of a planned 18) and about 130 pages. I have done most of the pathology now. But that is only half of his medicine. And there is still the whole political and anthropological aspect ahead of me. Virchow seems all of a sudden to have gained even a certain actuality, as in Russia unfortunately Speransky's opinion that neither Virchow nor Ehrlich ever contributed anything useful to medicine has become the official dogma, and a campaign along the lines "Down with Capitalist Virchowism", repeating the pattern of the campaign "Down with Capitalist Mendelism" has been started. I need not say that this whole thing is so far from any historical truth that it has had no impact whatsoever on my writing.

The semester is fortunately coming to an end. My six candidates for Doctor's theses fortunately all finished safely except for one who came down with a paranoic schizophrenia, a rather sad occurrence. You see I am remaining in the "great tradition"! I have also quite some work with a boy who does his Ph.D. in the History Department on the medical history of the Civil War.

Among medico-historical books that I have read recently a History of the Philadelphia Yellow Fever of 1793 "Bring out your Dead" by J. H. Powell stands out as a rather good job.

By-the-way, at the meeting it was announced that Jean Sabin had died. Nobody knew any details. I would not be surprised if it was a suicide. Poor girl.

In March we spent a week-end in Chicago with our friends with the old Anglo-Saxon names of Herskovits, Gourevitch, and Hsu. We went primarily to see a wonderful VanGogh exhibit, and a good Italian movie

(The Bicycle Thief). In April I was down in Baltimore and Washington. I had a meeting of a Committee of the National Research Council (on International Relations in Anthropology) and used the occasion to do some Virchow studies in the libraries of Washington and Baltimore. I was glad to see that the Institute is slowly coming back to life although it is still very far from being what it once was. I saw Temkin's little girl Judy for the first time. She seems to become the same intellectual acrobat as her progenitor (reads and writes at 5, selftaught) but otherwise quite natural. The older one is big, quiet, and pretty. The family here is O.K. I hope the same holds good for you all, and your personal health, work etc. are all satisfactory.

Kindest regards and best wishes.

Yours as ever,

Erwin

(Powell 1949).

New names:

Boyle, Robert (1627–1691) British natural scientist
Ehrlich, Paul (1854–1915) German immunologist and pharmacologist
Goldstein, Hyman (1887–1954) physician
Gourevitch, Victor, professor of philosophy
Mendel, Gregor (1822–1884) German geneticist
Sabin, Jean, probably Jean C. Sabine, a member of the AAHM
Speransky, possibly Aleksej Dmitrievich Speranskij (1887/88–1961) Soviet pathophysiologist

Names mentioned before:

Cohen, B.	A. to S. of 24 October 1946
Fulton	S. to A. of 26 February 1945
Galdston	A. to S. of 2 August 1944
Guerlac	A. to S. of 26 November 1947
Herskovits	A. to S. of 30 May 1949
Hsu	A. to S. of 22 October 1946
Kelly	A. to S. of 3 June 1948
Major	A. to S. of 10 May 1945
Sarton	A. to S. of 23 March 1945
Spector	A. to S. of 3 June 1948
Viets	A. to S. of 3 June 1948

My dear Erwin:

I am sure that you think that I have forgotten you but I can assure you that this is not the case, that I am thinking and talking of you often, and if I did not write sooner it is simply because I had a frightfully busy summer with one volume in the press, one that I was writing, 2 symposia in Pura, two weeks of lecturing in England, one in Copenhagen, and a steady stream of visitors from all sections of the Globe, plus one week in Geneva with conferences on international health with members of the World Health Organization. It is winter now, at least according to the calendar, the weather is still glorious and warm, but things are quieting down and I am trying to catch up with my correspondence. It will take some time, however, because I am without a secretary at the moment. The nice Mormon girl I had for the last two years went back to the States and I do not intend to replace her before the spring.

You will receive in the next few days an advance copy of my first volume. It was unduly delayed by the press, I do not know why. The book will not be for sale before the end of January but I heard that the Press has received some bound copies so I immediately asked them to send you and a few others copies as soon as possible. I had all kinds of difficulties with the Oxford Press and fought two major battles with, one of which I lost and one I won. I lost in the matter of footnotes. I wanted them at the bottom of the page but the Press declared that this was too expensive and that the footnotes would be at the end of each chapter. I think it is a perfect torture to read a book in which you have to turn pages after every few lines quite apart from the fact that you never know where the chapter ends. But all my threats and entreaties did not impress the Press and it seems that what can be done without any difficulty in the bankrupt European countries it [sic] not possible in America. I suppose that is the price for the high standard of living, the production of books becomes so expensive that nobody can buy them unless you cut down expenses wherever it is possible. The other battle fortunately I won. They wanted to omit the mention "Volume I" because it might scare retailers who might fear that they would have to buy Volume II also. But there I was adamant and the Press gave in. How could the book have been quoted if every volume had had a fancy title. Enfin, this is over and I am deep in Vol. II.

Urdang probably told you of our symposium in Pura. It was very pleasant and stimulating. Urdang himself was very good, he is such a nice and decent fellow. Genevieve and her mother were in Pura for almost six weeks. She had all kinds of difficulties with Guerlac in the beginning but seems to be better adjusted now. Personally I very much regret that the history of medicine is now more and more geared to the history of science even if it is done only nominally as in the case of the Leipzig Institute (under von Brunn). I always opposed this development because I feel as you do that the subject is a medical discipline first of all. I hope the introduction to my first volume will make this clear. I have no objection to medical science, anatomy, physiology, pathology etc. being discussed as part of general science but the history of medicine as such and as a whole is a medical discipline. I am anxious to see how Shryock will develop the Baltimore Institute. He was to come to Pura but in England he got the war jitters and went home. Gebrannte Kinder scheuen das Feuer. He was caught once before in Europe by war and now whenever he comes he thinks war is just around the corner. This deprived me of the pleasure of seeing him and of getting a first-hand account of his plans.

I must say, I had an excellent impression of England, the last tolerant and liberal country in the world. In all universities you find socialists, conservatives, communists and even fascists working peacefully side by side. While I was in London there was a partial taxi strike: the emplyd [sic] drivers struck and the owners of cars ran their cars – and every evening they share their earnings with the strikers. Where in the world would you find such a beheaviour [sic]? I attended meetings of Health Boards and Hospital Boards, talked with many doctors, patients and administrators. Every one had some criticism of the National Health Service but without exception all agreed that is [sic] was a great step forward and nobody would dream of giving it up. Copenhagen also made a very good impression, a highly cultured city, with excellent thatres [sic], museums a brilliant university, and also very liberal. The dean of the medical school, professor of anatomy, is a communist member of parliament and no one seems shocked about. One professor who thought he had to defend him, said as an excuse that he was a great idealist. Sounds different, does it not? I was invited to attend an old-fashioned doctoral disputation. The candidate who had written a thesis on the history of physiology of the muscle had to defend his thesis against a savage onslaught for three solid hours. I had to oppose him also but, of course, did it very tactfully. The best part came the following day when he gave a trmendous [sic] Doktorschmaus. Instead of a gown the doctors wear a large golden ring on the index with Minerva. I had six lectures in England, four in Copenhagen and this was about enough for this year.

Thank you so much for two good letters. Your Virchow must be finished or almost so by now. And I am anxious to hear about your candidates for the doctor's degree. Are their dissertations published? I heard from Hania whose husband seems to be in Switzerland at the moment. She still is a cause celèbre [sic]. How absurd the whole business is. The doctors everywhere seem to be the most disgustingly aggressive bussiness [sic] people in the world. The University of Zurich wanted an Austrian to fill the chair of obstetrics and gynecology. The faculty recommended him unanimously, the government offered him the chair enthusiastically and the the [sic] Medical Society let him know that he was not wanted and that they would make his life a burden. Of course, he declined the offer and a second-rater was appointed. Did you ever get my Letters of Jean de Carro? Months ago I asked the Hopkins Press to send you and a few others a copy, but I just heard that several friends did not receive the copy I had intendeed for them. The Hopkins Press as inefficient as it ever was.

I hope the family is well. I just became a gran-father [sic] as Nora gave birth to a son, Nov. 27. Do write me soon and I promise to answer without delay. We have no Christmas card this year and so, please accept our warmest wishes for the whole family in this informal way.

Yours as ever

[Henry]

"Mormon girl": Claire Bacher. Enfin = after all. Guerlac see A. to S. of 26 November 1947. Von Brunn see S. to A. of 14 May 1946. "Gebrannte Kinder scheuen das Feuer": Burnt children shun the fire. "Sounds different"from McCarthy's America. Doktorschmaus, Doctor's feast (with plenty of food). Hania Wislicka Ris see A. to S. of 12 November 1941. Jean de Carro (1770–1857) physician in Vienna and Carlsbad; (Sigerist 1950). The spelling errors are likely to be due to S.'s own typing.

Dear Henry,

Let's begin with the end of your good letter: the birth of your grandson. This is certainly good news! And we send to you and Emmy our heartiest congratulations and very best wishes at this occasion.

It is only one of the many pleasant aspects of your substantial letter of December 4 for which I thank you very much. Frankly speaking, I had wondered somewhat why you hadn't written for such a long time, but I should have been aware of the fact that, of course you were extremely busy this summer. Urdang has told us a great deal about your symposium with which he was extremely satisfied. Urdang is indeed a great blessing, a remnant of some better period, and I very much hope that he will still last for many years. He overdid it a little this summer, and was very tired when he returned (after all he is sixty-eight), but I hope he picks up again.

Apropos the Leipzig Institute, Richter, to whom I sent some old suits, wrote me that von Brunn had been retired in August at the tender age of seventy-five. The Institute is now under the provisary [sic] directorship of Boenheim who seems to have the policlinic. Boenheim also gives the indoctrination course in the medical faculty at Leipzig. He probably got the assignment because of his long party membership. He never exhibited any particular interest or knowledge in medical history. He was a third rate endocrinologist in Berlin before 1933. I'm afraid they will have a hard time to fill that chair again adequately.

I'm looking forward of course very much to the first volume of your history. I'm sorry that you lost the battle of the footnotes, but not surprised. My few contacts with American publishers have left me with a feeling of nausea. I apologize that I didn't acknowledge the Jean de Carro Letters. They must have arrived during one of my not infrequent health crises this summer. Since April my health went from bad to worse. Eventually I spent the better part of November in the Hospital, because apart from the local symptoms of my ulcer, I had become a case of malnutrition on account of the little and one sided food I took. I am now well again, but living a very dull life: no smoking, no more than eight hours of work a day, etc., etc. This means that I haven't touched my Virchow now for more than a month, which makes me very sad. All through the summer, even through the periods of pain I had kept working at the book and I would, without this accident, probably now be close to the end. I have done now 15 of 21 chapters, that is I am through with medicine and politics, and have started on his anthropological work, which fortunately proved to be more interesting than I had expected it to be. Except for a short trip that I undertook to Wichita, Kansas, where an old Swedish doctor (Thor Jager) has the only good Virchow collection in this country, and in addition a superb collection on the history of 19th century pathology in general, we stayed home. We had a great deal of visitors, mostly from Germany on government junkets, my sister included.

Of the six dissertations written this year under my supervision, I have placed one for publication so far, and I hope to place two more after editing. The trouble with these children is that they can't write english [sic]. This sounds very preposterous from me, but unfortunately my stuff is still more readable than theirs. This year I have only three students. Frankly speaking, I like this better. Six was a little bit too much. This "midwifery" takes up quite some time.

Your description of England and Denmark sounded attractive and fantastic in the depressing atmosphere in which we have been living here now for months. Eventually our different Macs have involved us into a war even more nonsensical than usual, that is with China, and God knows whether we will still be able to get out of something nobody, except the China lobby, ever wanted.

Kindest regards and best wishes.

Yours as ever,
Erwin

Richter and von Brunn see S. to A. of 23 February 1948 and 14 May 1946, respectively. Felix Boenheim (1890–1960) German physician. Carro see S. to A. of 4 December 1950 and (Sigerist 1950). Thor J. Jager (1882–1975) pathologist and collector. "Only three students", i.e., doctoral students. "Different Macs", probably General Douglas MacArthur or the anticommunists Joseph McCarthy and Pat McCarran, mentioned in connection with the Korean War and the involvement of China.

SIGERIST to ACKERKNECHT, Pura, 19 January 1951

Dear Erwin:
    Would you be interested in a chair at the University of Berne? The University of Zurich just created a full chair and institute for Bernhard Milt

who works mostly in the field of the Renaissance (Gesner, Vadian etc.). With the superb collection of Wehrli and with the University Library turning over all his old medical books, this is going to be a first-rate institute.

Now comes Berne. The [sic] are reorganizing the university[,] and the medical faculty is unanimous in its desire to have a chair of medical history. The dean wrote me about it the other day and they offered me the chair (this is the fifth chair and seventh job offered to me since I am in Pura: Zurich, Berlin, Jena, Leipzig, Berne; the History of Science Museum in Oxford and a very good position in the World Health Organization in Geneva; this is all off the record, of course). I am seeing the dean next week and will discuss the whole set of problems with him.

My own position is rather awkward. My appointment at Yale was for three years and expired last summer. It was renewed for three years by the university before they had the money for the salary. (Fulton was sick and this upset everything). In the mean time I had asked to be reappointed for years [sic] and had also mentioned what salary I expected (which includes a secretary, running an office etc.) Should for some reason or other Yale not get the necessary money I would have to accept Berne. However, according to latest news it seems likely that I will get all I was asking for. Of course, I would much prefer to stay where I am, where I now have a good workshop and where I feel confident that I will be able to continue my work successfully. I also must admit that I am rather scared of going back to a university job with all it implies.

Now, if I do not take Berne, whom shall I recommend. In Switzerland there is only Buess who is an awfully nice fellow, but a beginner and what Sudhoff used to call "nicht ein Ueberflieger". And so I thought of you although I have not the faintest idea of what your feelings are and whether you would ever consider coming back to Europe. Now that you have become a kulak you may prefer to stay in God's own country. I do not know yet any detail about Berne except that they will not create a chair unless they can get a good man. Let me know what you feel in a general way and I will let you have details later on.

Cordially as ever Yours
[Henry]

Bernhard Milt (1896–1956) Swiss medical historian. Conrad Gesner (1516–1565) and Joachim Watt called Vadian (1483?–1551) Swiss physicians and scholars. Gustav Adolf Wehrli (1888–1949) Swiss medical historian. Buess see S. to A. of 3 November 1949. "nicht ein Ueberflieger", not a top man.

Dear Henry,

Thanks ever so much for your letter of January 19th. I feel very honored that you thought of me in connection with a chair which has been offered to you. On the other hand I have moved around so much during the last twenty years that I would prefer to stay now in one particular place for awhile. It is also better for the children. Personally it does not matter very much to me where I am – the only country I would really like to live is France, and that is certainly out of the picture. Thus I might just as well stay here, where it is not bad, and I have been treated more decently than anywhere else. As to the farm, that is Lucy's baby. In general, the acquisitive tendency is not represented by me in this family.

I thanked you already shortly for your fine book. In spite of being very busy with exams and Virchow, I have already read half of it with great pleasure. (This was a repeat performance as I had read the manuscript of this part). I have eventually obtained the permission of my doctor to travel and have just returned from three days in the Crevar Library in Chicago. I have worked through 33 volumes of the Zeitschrift für Ethnologie, a horrible drudgery, but it had to be done, and now my Virchow material is more or less complete, and I can hope to finish at least the text part of the manuscript in not too far a future. Then there will be of course the job of revising, name glossary, bibliography, etc.

Hania eventually got her license. There is nothing like persistency. I have eventually succeeded in launching a journal club on the history of science which comprises such senior staff members on the campus that are interested in the history of science (about a dozen: a chemist, 2 biologists, a geologist, a psychologist, etc.). I had preached this idea for four years in vain to the other history of science people here. I feel this will give us more stimulation than a combination with philologists, historians, and philosophers for which my colleagues had greater inclination (or let's rather say into which the humanities people dragged them with great energy, while the science people have to be dragged).

Thanks again. Soon more. Kindest regards and very best wishes from all of us to you all.

Yours as ever,
    Erwin

"Your fine book": volume I of S.'s History (Sigerist 1951). Zeitschrift für Ethnologie, Journal of Ethnology. Hania see A. to S. of 12 November 1941 and 28 February 1950. A journal club is for discussion of the latest articles published in scientific journals.

SIGERIST to ACKERKNECHT, Pura, 11 June 1951

My dear Erwin,

I do not know if I shall still reach you at home. You may be on your way to Paris (I envy you). At any rate I wish to thank you once more for your good wishes for my birthday and for a splendid batch of reprints, your own and those of your students. I remember when you worked on the South American Indians, this was rather a long time ago and I am glad to see that the book is out by now. It was excellent news to hear that your book on Virchow is finished. Of course, I am looking forward to seeing it. Quite recently somebody asked me if there was such a book and I was glad to be able to annuncex [sic] your forthcoming volume. And now the Paris school! This is a very good and very worthwhile subject also.

We had a very pleasant time in Italy. First we spent two weeks in Amalfi. Emmy and I both had influenza in March, not badly, but I kept coughing for several weeks and Emmy had pains in the joints. So we decided that we needed a change of climate and a real rest and Amalfi was just what we needed. It was too cold for the season but still very nice. Then we had a week in Rome with beautiful sunshine. Rome had been cleaned up for the Holy Year but it was Rome nevertheless and we enjoyed every minute. I went to see Pazzini and his Institute but was very disappointed. The Institute is a huge junk store, a museum with some good pieces and a lot of rubbish, some originals and many copies, some good, some bad. The library is a typical "Zufallsbibliothek", old books, mostly 18th century, the gift of some old physician, some new books but few. Pazzini is a superficial worker, very active, a real busybody, but nothing solid. You'll find that his books are full of mistakes. He and his coworkers make huge bibliographies but I found that most of the books that they list on ten thousands of cards are practical [sic] all in the Index Catalogue of the Gurgeon [sic] General's Library. So what is the point of repeating the work? The department has practically no money at all and is located in the basement of the Department of Hygiene. In Florence I went to see Corsini and his

368

charming assistant Miss Bonelli. Corsini is a much more serious worker but his department is hopeless also. It is a "National Museum of the History of Science" and at the same time an Institute of the University of Florence. But there again they have no money whatever. The museum is extremely rich with instruments and apparatuses of Galileo and other member of the Accademia del Cimento but not a soul comes to see it. There is no instruction. The library is of the same type as that in Rome. Italy makes a brilliant impression on the surface, with good hotels, comfortable trains and superlative food – for tourist. Under the surface conditions are very bad. University professors went on strike while we were there because they just cannot mak [sic] ends meet and there is no wonder that the communist vote increased by 7 per cent in the recent elections. I wish you could come to Switzerland. If you feel like having a break just come to Pura. You can stay with us as long as you like, can work here in peace. Since Jack and Nora are in New York we have an empty room.

Warm wishes from house to house

Yours as ever

[Henry]

S. was 60 years old on 7 April 1951. A congratulatory letter (?) is missing. A. on South American Indians (Ackerknecht 1948c), his Virchow book (Ackerknecht 1953a), his work on the Paris school of medicine (Ackerknecht 1951b); his book on the latter subject appeared in 1967. Pazzini see S. to A. of 3 November 1949. "Zufallsbibliothek", an unsystematically collected library. Andrea Corsini (1875–1961) director of the Florence Museum of the History of Science. Accademia del Cimento, for the study of science, founded in Florence in 1657.

SIGERIST to ACKERKNECHT, Pura ?, 24 June 1952

Dear Erwin,

I am anxious to have the reprints of your papers bound, and we just made an inventory which is quite considerable. We found that two papers are missing, although I am sure that you gave them to me at the time, but I cannot find them. If you happen to have a spare reprint of these, I would appreciate receiving them.

Im memory of William H.R. Rivers. Bull. Hist. Med., 1942, 11: 477–480.

Problems of primitive medicine. <u>Bull. Hist. Med.</u>, 1942, 11: 503–521. There may also be papers that are not on our list. The supplement on <u>Malaria in the upper Mississippi valley</u> is a monograph and will not be bound; I have it here.

I never thanked you for your letter of March which was full of interesting news. You saw a Cezanne [sic] exhibit in Chicago, and I just saw a perfectly magnificent exhibit of Claude Monet in Zurich. Every few steps I recognised an old friend and then I found that they were paintings lent by the Metropolitan Museum in New York or the Art Institute of Chicago, and other American collections. It was the most representative exhibition of Monet I have ever seen, illustrating all phases of his work. I was vividly reminded of the novel of Zola in which he is pictured in his country place, in the midst of the roses, with the pond that he painted so many times, and with his long white beard. By the way, did you know that Lugano has one of the best picture galleries of Switzerland, certainly the best after Basle? It was a private collection of a Baron Thyssen who died a few years ago, and whose heirs, in order to escape inheritance tax, had to make it accessible to the public three days a week. The collection has four magnificent El Grecos and about every school from the late Middle Ages to the 18th century is represented with good pieces.

You wanted to know what new chapters I am adding to the <u>Great Doctors</u>. Well, I thought to bring in neurology by having sketches of Ramon y Cajal, Pavlov, and Cushing. This would illustrate the anatomy, physiology and surgery of the nervous system. Then the publisher asked me to include Hahnemann to which I had no objection, and finally he suggested also Friedrich Müller and Sauerbruch. They were both my teachers and I thought to end up the book with sketches of these two men who were very different, but both very good teachers, and I could write them in a more personal way than the others, as I knew them both rather well. Schuman plans to make a new American edition with the new chapters added. I am just rereading the <u>Great Doctors</u>, and I think it makes quite a good introduction into the subject for students.

Have you seen the autobiography of Sauerbruch published under the title <u>Das war mein Leben</u>. If not, try to get hold of a copy of it, because it is great fun. It is a huge success, and the book has been serialised in a number of popular magazines.

It was excellent news to hear that your Virchow book will be published by your University Press, and I am looking forward to seeing it. There is much need for such a book, and many people have a completely wrong idea of Virchow and what he stood for. I was also very glad to know that you are continuing your work on the history of diseases. Pazzini's book is very disappointing. I saw him in Bologna not long ago, when I attended the meeting of the Italian Society of the History of Medicine at which Jerome Webster was given an honorary degree for his superb book on Tagliacozzi. Following the meeting we spent a very pleasant week in Florence.

I was very happy to hear that you still liked the first volume of my History. It had excellent reviews, but was attacked from two quarters. One came from Frans Jonckheere who read only the chapter on Egypt, so that he did not know at all what the book was all about. He criticized that I did not quote certain books which I knew as a rule, but did not quote because they did not add anything to our knowledge. He also criticized that I did not list the 14 names that the Egyptians have for testicles. I knew that there were that many names and even more for the heart, but I did not see the point in listing these names for readers who are not Egyptologists. He also found that I should have begun the chapter with anatomy and physiology, while I find that in archaic medicine the emphasis is on the sick man with his symptoms; anatomy and physiology come last. Jonckheere has a strange reputation. René Sand told me that he was divorced from his first wife for physical and mental cruelty, and that his second wife died while he was operating on her. He is a surgeon but undoubtedly knows a great deal about egyptology.

Another critique came from Bernard Stern in Science and Society, who disagrees with some of my anthropological statements. You know best what social anthropologists are like; I do not think there are two in the country who agree on anything.

It must be summer by now in Wisconsin. I am sure you had a big celebration for Urdang who certainly does not look his seventy years. I am glad to know that he will still continue with the Institute.

With all good wishes to yourself and family,

 I am,

  Yours as ever,
   [Henry]

A.'s letter of March 1952 is missing. Great Doctors is the Englisch translation of (Sigerist 1932). "Das war mein Leben" = Such was my life, (Sauerbruch 1951). (Pazzini 1950). (Gnudi / Webster 1950). Urdang's Institute for the History of Pharmacy in Madison.

New names:

El Greco (1541–1614) Spanish painter
Hahnemann, Samuel (1755–1843) creator of homeopathy
Müller, Friedrich (1858–1941) German professor of medicine
Pavlov, Ivan P. (1849–1936) Russian physiologist
Ramon y Cajal, Santiago (1852–1934) Spanish histologist
Tagliacozzi, Gaspare (1545–1599) Italian surgeon
Thyssen, Heinrich (1875–1947) art collector
Webster, Jerome P. (1888–1974) surgeon

Names mentioned before:

Cushing   A. to S. of 12 April 1946
Jonckheere S. to A. of 23 February 1948
Pazzini   S. to A. of 3 November 1949
Sand   S. to A. of 18 July 1946
Sauerbruch A. to S. of 23 May 1945
Stern   A. to S. of 23 March 1945
Zola   A. to S. of 5 May 1938

ACKERKNECHT to SIGERIST, Madison, 27 June 1952

Dear Henry:

Thank you ever so much for your letter of June 24th. A letter of yours makes me always very happy. I feel very honored that you want to bind my reprints, and I am sending you under separate cover ten items which you do not seem to have yet; some of them are my last copies. But I am very glad to give them for such a purpose. I also include my own list of publications as of today for the sake of checking.

The Monet exhibit must have been magnificent. My father, who was for a few days in Zurich, wrote me about it. Your reference to the novel of Zola reminds me of a fact that unfortunately you have never worked up the material you collected on Zola. I knew about the Thyssen Gallery (they had an illustrated catalogue published) but I did not know that it had become more or less public property.

Thanks ever so much for telling me about the new edition of the "Great Doctors". It is indeed a very fine introduction into the subject for students, and I always recommend it to my students. It will undoubtedly gain through the additions. If only Cushing had not been such an extremely mean character. As to Pawlow [sic] one could say of him, like of Freud, Marx, and other great men (especially in view of Speranski): God

372

protect him against his heirs. A friend here, another ex-German, gave me the autobiography of Sauerbruch. I have not yet read through it, but what I read I found highly illuminating and amusing.

I read the Jonckheere criticism of your book, and found it somewhat unfair, too much written from the point of view of the Egyptologist. In seeing him once I had rather thought he belonged to the species who never marry. At least women. I have not read Stern yet, but I suppose I did not miss much.

The Urdang celebrations here seem indeed to have been very nice. I personally was unfortunately not present as I had to assist a giant two week's symposium on the present state of anthropology in New York City from which I have just returned. Urdang is still doing all right, but he has strangely aged since his visit to Germany which seems to have been not only a very heavy physical but also psychological strain.

Since I wrote you last I gave my Davis lecture in Chicago. God knows when it will be published. I hate these lectures. And yet it is difficult to refuse. They interrupt your research work, and afterwards they are published in such a way that they are practically lost. I also was in Kansas City for the Association meeting. Gave a paper on Virchow. The meeting was very well organized, but unfortunately the papers were even weaker than usual. Sarton gave just a couple of classroom lectures. We gave Temkin the Welch Medal which I think he deserved, but might never have gotten in view of American prejudices except for the accident of the composition of this year's committee.

Then I re-wrote completely my old series on the history of malaria for Ciba Zeitschrift, a heavy and not very amusing job. Then I prepared myself for the abovementioned Symposium in reading the fifty papers that were discussed. That is my stupid German obsessional "Pflichterfüllung". I should have read only ten. The others do not mean anything to me anyhow. This Symposium was quite a show (I have invented several names for it like "Organized Schizophrenia", "Anthropology in the melting pot", "Symposium on mythology" – some of these guys like Mead and Linton did an awful amount of misrepresentation). The meetings actually did not produce anything but boredom and fatigue, but there were fifty representative people from this country and thirty from other countries (Great Britain, France, Japan, India, Scandinavia, Turkey, Siam, etc.) and the personal contacts, and the evenings off which I spent with old friends in French restaurants made the horrible strain (it was also very hot) worth while. There was also a Nazi, of course, but we smoked him out. He left after a week. The best thing that happened to me during my sojorn in New York was that I was told that there is a faint hope that I will be sent as a U.S. delegate to the Anthropologist meeting in Vienna from Sept. 1st to Sept. 8th.

I do not care a hang for Vienna but this will give me an opportunity to stay one week in Paris while going and one week in Paris while returning. I had been really rather desperate that all my plans to go to Europe this summer had failed because I feel so damned lonely here, and this has really improved my moral tremendously, although the voyage itself will probably be regrettably short. The reverse of the medal is that I will have to work now awfully hard because I am also going on a three week's vacation with the car with the girls – I promised it to them – and I absolutely have to polish the Virchow manuscript before September when it is supposed to go to the printer. Never mind. Better to work this way with some hope than to work merely in order not to feel too unhappy.

While I was doing all that mechanical work in Spring [sic] I read as a relaxation dozens of biographies of politicians and writers of the period (Paris 1800–1850) with which I am so much concerned in medical history. I found it considerably more rewarding than reading novels. Most of these biographies are quite extraordinary like the youth of Victor Hugo, George Sand, Flora Tristan, etc. The one that puzzles me most was Benjamin Constant.

Wishing you all a pleasant summer I remain with my kindest regards
Yours as ever
Erwin

"Association meeting" of the AAHM. "Pflichterfüllung" = performance of one's duty.
New names:
Constant, Benjamin (1767–1830) French politician and author
Freud, Sigmund (1856–1939) Austrian psychiatrist
Hugo, Victor (1802–1885) French writer
Linton, Ralph (1891–1953) anthropologist
Sand, George (1803–1876) French novelist, real name Aurore Dupin
Tristan, Flora (1803–1844) French socialist writer and activist
Names mentioned before:
Cushing   A. to S. of 12 April 1946
Jonckheere S. to A. of 23 February 1948
Marx   A. to S. of 17 September 1948

Mead	A. to S. of 23 March 1945
Pavlov	S. to A. of 24 June 1952
Sauerbruch	A. to S. of 23 May 1945
Speransky	A. to S. of 26 May 1950
Stern	A. to S. of 23 March 1945
Thyssen	S. to A. of 24 June 1952
Zola	A. to S. of 5 May 1938

SIGERIST to ACKERKNECHT, Pura ?, 10 July 1952

Dear Erwin,

Thanks for your long letter. You mentioned that you were puzzled by Benjamin Constant. Have you seen his autobiographical novel Cécile that was published quite recently by Gallimard? If not, I shall send it to you. It is an extraordinary piece of work.

I was delighted to hear that Temkin was awarded the Welch Medal. He certainly deserves it, and I am glad your committee gave it to him and not to one of the highly advertised amateurs of whom we have more than enough.

O'Malley and his wife were here recently, and I had a very good impression of both. He is a good historian and a good latinist, knows the Renaissance inside out, and is now on a Guggenheim Fellowship, looking for Vesalius material in European archives. So far with little result. It seems that there is not much unknown material available. Moritz Roth got hold of the most important documents long ago. O'Malley's wife is a very successful dermatologist, and together they make $ 25,000, which for a historian's household is not so bad.

You probably heard that the Swiss edition of the Ciba Zeitschrift will be discontinued, but they will continue in Germany and also in Italy. Dr. Reucker, who founded all these journals, has just retired and is moving to Pura where he built a very nice house.

I am going to hear more of the anthropological symposium, because Esther Lucille Brown, the sociologist of the Russell Sage Foundation, will be here next week, and I also just received a mimeographed copy of William Caudill's paper on Applied Anthropology in Medicine which, however, I have not read so far. I can well imagine what such a monster meeting must have been like.

I wish we could manage to meet if you go to Vienna, but I have a very full schedule myself this summer.

I am looking forward to receiving your reprints and with warm regards,

I am,

Yours as ever,

[Henry]

Constant see A. to S. of 27 June 1952 and (Constant 1951). Charles D. O'Malley (medical) historian. Vesalius see A. to S. of 23 February 1946. Moritz Roth (1839–1914) Swiss pathologist and medical historian. Reucker see S. to A. of 10 July 1948. Esther Lucille Brown wrote on nursing education. William A. Caudill (1920–1972) anthropologist.

ACKERKNECHT to SIGERIST, Madison, 31 July 1952

Dear Henry:

Thanks ever so much for your letter of July 10th, and your kind offer to send me Cecile [sic]. I bought it last summer in Paris, and was also extremely fascinated by it.

I am glad you feel the same way about Temkin and the medal. We saw him by the way about ten days ago in Baltimore when we came through on a three thousand mile trip East in the car, undertaken mostly for the benefit of the children, and I was delighted with the improvement in hearing that has resulted from the operation, and not only in hearing, but also in sociability. I had known him, of course, in his better days, but Lucy who had known him only in his paranoid phase was quite surprised.

No, I had not heard that the Swiss Ciba Zeitschrift will be discontinued too. I am very sorry that there is one more fine medico-historical journal that disappears.

The William Caudhill [sic], who sent you his paper on applied anthropology in medicine, is quite an original young man, and I got rather chummy with him. Unlike the older generation of anthropologists who talk so much about psychiatry without knowing anything, he really does know the subject, even from the other side of the barricade, having had himself locked up for several months in a psychiatric clinic as a patient, only the director knowing that he was "normal". He produced what he

376

thought to be a personality disorder, but was diagnosed as a schizophrenia. It is, by the way, a nice projective test to think what psychosis one would imitate.

My Vienna mission has collapsed as government projects so often do, and I was really quite depressed. I hope, nevertheless, to go next summer again to Europe. I can not see how I can stand it here without doing so. The above mentioned trip through Ohio, New York State (rather beautiful in the lake region), New York City (which is interesting even with children), Philadelphia, Baltimore, Washington, the Virginia mountains, and Kentucky (where we have friends) was interesting, but a poor ersatz for a Europe trip. I will go back now to my studies on French medicine. There is also, of course, quite some work to do with the Virchow which is processed. Do you by any chance know anybody who would be in the possession of a few good original photographs of Virchow? I have a collection of very interesting photographs but as they have been reproduced already once they reproduce too badly the second time.

A few weeks ago a very strange individual who is now associate professor of clinical medicine at the university of Illinois, called Frederick Christ Lendrum, looked me up with some crackpot idea on the history of leprosy. He referred to you as his friend, I suppose without your authorisation. I was also looked up by an English chemist DeLaszlo who is looking for a contraceptive drug and tried to get me drunk so that I should tell him primitive secrets. He could have saved his whisky. I told him anyhow what I knew. This is another adventurer to beware of.

Baltimore has really much improved since the time we lived there. They have built a great deal, cleaned up a great deal, and in the Museum they have now a magnificent collection of French post impressionists, due to the Cone and several other donations. But the climate is as dismal as ever.

Kindest regards and very best wishes to you all

Yours as ever

Erwin

Cécile see (Constant 1951). Caudill see S. to A. of 10 July 1952. Frederick C. Lendrum published on leprosy. Henry Delaszlo published on contraceptives, however, the first oral contraceptives were introduced in the late 1950s.

Dear Erwin,

Many thanks for your letter of 31 July. I have written a few letters trying to find somebody who had original photographs of Virchow, my special hope was Edgar Goldschmid in Lausanne, formerly of Frankfort, who is a historian of pathology and pathological illustrations, and who might have had original photos. But now I just hear that this is not the case. The Berlin Pathological Institute would undoubtedly have pictures, but as it is in the Eastern Zone, there is little hope of getting anything; although I am glad to say that the Leipzig Institute supplies me with everything I need. Thus they gave me a complete set of portraits for the illustration of the <u>Great Doctors</u>, as the original plates were altogether destroyed. Have you tried the various collections in the States, New York Academy of Medicine notably, the Baltimore Institute of the History of Medicine as well as the one of pathology, the Boston Medical Library, the Armed Forces Medical Library, etc? I shall keep an eye open, and if I can think of any possibility, will let you know.

I have not the faintest idea who "my friend" Frederick Christ Lendrum may be, although the name sounds vaguely familiar. I probably had some correspondence with him while I was in Baltimore.

I am glad that you wrote me about DeLaszlo. He wrote me several letters and I could not make out who he was. I stopped answering his letters and I hope this is the end of it. It would be fine to have a pill that would render a woman sterile for a month, but I am afraid it will not be quite so easy to find.

I had heard that Miss Cone had given her perfectly superb collection to the Baltimore Art Museum. It is unique in its way and certainly greatly adds to the art treasures of Baltimore.

That Baltimore has greatly improved I heard from various sides. Just two days ago we had the visit of Bertram Bernheim and his wife. You may have met him actually. He is a surgeon of the Halsted School, now emeritus, very liberal, who wrote some peppery books on medicine at the cross roads, surgery, Johns Hopkins, etc.

Next week I must go to Berne and swallow a number of papers read before the Swiss Society of the History of Medicine and Science. As I am one of the few founding fathers of the Society left, I cannot escape these meetings where I shall have to take benzedrine to keep awake.

With warm regards, I am,

Yours as ever,

[Henry]

Edgar Goldschmid (1881–1957) German pathologist and medical historian. Lendrum, Delaszlo, and anticonceptive pill see S. to A. of 31 July 1952. Claribel and Etta Cone collection. Bertram M. Bernheim (1880–1958) surgeon. William S. Halsted (1852–1922) first head of the Hopkins Deparment of Surgery. Benzedrine = Amphetamine.

ACKERKNECHT to SIGERIST, Madison, 21 August 1952

Dear Henry:

Thanks ever so much for your letter of August 14th. I am very grateful to you for your tips concerning possible sources for Virchow photographs. I had not yet consulted all the American institutions you mentioned. The main trouble with those I consulted so far is that they (even the great collector Thor Jager) have only photographs of Virchow with that long dismal beard which makes the face more or less meaningless and are historically misleading. Because the great discoveries were made ante barbam, I want to bring of that as little as possible. For years I have been collecting as a hobby beardless pictures of famous bearded men, and I have now amongst others such of Virchow, Helmholtz, Koch, Pasteur and Darwin. The difference is amazing, esthetically and psychologically. I have looked in vain so far for a beardless picture of Freud which also should be quite revealing.

Your "friend" Frederick Christ Lendrum is one of the worst stutterers I ever met in my life. He is also associate professor of medicine in the university of Illinois, and it is a complete mystery to me how he handles patients or teaches. De Laszlo is the son of a Hungarian painter who was once very fashionable in the English upper crust. He himself pretends to be a chemist. He lives in London, while his wife lives in New York.

While you had the visit of Bertram Bernheim (a literate surgeon is quite a rare thing, at least in these regions; I do not know Bernheim but his writings) I met Canby Robinson at a dinner out on Long Island during our trip. It seems to me that in many ways he belongs to the same generations [sic] as Bernheim. By the way, he spoke with great warmth of you and wants to be remembered.

I hope you have survived the ordeal of the Swiss Society Meeting. It sounds kind of strange that you should be already in the generation of the Founding Fathers. I am right now working my way through 80 volumes of the Archives Générales de Médecine. (Up to 1850). It is a very tedious job, but it has been my experience that this method provides one with a much clearer view of the actual level and dynamism of medicine in a period, than if one only studies selected articles, or [?] the books of those who have survived through the greatness of their work.

Do you know the little book by Charles Richet, "Le Savant"? It is a kind of counterpoint to the more serious discussions of Claude Bernard or Arthus of the same subject. It also contains a few good anecdotes. I found it amongst second hand books in New York when I was there in June. I also found there one of the novels of Charles Nicolle, the bacteriologist. Nothing of great literary importance while his letter to the deaf (republished in the little biography by Fernand Lot, Paris 1946 – he was deaf himself –) is one of the most powerful documents I have ever read in my life.

Here it is more or less peacefull [sic] and dull. Fortunately my friend Marshall Clagett (one of the two history of science men here, and the only good one, and a very lovable person) has returned from his Europe trip. And last weekend we had the visit of two young French anthropologists. Their conversation was quite a relief. Do you remember the wonderful passage in Mme. de Stael's "De l'Allemagne" on the French art of conversation versus the German one? One could write an even more depressing parallel on French versus American conversation.

Thanks again for the information.

Kindest regards and very best wishes

Yours as ever,

Erwin

Herrmann Ludwig F. Helmholtz (1821–1894) German physiologist and physicist. Charles R. Darwin (1809–1882) British natural scientist. (Richet 1926). (Lot 1946). Germaine de Stael (1766–1817); her famous book on Germany was first published in London in 1813.

Names mentioned before:
Arthus   S. to A. of 12 February 1946
Bernheim   S. to A. of 14 August 1952

Clagett   A. to S. 17 August 1947
Delaszlo   A. to S. of 31 July 1952
Freud   A. to S. of 27 June 1952
Koch   A. to S. of 14 April 1945
Lendrum   A. to S. of 31 July 1952
Nicolle   A. to S. of 7 February 1947
Pasteur   A. to S. of 25 November 1946

SIGERIST to ACKERKNECHT, Pura, 16 April 1953

Dear Erwin,

I just read your very interesting paper on Villermé and Quetelet, and your name was mentioned so often during the last few weeks that I was reminded of the fact that I had not written you for a very long time. Your "friend" deLaszlo was in Pura for two days and took up a lot of my time. He is slightly crazy and now claims to know one hundred drugs that will prevent conception. Of course he has not tested them yet. Do you know that he is the son of the painter who painted all the millionaire women of America a generation ago? He said that his father made at least $ 4 million painting these women, but he also spent them. His wife is a psycho-analyst in New York, she is from Zürich and I knew her as a child.

Then we had a visit from Gregory Zilboorg, who saw you at Iago Galdston's Institute in New York. Do tell me what your impression of this Institute was, I had many reports, but some were rather contradictory.

Next week we are expecting the Edelsteins. You probably know that he is teaching at Oxford for one year and they are spending their spring vacation in Greece and will be here on their way back to England.

Here little is changed, I am as busy as ever struggling to get three books out this year: the second volume of <u>The History</u>, a series of lectures I gave last November at the London School of Hygiene and Tropical Medicine on the history of hygiene; there were five lectures and the series was called <u>Landmarks in the history of Hygiene</u>, the London branch of the Oxford Press will publish them, but they are not written as yet; I have a lot of material ready, but still need to do some additional research, and thirdly a new enlarged edition of the Great Doctors.

Last December I spent a week in Nancy. Have you ever been there? It is a fascinating city and the food is very good. I was attending a meeting of the Committee on the Teaching of Social Medicine of the WHO and our report is going to be published in May. I do not know how much we achieved but I hope we will stir up some discussion in Europe where the professors of hygiene are bacteriologists or serologists or engaged in virus research and are never interested in Hygiene or social medicine. This is the heritage we have from Robert Koch. By the way have you seen the Koch biography by B. Möllers? It is a huge and frightfully dull book, but contains a lot of material from many letters and is useful as a reference book. Schuman thought of publishing an English edition but I dissuaded him.

Are you coming to Europe this year? If you do I wish you could manage to come to Pura. Six years is a long time, and I do not know when I shall be able to come back to the States for a visit, I have become such a country bumpkin that large cities frighten me. I had hoped to go to Rome this spring, but I am so busy that I have to postpone the trip to the Autumn.

With warm regards to you and the family,

    I am,

        Yours as ever,

          [Henry]

Villermé and Quetelet (Ackerknecht 1952a). Delaszlo and Zilboorg see A. to S. of 31 July 1952 and 5 August 1941, respectively. Galdston and Edelstein see A. to S. of 2 August 1944. Galdston seems to have moved to the Department of Mental Health of the State of Connecticut. In Pura S. was flooded by visitors; in the years 1951–1953 there were 50 to over 100 per year (Bickel 1997). *Landmarks* (Sigerist 1956a). The German version of *Great Doctors* was published in its 3rd edition in 1954. Koch see A. to S. of 14 April 1945; his biography (Möllers 1950).

Sigerist to Ackerknecht, Pura, 24 April 1953

Dear Erwin,

Just a short line to congratulate you most heartily on the Welch Medal. I was perfectly delighted to hear that it had been awarded to you. It seems that the medal is remaining in the family, as the only recipients so far were you, Temkin and I.

Thanks also for your recent publications. The Malaria number made me feel a little sad because it is the last number of the Ciba-Zeitschrift. Brodbeck and Hartmann both General Directors of Ciba who were vitally interested in the Zeitschrift are dead. Reucker, who founded and edited the journal is retired and so the Company decided to discontinue the Zeitschrift and to publish a little sheet instead, with clinical papers that could be published in any other Medical Journal just as well. A hundred years from [now] the Ciba-Zeitschrift will still be read, used and quoted, when all these clinical rags will have been forgotten for a long time.

Cornfield's [sic] dissertation [?] is a very creditable piece of work and I learned something from it as I had never heard the name of Burnett before.

I had various reports about the meeting at Columbus, Ohio, I know the place and do not think it was particularly inspiring, [sic] It also seemed to me that the programme was flooded with papers on local history.

With all good wishes,

I am,

Yours as ever

[Henry]

History of Malaria (Ackerknecht 1952b). Reucker see S. to A. of 10 July 1948. Cornfield, most likely Paul F. Cranefield (1925–2003) physiologist and medical historian, (Cranefield 1951), A.'s doctoral student. There were several physiologists named Burnet(t).

ACKERKNECHT to SIGERIST, Madison, 28 April 1953

Dear Henry:

Thanks ever so much for your good letters of April 16th and 24th which I found today on my desk, returning from a week's vacation in the Ozark Mountains with the family. We were so completely fed up with the eternal winter here that we made the little trip into the Spring. I appreciate very much your kind congratulations for the Welch Medal, and I am of course extremely proud to have received an honour which once went to you. You have seen the Columbus program, and you can easily imagine what it was. Genevieve gave a good craftsmanlike paper, but she is no speaker. Neither was anybody else. Suffice it to say that, so far as I am concerned, the "most stimulating" paper was that of Ralph Major on Etruscan Medicine, probably on account of my total ignorance of the subject, and because it forced me to rethink somewhat my ideas concerning Romans.

I was very happy to hear more about your work. I hope you have not taken on too much. Your book on <u>Landmarks in the History of Hygiene</u> should be most welcome, as nothing good exists in this field.

I have unfortunately never been in Nancy, although I am most interested in the place on account of Liébéault and Bernheim. I have always been very much interested in the Problem why Bernheim, trained by Kuess [?] and Virchow, and originally a specialist in infectious diseases, turned to psychotherapy. I think I found the answer in the fact that when he arrived in Nancy after leaving Strassburg for patriotic reasons (1871), there was absolutely no equipment to continue his laboratory studies, and there was the example of Liébault. I was quite intrigued to learn recently that there was even earlier interesting psychiatric goings on in Nancy, in so far as Morel worked nearby for several years. Morel, the inventor of the modern concept of degeneration, is a most fascinating personality, the friend of Claude Bernard and Lasègue, and of Lammenais [sic] and Buchez at the same time. While degeneration became later on an evolutionist concept, with him it was still a biblical one! Which all seems to prove that if a concept is in the air, people will rationalize it in the queerest ways. The degeneration concept corresponds, as far as I can see, to the spasmodic search of the 19th century psychiatrists for an anatomical basis of mental disease. I am just giving a seminar on the History of Psychiatry where we are discussing all these things, and which I am enjoying very much, inspite of the fact that the subject was not of my choosing, but was picked by my students.

The Galdston Institute was a tedious affair. Fifty percent of the people were interested in medical history, and there was therefore no need to tell them how beautiful it is. Fifty percent were to be interested (because Iago wants to create an Institute of the History of Medicine in connection with the New York Academy of Medicine – not a bad plan) and I do not believe that you can get them interested that way. To me the best way is in presenting a good piece of medical history. But Iago should know himself best about his politics. It was kind of queer. All the speakers were foreign born. I have never had as lively a feeling to assist a session of Romans, fat, rosy, strong, and bilious and [sic] legislators, who do not know anything about philosophy, listening to some Greek slaves and enjoying in a way their whisperings without understanding it.

I have just received my passport and I think I can say now that I will be coming to Europe this year. And I will do my utmost to see you. I will be, roughly speaking, from the middle of June to the middle of September in

Paris. I will have to go for a few days in July to London for the International Medical Librarians Meeting. I will have to go in August to visit my parents for ten days. At this occasion I would very much like to pass on my way back through Pura, and spend a couple of days with you. Would this time agree with you? I am very eager to see you again after these long years of separation, and I hope I can swing this year a financial deal in Germany (radio-lectures or newspaper articles) which will make the trip financially possible for me.

I am right now overwhelmed with work, and in a rather rundown condition. There is not only the usual teaching and committees, and mammoth correspondence, there is also the out-of-town-lecturing, and on top of all of it I have to read the proofs for the Virchow book rather hastily as I have to finish the index before I leave. It should be on the market in Fall [sic].

In spite of all disturbances I have nevertheless succeeded to write in the beginning of this academic year an article on Broussais, which I hope will be of some interest. As I had to write a paper for a Festschrift (for Wilson D. Wallace) on Method in Anthropology, I have written a short thing which actually boils down to the influence of comparative anatomy on several other disciplines in the first half of the 19th century. One usually thinks in this respect only of Darwin. But Cuvier was even far more important. The paper does not amount to much, but I enjoyed very much preparing it. The short moments that are left now to me I am working on Gall. This subject is none of my choosing, but the only way to get a grant for me this year was to make a study of the Gall collection at the Museum of Natural History in Paris. And I must say the subject is interesting. In order to be in the same rat race when I come back I have signed up for a short text book of medical history, deadline January 1st, 1954.

Kindest regards and very best wishes from all of us to you all

Yours as ever

Erwin

Columbus program see S. to A. of 24 April 1953. *Landmarks* (Sigerist 1956a). In 1871 French Alsace with Strassburg came under German rule. A.'s History of Psychiatry (Ackerknecht 1959), article on Broussais (Ackerknecht 1953b), book on Franz Joseph Gall collection (Ackerknecht/Vallois 1956), short textbook (Ackerknecht 1955a).

New names:

Bernheim, Hippolyte (1840–1919) French neurologist.

Cuvier, Georges (1773–1838) French zoologist and comparative anatomist

Buchez, Philippe-Joseph-Benjamin (1796–1866) French physician and psychologist
Kuess not identified
Lamen(n)ais, Robert F. de (1782–1854)
Lasègue, Charles (1809–1883) French psychiatrist
Liébault, Jean (1823–1904) French physician
Morel, Benedict-Augustin (1809–1873) French psychiatrist
Wallace, Wilson D. is likely to be misspelled for the anthropologist Wilson D(allam)
    Wallis (1886–1970)
    Names mentioned before:
Bernard   A. to S. of 21 August 1952
Broussais A. to S. of 2 October 1947
Darwin   A. to S. of 21 August 1952
Gall   A. to S. of 2 October 1947
Major   A. to S. of 10 May 1945

SIGERIST to ACKERKNECHT, Pura, 5 May 1953

Dear Erwin,

It was marvellous news to hear that we may see you this year. I am planning to be here the whole summer so that any time in August would suit us. We have a guest room and just let us know when you are planning to arrive in Lugano so that we can meet you there with the car.

Speaking of psychotherapy, do you know that Raymond de Saussure who used to practice psycho-analysis in New York is back in Geneva and is writing a four volume History of Psycho-Therapy from Mesmer to Freud? He lives in a palatial family mansion and plans to found a museum and a journal of the History of Science in Geneva. There are thousands of letters and other manuscripts in the old Geneva families, and there is always the danger that the dealers will get hold of them. Saussure was here in March when the medical historians met in Pura and I do hope that he will get a chair at the University and will be able to get his museum established in one of the old Geneva mansions.

There is so much I would like to discuss with you, but I am postponing everything until we meet.

With all best wishes, I am,
    Yours as ever
        [Henry]

De Saussure see A. to S. of 23 March 1945. His book was co-authored and single volume (Chertok / Saussure 1979). There are several journals of psychotherapy, founded toward the end of the 20th century. The Geneva Museum of the History of Science was founded in 1955 by de Saussure, Marc Cramer and others. In 1973 the Raymond de Saussure Psychoanalytic Center was founded. De Saussure was lecturer at the University of Geneva. Pura Conferences of Swiss medical historians see S. to A. 22 February 1950.

Ackerknecht to Sigerist, Madison, 12 May 1953

Dear Henry:

Thanks ever so much for your kind letter of May 5th, and your kind invitation. I will let you know more details about my visit, when in Europe.

I had not known that Raymond de Saussure has left the U.S. It is a good thing that he will write a history of psychotherapy from Mesmer to Freud, as he is considerably more learned and honest than Zillboorg [sic]. It is on the other hand regrettable that he wants to limit himself to that period – and to psychotherapy – there is more in psychiatry and even 19th century psychiatry than just psychotherapy. Eventually his psychoanalitic [sic] bias will probably not make it the history of psychiatry, which we so badly need, and do not have. His work in Geneva should be very promising, as Geneva is extremely interesting, and has been so badly neglected by medical historians.

Now that I am reasonably certain of seeing you soon, I also prefer to postpone most other items to oral discussion. Not much has happened here since I wrote you last. We spent a weekend in Chicago where I gave a lecture, and saw an interesting piece by Brecht, and an agreeable Fernandel movie. I go on suffering from Virchow, and working on Gall.

Kindest regards and very best wishes and see you soon

Yours as ever

Erwin

De Saussure see A. to S. of 23 March 1945 and S. to A. of 5 May 1953. Zilboorg see A. to S. of 5 August 1941. Bertold Brecht (1888–1956) German dramatist. Fernandel, French movie actor.

Dear Henry:

I made it. I will be here till Sept. 13. I will go to London for three days in July (19–22) for the Med. Librarians Meeting. And to Ludwigsburg Aug. 9–19 (approximately). It's on my way back that I intend to come through Pura, where, if this suits you, will probably be on Aug. 20 and 21. My address here is:

Musé de l'Homme
Palais de Chaillot
Paris XIIᵉ
(Tel. Passy 7446)

Hope you are doing all right. Everything else by word of mouth. Kindest regards and best wishes to you both.

yours as ever
Erwin

ACKERKNECHT to SIGERIST, Ludwigsburg, 10 August 1953

Dear Henry:

I just found out about train connections which unfortunately are poor. Thus I will arrive in Lugano on Wednesday Aug. 19 at 17₂₂. Will have to leave Lugano on Thursday Aug. 20 at 19₀₇, as I have an appointment in Paris next evening with Jim Tanner (I think you know him too – from London – we became friends last summer in New York)[.] I wish I could stay longer. But "c'est la vie". The country here is beautiful, the reconstruction stupendous, the people neither. My parents are unfortunately very much reduced. Paris is still the best. Even work is fun. Found a lot of Gall material. More about that orally. Looking forward to seeing you both soon

I am with my kindest regards and best wishes

yours ever
Erwin

Jim Tanner not identified. "C'est la vie": such is life. Gall see A. to S. of 2 October 1947.

ACKERKNECHT to SIGERIST, Paris, 26 August 1953
(Original in French)

My dear Henry,

Here I am back in Paris. I arrived yesterday 9 o'clock after a rather tiring ride and with a nasty cold. Once more, let me thank you for these wonderful days. I cannot say more because I am not a writer, and ill-chosen expressions might spoil memories and feelings. You know I sincerely mean it.

In the train I have wondered why I had left this paradise (with a God father and an Eve and all — myself likely to be a silly Adam prior to the distribution of the apples). But when I heard the chirp of French women and when I saw the glorious blue sky above the roofs of Paris I understood why I had left. At the Museum I found a lot of dull business letters, but also the announcement that my Virchow had definitely appeared. Thus, you will have a copy in a couple of weeks. I hope you will not be disappointed by the dry tree which came out of the seed you planted into my poor brain 25 years ago in Leipzig. This is duly mentioned in the Foreword.

Take good care of yourself (days of rest!) best regards and wishes
Yours as ever
Erwin

My best to Evita. I have returned to the same hotel, same room, but my address remains Musée d'Homme – until 13 September, damned day among us.

"Evita" is Eva D. Stiasny, S.'s new (British) secretary. "Mentioned in the Foreword": "… the stimulating influence of H. E. Sigerist".

ACKERKNECHT to SIGERIST, Paris, 5 September 1953
(Original in French)

My dear Henry,

I was so happy to have your note of 2 September, but sad that the casa once more has become too serena. Nine days from here I shall be in the same situation. – At the moment I am still defending myself. Not only have I survived the lunar rites but also two weeks with almost no sleep. It is so unbelievably beautiful that I cannot bring myself to go to sleep. Truly, this beauty from time to time gives me funny nightmares in view of my departure. The rope around my neck is drawing together. I often think of you, how wonderful it was, how wonderful you were. It would be great for me and for you, my friend, to be here. Last night for instance, we've been at [...] with my friend from student days 27 years ago who is now Cuban, and in pleasant company. It's always nice.

I am no longer very busy. But you will soon receive my Virchow in order to remind you that I can be very serious too. According to my publisher it has been sent ten days ago. I hope you won't be too disappointed. It's dull.

I am not very proud of my little photo. But then it is a memory of happy days.

> Best wishes
> > Ever yours faithful pupil (in all branches)
> > Erwin

My love to the ladies

S.'s letter is missing. Unclear passages in A.'s letter. "The ladies": Emmy Sigerist and Eva Stiasny (see A. to S. of 26 August 1953).

SIGERIST to ACKERKNECHT, Pura, 11 September 1953
(Telegram, original in French))

JUST RECEIVED VIRCHOW, SINCERE CONGRATULATIONS, BON VOYAGE AND HAPPY RETURN
HENRY, EVITA

ACKERKNECHT to SIGERIST, Madison, 18 September 1953
(Original in French)

My dear teacher and friend,

Let me thank you for many things: your good letter of 9 September, the excellent photographs (you're still a master of the art), the telegram (I was happy to see Evita's name on it – after all, we had a good time), and finally the reprints which arrived today. I have immediately read the Sudhoff article and "the autonomy", and I liked both very much. I hope that you have survived the sessions of the Society, that you could also rest, and that you find life agreeable nevertheless.

The end of my time in Paris contained some unforgettable days and nights. Also a day in Rouen which despite the destructions is still a beautiful and interesting town. Yet, Sunday night was the end, and Monday evening saw me in Madison again, with a hangover and a bad cold. I am almost voiceless – too bad for my classes – and totally confused by the rapid change as well as by the fact of "returning" into a new house (2133 Fox Ave) where Lucy had done good work. It's a very good house. I have tried to read the mail of three months, and I had already a committee meeting. I am still too busy to be melancholy, and the weather is fine, the kids charming, and […] makes an effort to be agreeable which is commendable ("pourvu que ça dure" said Laetitia, Buonaparte's mother). Looking at the pokerfaces of my colleagues and the natives in general gives me a headache. This is my last letter in French, of this happy summer with Pura as a highlight. And now "hibernation". But summer will return, and so will I!

Yours as ever
Erwin

P. S. I have seen poor Urdang. He goes from bad to worse. Apparently bulbar hemorrhages with symptoms of Parkinsonism (salivation, impaired swallowing etc.). He sends his regards.

S.'s letter is missing. Evita see A. to S. of 26 August 1953. The two reprints are (Sigerist 1952 and 1953).

ACKERKNECHT to SIGERIST, Madison ?, 30 September 1953
(Original in French)

My dear Henry,

Many thanks for kindly sending the beautiful poem. How interesting, that the country which inspired Hesse to Chinese imitations led you in the same direction. I will send you one of his short stories containing the water colors which you may ignore. I hope you like them.

In addition of classes, students, a new house etc. I am busy preparing a bad lecture I will deliver tomorrow in Milwaukee on "Medical art as a psychological safety valve". The site will be a poor exhibition "The Story of Medicine in Art", one of those typically American enterprises with 750 mediocre pictures instead of 150 well chosen and well presented ones.

Damn these lectures. What a waste of precious time! I would prefer to give one on "Lectures as a psychological safety valve". One of my colleagues asked me meaningfully: Do you know what my wife and I did in Paris. We spent every evening in the hotel playing Canasta. I told him they should have shot you at sunrise. They didn't know that what they called their "moral fiber" was in reality their " moral fibrosis".

Now I have to deal with my little textbook. I will go to Chicago on 20 October and to Washington on the 24th. A bit travelling will be good because I am about to wake up from my dream and to become aware that I am back again.

I hope everything is fine with you. Best wishes

Yours as ever

Erwin

My best regards to Emmy and Evita

S.'s poem is again missing. A possible explanation for a series of missing letters is that S., like A., wrote these French letters in long-hand and without making copies. Hermann Hesse see A. to S. of 1 July 1946. Added to the letter is a short French poem.

Dear Henry:

I apologize for not having thanked you earlier for your very beautiful poem, but I was still waiting for that letter in prose which was to follow soon, and also I lacked inspiration for writing, nothing important ever happening here. Except for a trip to New York (I had a committee meeting in Washington) and one to Chicago, where there were good theatre, movies, museums, French records and books, and friends, more interesting than the people here, it has been, in spite of the wonderful fall weather, one pretty gray long routine. I am working on the textbook, and I do not like this pretended omniscience very much, but if at least they would leave me alone, and there would not be the usual courses, lectures, and worst of all, committee meetings, and so called small town university social life.

I am looking forward to work on Gall, when I am through with the text book. There will also be a paper to be presented at the association meeting in spring (Lloyd Stevenson asked me for it), and Shryock is preparing a symposium for June. I have not yet committed myself to attending the latter, as I want to see first the program. If this is to be another accumulation of common places on the teaching of medical history, as was the New York Academy thing, and another one of the AAAS, I will not go. Fejos also wants me to organize a symposium on primitive medicine. I do not believe in all these symposia, and one on primitive medicine fits in very badly now with my work, but it is hard to refuse something to one's financial angel. I still hope to kind of slip out from under it.

Occasionally I read a novel, but most are no good. I liked very much Uranus by Marcel Aymé, and <u>The Catcher in the Rye</u> by a certain Salinger. The latter is not a great work of art, but interesting documentary (slang and mentality of an American adolescent – I have not passed through this stage here, and almost exclusively had contact with so called grownups; it has taught me a few things concerning my own children.)

Koyré is here for the first semester as a guest professor. He seems to get already pretty melancholic in the Mid-western atmosphere (though it pays well). It is a pity that with all the due respect for his intelligence and learning, I have not much in common with him personally. Also he speaks French with a heavy Russian accent.

I hope you are doing well. I have one of the Pura pictures on my desk, and occasionally escape to the warmth of the beautiful memories of the last summer.

> Very cordially
> Yours ever,
> Erwin

"Textbook": (Ackerknecht 1955a). Gall see A. to S. of 2 October 1947. Stevenson see S. to A. of 3 November 1949. AAAS: American Association for the Advancement of Science. Fejos see A. to S. of 17 July 1945. *Uranus* (Aymé 1951); *Catcher in the Rye* (Salinger 1952). Alexandre Koyré (1892–1964) Russian-born French philosopher and historian of science.

SIGERIST to ACKERKNECHT, Pura, 4 December 1953

My dear Erwin,

This is the prose letter I promised, it comes late but "mieux vaut tard que jamais". I have to thank you for several letters, for a very delightful poem and for two reprints that I just read with great pleasure. Broussais certainly was a character and I like the statistics of the leeches imported by France in those years. I also read you [sic] radio talk on Gall long ago. There is certainly much work to be done on him and nobody could tackle that better than you. I am reviewing your <u>Virchow</u> for Isis and I had hoped to add a carbon of the review to this letter, but it is not quite ready yet but is however on this month's list. The book is very good and is the first full sized biography of the man.

You will receive a copy of the new edition of my Grosse Aerzte. Lehmann, who by the way is dead, was a Nazi to be sure, but how much more pleasant it is to deal with a German than with an American publisher. The [sic] do not edit your text, they follow all your wishes, they pay for the right of reproduction of illustrations and I got forty free copies while the Oxford Press gives me six. You remember that I was slaving on the book while you were here and now thank God I have one worry less.

In October I attended the Annual meeting of the Italian Society of the History of Medicine which was held at Verona and centered around Fracastoro. The Italian colleagues are charming people and I must say that the general standard of the papers is infinitely superior to what we hear in

America on similar occasions. I would have liked to stay a few days longer in Verona and go home by way of Mantua and Cremona, cities that I had never visited, but it was raining day and night, so I went home as soon as I could.

Now I am just back from England, where I spent a very pleasant week in London. I managed to be incognito for a few days, went to museums and saw superb performances of Hamlet, Peter Grimes and even Fledermaus. I gave a lecture on "Science and History" to the British Post-Graduate Medical Federation and the following day I received an honorary D.Sc. on the occasion of the Foundation Day of the University of London. It was a very colourful and dignified performance, but in no way pompous as it would have been in America. The orator who sang one's praise always did it with a touch of humour.

I flew home for my mother's 88th birthday, but found her in bed with pneumonia. However, she seems to be making a good recovery. And now I am back at the grindstone, grinding out books and to make matters worse I began writing an autobiography of which I am sending you a copy of the introduction. There will of course be serious chapters, but I thought I would begin in a light vein to capture the reader's attention. I will not follow a chronological order, but will write the way one reminisces. The next chapter will deal with Paris, the way I see the city and what it meant to me and incidentally I will recollect my childhood there in the nineties. I could write the book in one year if I had nothing else to do, but with eight volumes of the <u>History</u> on my neck it will take more time. It is great fun writing such a book.

Soon you will be buried in snow while we had a most gorgeous Indian summer with violets and snow drops in the garden. I count on your visit next year and do plan to attend the congress in Rome and Salerno, you will find the whole international medical-historical ménagerie there together. I have one of the main addresses on the Influence of Medicine upon civilisation. Each such subject will be discussed by two people with opposite philosophies, thus my partner will be Lain Entralgo who is a Catholic Spanish Fascist.

Our Christmas Card will I am afraid be late this year, so I take advantage of the opportunity to wish you and yours a good holiday and a good 1954.

Yours as ever,

[Henry]

"Mieux vaut tard que jamais": better late than never. Broussais see A. to S. of 2 October 1947. Isis, a journal for the history of science. *Grosse Aerzte* = *Great Doctors* (Sigerist 1932). Lehmann, German publisher. Fracastoro see A. to S. of 26 November 1947. S.'s D.Sc. from the University of London was his fourth honorary degree. S.'s autobiography remained a torso; his daughter Nora included the existing first chapters into the *Autobiographical Writings* (Sigerist Beeson 1966). Lain Entralgo later became the editor of a 7 volume history of medicine (Lain Entralgo 1972).

Ackerknecht to Sigerist, Madison, 11 December 1953 (Original in French)

My dear friend,

I should write a chapter of my little textbook, I should write my dad for his birthday, I should … but first, let me thank you for your good letter and above all for the "Prelude" which I must not do in my professional English but rather in the language of my heart. The "Prelude" is amazing, it's excellent, it's splendid. I have read it with so much pleasure, and I am anxious to read the next chapters. You absolutely must write this book. And soon. When you mentioned the plan last summer I knew you would do a good job, but I did not realize your talent to do precisely this. It will also relieve you from the hard work at big history. It is so full of atmosphere (e.g., the description of rural Maryland in two lines or the summer of 1940), it is so spiritual (e.g., the centenary of Penn. Univ.). I am really delighted. I think some humor is appropriate. After all, laughter is one of the most unique inventions of "homo sapiens". I would like to leave this world with a roaring laughter. As to the writer's art you are going to face interesting problems which, I am sure, you will handle perfectly.

I was very happy to learn that you were able to escape to Italy and to London. I am anxious to receive the "Great Doctors", and I hope your mother will recover without too many difficulties. Here we had snow since Thanksgiving after a long and hot Indian summer. And still boredom, a reason to work a lot. We have now a Swiss at our Medical School: Akert from Zurich, a brilliant young physiologist (three kids already, my God), personally nice and interesting. The poor nervous products of the American university career are surprised of his independent ways. You have certainly heard of the death of our old "friend" Laignel-Lavastine. He was a victim of the Congress in Jerusalem and of the August strike. Instead of waiting for the end of the strike he returned to Marseilles, boarded a truck and died of a cardiac attack on the way to Paris. He was 79, and I had seen him in Paris in July. He looked much younger than before the war as a result of having cut off his beard. It was Delaunay who wrote me the whole story. He is a fine old man, touching in his extreme, old-fashioned, provincial politeness (he spent all his life in Le Mans). – Have I written you that Marcel Aymé's novels have impressed me?

Best wishes for Christmas and New Year! My regards to Emmy, my best to Evita (is she still in Pura?). All my best feelings for you

Yours as ever

E…

Prelude is the first chapter of S.'s autobiography. Konrad Akert (born 1919) Swiss neurophysiologist in Madison and Zurich, became a friend of A. for the rest of his life. Laignel-Lavastine see S. to A. of 11 May 1949. Paul Delaunay (1878–1958) French medical historian. Aymé see A. to S. of 24 November 1953.

ACKERKNECHT to SIGERIST, Madison, 17 December 1953

Dear Henry:

This is to thank you in haste for the "Great Doctors" which just arrived. It is a beautiful book, and the new chapters which I read immediately, and which are particularly dear to me, as you wrote several of them whilst I was with you, are worthy of their predecessors.

Nothing new happened since my last letter. That is, my dean broke his leg in playing ball (oh these Americans). He is 64, but I hope he will pull through all right. It is only the ankle.

Kindest regards and very best wishes

Yours ever,

Erwin

SIGERIST to ACKERKNECHT, Pura, 30 January 1954
(Original in French)

My dear Erwin,

Let me thank you for two letters and for the translation of Breuer's CV which is really interesting since he was in fact the one who initiated the psychoanalyst movement. I am happy to know that you like the idea of my autobiography, and I hope to finish the first chapter soon which may be titled "Paris as I Remember it". It will deal with my childhood but also with the "front populaire" and the crisis of Munich. The second chapter will be "Education in Zurich" in which I shall try to show the difference between a humanistic "Gymnasium" in Europe and a High School or College in America. I shall send you all the chapters as soon as they will be done but, of course, they will be a first draft, and I can see the American editor with his red pencil eliminating whole paragraphs "for being of no interest to American readers".

It is good to know that you liked the "Grosse Aerzte". Lehmann made it a fine book. He sold 1,525 copies in the first five weeks which resulted in 3,200 Marks for me. The sum will be used for Emmy's trip to the U.S. where she intends to spend the summer with Nora and her family. Evita will stay here until fall and will look after me. It goes without saying that we expect you, alone or with your family. We have space for all of you.

No news otherwise. In May I shall spend two weeks in Yugoslavia in order to study their public health system and to give a few lectures. I have recently received a personal invitation from the USSR Minister of Public Health to spend six weeks in his country, however, in February and March it will be too cold in Russia. I prefer to do the trip next year. Let's wait and see. In the meantime I shall write my other books. We do not have snow, but it is cold at the moment after a very mild winter.

Yours as ever

[Henry]

Josef Breuer (1842–1925) Austrian physician and physiologist. "Crisis of Munich" 1938. *Grosse Aerzte*, the new edition of (Sigerist 1932). Lehmann see S. to A. of 4 December 1953. "Nora and her family", i.e., husband Jack Beeson and son Christopher in New York. Evita see A. to S. of 26 August 1953. The planned trips to Yugoslavia and Russia did not materialize.

Dear Henry:

Thanks ever so much for your letter of January 30th. I am very grateful that you will let me have the chapters of your autobiography as they come, and I am looking forward very much to "Paris as I remember it". You remember that we were walking the streets of Paris together during the Munich crisis? I think it was not yet at its height. I was also very glad to hear that the Grosse Aerzte is such a financial success, and Emmie thus can go to the United States. But the trouble is that we can not go to Europe this summer, and will come only in 1955. I very much hope that this trip then will not coincide with your trip to Russia, as I had already nice plans of sending our womenfolk to Italy, as they seem to enjoy travel, and stay with you for a while in Pura, as I am so lazy.

Needless to say that we never have much news here, especially in winter. Next week Temkin will come for a lecture. That is already an exciting event. After having finished my textbook manuscript according to plan, I took off a few days with disease and French novels (The ten volumes of the Thibaults of Roger Martin du Gard, still more Marcel Aymé, and a novel of André Chamson "La Galère" on the 6 Feb. 1934 which brought back an important episode in my life rather vividly). But soon I had to settle down again on Gall who is fortunately rather interesting, and to the usual futilities of my existence here. We were rather depressed by the tragic suicide of the wife of a colleague and friend here (H. H. Gerth, a sociologist) a former Countess Reventlow who cut her throat. Well, to speak about something more gay, I just received a letter from Iago Galdston who seems to have read for the first time something written by me and accuses me out of a clear sky of a lot of sins [?] like lack of tolerance and penetration, supercilious treatment of the Vienna School, Wunderlich, etc., and above all of "disparaging remarks" about the concept of the epidemic constitution. As to the latter point he is perfectly right. I have never had much sympathy with vagueness and mysticism, so dear to my ex-countrymen, and apparently to him too. For whatever intestinal or political reasons he attacked [?], I guess he ran into the wrong person. I am no Shryock. Neither will I waste much time in polemics nor will I on the other hand cuddle up to the mighty judge. It is not in my temperament, and besides he needs me more than I need him. Well, that brings a little warmth and excitement into the greyness and coldness of this Wisconsin winter.

Kindest regards and very best wishes
Yours ever
Erwin

ACKERKNECHT to SIGERIST, Madison, 6 March 1954

Dear Henry:

Thanks ever so much for the carbon of your review of my Virchow, and the most magnificent buildup you gave me. It is as good as a medal! – I hope you are doing well. Nothing particularly new here, as usual. I have just now moved into two large new rooms, where we have concentrated all our books prior to 1850, and all books on medical history. (about 5000 volumes). I am very much pleased with the new arrangement, which almost looks like a little institute, and regret that I can not show you my new installation. – My seminar on medical autobiographies from Cardano to Sauerbruch is also proceeding [sic] quite satisfactorily. We have a rather agreeable and able young physiologist from Zurich (Akert) on the staff (his wife cooks superbly), and for a year a Parisian psychiatrist called Rappaport who is not without interest. But it is still rather dull here. I am going on with my Gall, and I got myself a very nice series of chansons by George Brassard [sic], sung by Patachou. – In summer not having enough money to go to Europe, we will probably go to Mexico, where also my friend Boris Goldenberg is supposed to come from Cuba. His Spanish and his company should make this an agreeable venture. We replaced the 1940 chevrolet by a 1949 chevrolet, which should carry us without too great difficulty to and from Mexico. Thanks again.

Kindest regards and best wishes
Yours ever,
Erwin

Carbon: carbon copy of typescripts. Geronimo Cardano (1501–1576) Italian physician and philosopher. Sauerbruch and Akert see A. to S. of 23 May 1945 and 11 December 1953, respectively. Georges Brassens (1921–1981) French composer. Patachou (born 1918) French female singer. Boris Goldenberg (1905–1980) Russian-born socialist, politician, and historian.

ACKERKNECHT to SIGERIST, Madison, 13 May 1954

Dear Henry:

I have just returned from the New Haven meeting of the Association. As far as I can see nothing sensational happened. The program was much better than last year, but still too much rehash. The good performers are still the same old men, Temkin, Rosen, etc. Of the many young men who have passed through the Institute during the last years, and some of whom are of very poor quality, one, Multhauf, seems to be rather good. I drew again the wrath of Iago, the perennial paranoiac, when in a private conversation I modestly suggested to him that neither Griesinger, Wunderlich, nor Henle, nor the Vienna School were romantics, as he always affirms. His Geschichtsklitterung was so bad that even Temkin rose in the […]. Bruno Kisch, the former physiology professor in Cologne, proved to be a very agreeable man. And a good speaker. After the thing was over I had at least twenty-four hours in New York with good French friends, food, records, and movies. I hope to have the same this week-end after a National Research Council meeting in Philadelphia. In June I will go to Baltimore to the Shryock symposium, rather out of loyalty to the place than out of sympathy with the program which I fear will be the usual educational bunk. Why can't he go on doing the seminars as you did them.

At the end of June we will go for four weeks to Mexico. In case you know of anybody worth while seeing there, please let me know. It is also time to think of financing next summer's trip to Europe. It seems that one of the possibilities is to get a lecture with the Ciba Foundation in London. Do you know anybody there, or do you know whom to approach there?

I have eventually finished my little Gall monograph, and will see now what Vallois will do with it in the way of changes and publication. I wrote it in French which was foolish, as it takes me now about twice as long to write in French than in English, and the French is probably bad. I am engaged in the usual row with the publisher of my textbook who, like all

American publishers, has the obsession of editing what he could leave to me, that is bibliography, etc. The MD theses of this year are coming in now. Of the five some promise to be not bad. Especially one on Rasori.

We had Guthrie here for a lecture. We had to take him as Major was his manager, and is a close friend of our dean. What a pretentious mediocrity. Our dean is by the way retiring next year, and the usual row for the succession is going on. My position here is secure, but still I will miss him. We will not find so easily a man of the same qualities, and with a similar interest in medical history.

You know from the newspapers about our political situation here. I am extremely pessimistic. Even if our senator's stock is declining at the moment, the collective psychosis upon which his activities are based, goes on unabated. For fun I read through Les Misérables. In the beginning I found it only grotesque, but going on I was more and more charmed. In the seminar on autobiographies we are now dealing with Ramon y Cajal. Of all the autobiographies this is perhaps the strangest and most interesting one. Medieval thought in terms of modern neuro-physiology. What a nation these Spaniards. No wonder that they have fascinated so many since the time of the French romantics. Recently I had a dream I was in Pura with you on the terrace, your grandson playing around. Outside it was all full of snow. Typical dream world. It is of course not you, who have the snow, but we. As late as last sunday [sic]. I hope you are all doing well.

Kindest regards and very best wishes
    Yours ever,
        Erwin

How is the autobiography coming?

Association, American, for the History of Medicine (AAHM). "Iago" Galdston. Geschichtsklitterung: Falsification of history. A.'s Gall monograph with H. V. Vallois as coauthor was published in French in 1956 and in English one year later (Ackerknecht/ Vallois 1956). W. S. Middleton was Dean of the University of Wisconsin School of Medicine from 1935 to 1955. "Our senator": Joseph McCarthy, senator of Wisconsin, was censured by the Senate in 1954. Les misérables, a novel by Victor Hugo (1802–1885).

New names:
Griesinger, Wilhelm (1817–1868) German professor of psychiatry
Guthrie, Douglas James (1885–1975) British medical historian
Henle, Friedrich G. J. (1809–1885) German anatomist and pathologist
Kisch, Bruno (1890–1966) German physiologist

Multhauf, Robert P., Ph.D. 1953, published on history of chemistry
Rasori, Giovanni (1766–1837) Italian physician
    Names mentioned before:
Galdston   A. to S. of 2 August 1944
Hugo   A. to S. of 27 June 1952
Major   A. to S. of 10 May 1945
Middleton   A. to S. of 7 October 1946
Ramon y Cajal S. to A. of 24 June 1952
Wunderlich   A. to S. of 6 February 1954

SIGERIST to ACKERKNECHT, Pura, 23 June 1954

Dear Erwin,

I know that you are in Mexico at the moment but I am writing you nevertheless as I owe you an answer to two good letters and if [?] I do not write now I do not know when a letter will be written. If the letter is forwarded to you to Mexico I would advise you to look up Joaquin Izquierdo who is Professor of Physiology at the University. I do not know him personally but he seems to be the best they have in medical history, he wrote about Harvey and Claude Bernard, translated Walter Caron's book and I have just written the preface to a book of his on Montana [sic] one of the early pioneers of the social and scientific movement in Mexico. I am sorry I never had a chance to visit that country which is so close to the States and is so interesting historically as well as socially. The new University buildings must be fabulous and Mexico has a school of painters at the moment such as no American and very few European countries have.

I was amused by what you wrote about Galdston's antics. He has a strong feeling of inferiority, which he over-compensates a little too spectacularly. I had various reports about the New Haven and also the Baltimore meetings, they all agree that there was an improvement in the Programmes compared with the last few years, but I know well enough what these meetings are like and how tired one gets of them. I shall however, attend the International Congress at Rome and Salerno, not to listen to papers, but to have an excuse to see Rome and Salerno again. The attraction is infinitely greater than that of Nice and Cannes, where it would be delightful to be, but not with a crowd of colleagues.

Guthrie is a frightful bore and beastly pretentious at that. His book was translated into German by the Guttenberg [sic] Gilde and they produced a beautiful book. Unfortunately it is full of mistakes.

You have been very productive this winter, finishing the text book and a monograph on Gall. I am sorry to say that I cannot say the same of myself. I work all the time and achieved very little. One reason has been that my health has not been so good recently, I had several attacks of angina, minor ones, but unpleasant enough. I am being fed with Serpasil and a few other drugs and my chief difficulty of course is that I am constantly overweight. I have taken off 10 lbs, which does not improve one's morale and I have 10 more lbs to go. I have no objection to tomatoes and cucumbers, but I prefer French or Chinese cuisine.

I also had a great deal of worry about my old mother who is 89 and is just about falling to pieces physically and mentally. With these new drugs old people no longer die peacefully of pneumonia as they used to do in the past, but one keeps them alive until they are complete wrecks. […] So I am going to Basel.

Being a realist at heart I have taken a heroic resolution to make my History of Medicine from Volume IV on if not sooner a co-operative undertaking. There is decidedly a need for a detailed book and I have just not the time left, nor the strength to do it all myself. If we make it a handbook and if all co-operate the 8 volumes could be out in a few years. Otherwise I shall be repeating what Neuburger did, begin a book and get stuck at the end of the Middle Ages. I shall work out a plan during the summer, and will be very anxious to have you [sic] opinion. I also would like to launch the Sociology of Medicine that I had planned originally and I think there are people who could be called upon to colaborate [sic].

I am sending you the Paris chapter of the autobiography by surface mail. It will give you an idea of the style and the method. Please remember that this is a very rough first draft, there are repetitions and lengthy passages that will have to be edited carefully, but I write as it comes. At the moment I am working on the Chapter that deals with Zürich in which I talk of school days but also of Georg Büchner and Lenin and of the now defunct liberalism of Switzerland. Before World War I the old democracies felt secure, the socialists were noisy but harmless, but the present state does not tolerate any opposition or even criticism.

Genevieve Miller could give you information about the Ciba Foundation in London. She spent a week there as guest of the Foundation. I do not know anybody there, but it should not be too difficult to be invited to give a lecture. Any Professor can stay there by simply writing, provided that rooms are available. I will enquire into the matter further because I would like to make the Ciba Foundation my Head Quarters when I am in London and I go there almost every year now. I was to have been there a few weeks ago because the Royal College of Physicians made me a Fellow, but I did not feel well at that time and also cancelled, or rather postponed my Jugoslav [sic] Tour.

Have you read Victor Hugo's Diaries? Two volumes have been published recently and they make fascinating reading. These romantic poets had guts, Hugo as well as Lamartine. When they believed in something they stuck to it. The second volume is a scream because the old fellow was still going to prostitutes regularly and kept book of whatever he paid them.

I have been doing an infinity of minor affairs recently, prefaces, book reviews, a few essays, now I must finish the Heath Clark Lectures that have been dragging out for almost two years and then of course must finish volume II of the History where I have simply got stuck in India.

Of course I count on your visit next year and I hope you can stay with us as long as possible. My travelling plans are as vague as can be, chiefly on account of my health. The old heart is not getting better with the years.

With all good wishes,

I am,

Yours as ever

[Henry]

William Harvey (1578–1657) British physiologist. Claude Bernard see A. to S. of 21 August 1952. Walter Caron's book not identified; possibly a misspelling. Joaquin O. Izquierdo: Mexican physiologist. Luis Montaña (1755–1820) Mexican physician and medical historian, see also (Sigerist 1955a). Guthrie see A. to S. of 13 May 1954. Gutenberg Gilde: a German publisher. Serpasil, generic name reserpine. Neuburger see S. to A. of 14 February 1947 and (Neuburger 1906).

Cooperative undertaking: By 1954 S. realized that progress on his *History* was so slow that he would never finish it on his own. The idea that coauthors would finish it was near at hand but maybe not realistic. Georg Buechner see A. to S. of 15 July 1948. Lenin (1870–1924) Russian revolutionary. S.'s study tour in Yugoslavia did not materialize. Victor Hugo see A. to S. of 27 June 1952 and (Guillemin 1954). Alphonse de Lamartin (1790–1869) French poet. Heath Clark Lectures (Sigerist 1956a).

Dear Henry:

I was so happy to have a letter of yours before leaving for Mexico (thanks ever so much), and so unhappy that your health has not been good. Even when these angina attacks do not mean much in the sense of survival – you know yourself that one can live with them for twenty years – they must be very trying, and living on a diet is not very funny either. Do you know by the way that this Serpasil is a primitive drug, one of those George Harley brought back with him from Liberia fifteen years ago, and which the […] men of Colombia threw into the ashcan. Now that the Indians (!) developed it, the pharmaceutic industry seems to have seen the light. I am looking forward so very much to your chapter on Paris. All my sympathies are with you in this situation with your mother, as I know it only too well from my own parents.

I will follow your advice and look up Isqaiedro [sic] in Mexico. I read a few of his things, and they seem to me pretty good. I am looking forward very much to Mexico. I know that it will not be like Europe, but it should give some relief from the stifling climate here. I hope you will have a good time in Rome and Salerno. I will look back a lot this summer to the beautiful days in Pura (I have still one of the pictures on my desk) and I am looking forward already eagerly to our next reunion next summer.

I think your decision to transform the later volumes of your history into cooperative ventures, is a very sound one, and am looking forward to your plan. – If Vallois is reliable, his additional chapter should soon be written, and the Gall monograph should be printed by the end of the year. If … I have indeed been rather productive this winter in a […] way, but I am not satisfied at all. It is all so dry and pedantic. My dream is to write once something which is scholarly but has also the qualities of a novel. Perhaps I can do it on the Paris School. My greatest handicap in this respect is the language. Even if I would fall back on German for this purpose, it would be no longer good enough either. I am now reading again French material. But I do not know whether I will work on it in the Fall or on my short history of diseases which is partly written.

I will try to read the diaries of Victor Hugo. To judge from what little had been published so far, they ought to be very good. As a matter of fact they seem to me much better written than the novels. – I have found Koestler's autobiography (Arrow in the Blue) quite amusing (without endorsing his philosophy). I am now reading a seven hundred page book by Lucien Rebatt [sic] "Les Décombres". This is a stinking Fascist, and rightly in prison, but unfortunately, in spite of having only the most rudimentary and most barbaric ideas (antisemitism) he can write excellently. He gives a picture of France 1939–41 as I have never seen it elsewhere. I have wasted the last weeks with the last spasms of the scholastic year: exams, committees, commencement, etc. We are now living in the country, as we have rented the town house, and I find it rather uncomfortable and boring. Fortunately the rest of the family enjoys it, and we will soon leave. Wishing you a very good summer, and the best of health, I am

    Yours ever,
      Erwin

P.S. In case Evita is still with you, please give her my regards

George Harley (1894–1966) missionary and physician. "Chapter on Paris" of S.'s autobiography. Izquierdo see S. to A. of 23 June 1954. Vallois se A. to S. of 13 May 1954. "Paris School" of medicine. Victor Hugo see A. to S. of 27 June 1952. Arthur Koestler (1905–1983) British anti-communist, (Koestler 1952). (Rebatet 1942). Evita see A. to S. of 26 August 1953.

ACKERKNECHT to SIGERIST, Madison, 25 August 1954

My dear Henry:

When I returned yesterday to my office, the first thing I found on that frightful pile of accumulated mail was your chapter on Paris. I immediately read it, and enjoyed it tremendously. Thanks ever so much. This ought to become a very interesting book, and I hope it proceeds to your satisfaction. Later on, going to the same awful pile, I found the heart-warming postcard of you and Evita. Thanks too. Till I can come again and adore with you Luna, I will have to live on my melancholic but beautiful memories, und marschiere im Geist bei Euren Feiern mit. Well, your summer will be soon over too.

We came back yesterday from Mexico, sound in mind, body and car. It was a beautiful summer, except for the twice four days driving from and to the border. Everything is very pictorresque [sic] and beautiful in Mexico: the mountains, the plants, the animals, the humans, the pre-Columbian pyramids, the Spanish buildings, and last but not least, the ultramodern buildings, especially in Mexico City. The climate is ideal. But it is a hard and serious country (Spanish plus Indian seriousness) with lots of cruelty, corruption and poverty. It reminded me very much of the Balkans of my youth in every respect. Only the prospects are less hopeless than they were for the Balkans. We stayed three weeks in Mexico City, a very hectic place, and in the beginning somewhat difficult to get used to the high altitude, and the driving habits, but a very fascinating place. Then we put the children into a children's home, and drove one week into the cities and sites of the north-west, then one week to the cities and sites of the south-east, which is, as in Germany and France, the more gemuetlich part of the country. It was very cheap, and no trouble with the language even if we had not had with us my "Cuban" friend Goldenberg, who speaks Spanish fluently. Of course, all impressions from such a short trip, and from people who do not talk Spanish, are necessarily very superficial. We did not go there as students, but to enjoy ourselves, and breathe some different air, and this we succeeded in doing. […] this remains America too, though a very different America, and can never replace Europe. It was good, but my nostalgia for Paris is now even greater than ever, and I absolutely have to go next year.

As far as medical history is concerned, I saw Chavez and his wonderful Institute (with fine murals of Diego de Rivera). I also saw Izquierdo. Both spoke with much respect and sympathy of you, and as your pupil I was immediately welcomed by them. (By the way my Papa recently heard a radio address of yours, and also writes very enthusiastically about it). Izquierdo insisted on arranging a meeting where I spoke in French about the Paris Clinical School. He gave a little paper on Montaña [?]. It was a nice group of mostly older men (the younger ones speak only English). I met there a third worth while medical historian Fernandez del Castillo [?], and humanly perhaps the nicest of them. One of these lovely oldfashioned enthusiastic old fools. (Chavez and Izquierdo are both very good men, but also big operators.) Speaking of nice old men, the book of Bruno Kisch "Forgotten Leaders in Modern Medicine" (Valentin, Grub [sic], Remak, Auerbach) has just appeared, and seems to be very good, although Kisch is of course a defender of Remak (and Remak deserves one) rather anti-Virchow, and his English is clumsy.

In view of that unsettled pile of mail, I have to close now. Many, many thanks again, and very best wishes for your trip and your health.

Kindest regards

Yours ever,

Erwin

The postcard is missing. "Marschiere im Geist bei Euren Feiern mit": I am thinking of you and your celebrations. Balkans: A. had been in Bulgaria as a student. "Gemüt-lich": easy, cozy. Goldenberg see A. to S. of 6 March 1954. Chavez see S. to A. of 9 September 1947. Diego de Rivera (1886–1957) Mexican muralist. Izquierdo and Montaña see S. to A. of 23 June 1954. Bruno Kisch see A. to S. of 13 May 1954 and (Kisch 1954). David Gruby (1810–1898) Hungarian Physician in France. Robert Remak (1815–1865) German embryologist, physiologist, and neurologist.

ACKERKNECHT to SIGERIST, Madison, 30 October 1954 (Original in French)

My dear teacher and friend,

I am absolutely distressed to learn from Temkin that you are in the hospital and seriously ill. I hope the news is exaggerated and that you will recover quickly. If I could pray I certainly would do it for you and with all my power. But since I cannot pray let me simply send you my very best wishes and express my friendship and devotion. I do hope that you are well taken care of and that you do not suffer too much, physically and morally. Above all, do not worry about things left unfinished. These will be taken care of in the near future. After all, you've made so good and beautiful things that you don't have to worry and you can be reassured that your name will always be loved and honored even if in the future your working capacity should be reduced. Today I lack the courage to write you about my usual doings. Since our return from Mexico I have dealt with Alexander Humboldt. I will tell you more about that in coming letters or from person to person next summer. And I will make you laugh. Once more, my sincerest wishes and all my friendship.

Yours as ever

Erwin

In October 1954 S. had an apoplexy and was brought to a hospital in Lugano where he stayed for several weeks.

Dear Henry:

Emmy was so good as to write us twice concerning your situation, and we were very glad to learn that a certain improvement has occurred. We hope it will speed up in the weeks to come, and send you again our very best wishes, and our heartfelt sympathy in the misfortune that has befallen you.

I think I wrote you already that after my return from Mexico I started work on Alexander von Humboldt. It is so fascinating that it helps me most of the time to forget my rather drab surroundings (what a country!, we had already two days of snow at the end of October.) The life of Humboldt is so incredibly rich, it leads into so many avenues. The poor man, after the wonderful years in South America and Paris, he had to go back to Berlin. But even then he succeeded in writing Kosmos. At the occasion of Humboldt, I also bacame very much interested in the history of Goettingen. I read d'Arcy's last book, and found it much better than his earlier works. Though even those were not bad. Unfortunately I will not be able to stay too long with Humboldt. When I have finished a paper on "Humboldt, George Foster [sic] and Ethnology" I will have to go back to that half finished manuscript on the history of diseases, which by now bores me.

Otherwise its [sic] the usual stuff here: courses, lectures, committee metings, etc. I have unfortunately not been able to get away from here since our return from Mexico. I am having a lot of work as the chairman of the program committee for the next association meeting. Genevieve is the only person who helps me generously in this grateless [sic] task. I have a lot of trouble with my text publisher. American publishers are really the worst on earth. My Gall book in French seems to come out without great difficulties at the beginning of next year. Dean Middleton will unfortunately retire on July 1st. Thus one candidate after the other is passing through here inspecting us and we are inspecting him, and one looks worse than the other.

Excuse me for bothering you with all this small talk. At least it should not tire you.

Again very, very best wishes and cordial regards
    Yours ever,
        Erwin

Alexander von Humboldt (1769–1859) German naturalist, *Kosmos* is one of Humboldt's main works. D'Arcy Power (1855–1941) British medical historian. A.'s Humboldt paper (Ackerknecht 1955b); Georg Forster (1754–1794) German naturalist. Middleton see A. to S. of 7 October 1946.

SIGERIST to ACKERKNECHT, Pura, 5 February 1955 (Original in French)

My dear friend,

Let me send you a report on the present state of my health, and let me also thank you very much for your reprint which I have read with greatest interest. So here comes my report:

Right leg completely restored; right arm and hand not completely restored, I keep working at it. The difficulties of speaking will require more time, but I dictate letters and book reviews. Well, I got away once more.

All my best
[Henry]

ACKERKNECHT to SIGERIST, Madison, 17 February 1955

Dear Henry:

Thanks ever so much for your "Bulletin" of February 5th. I had already heard about your miraculous recovery, but it was of course a particular joy to have direct evidence of it. Let us hope and wish, and there is every reason to hope, that your recovery will continue.

From us here not too much to report. Since I have finished my Humboldt paper in December, I have wasted my time on silly administrative adventures like preparing the program for the Detroit meeting of the Association, preparing a medical-historical column for the Journal of Medical Education (my new Dean Bowers is the editor – old Dean Middleton showed how tired he was in accepting the direction of 170 veterans' hospitals), in developing a plan for a drug firm for a history of medicine in pictures, etc. etc. Besides I have taken on more teaching than usual. Besides my regular course and seminar I am giving a seminar on primitive medicine in the department of anthropology, and numerous lead-off lectures for other courses where I think they have me mainly come in order to say a few unpleasant truths in which these good professors believe but which they do not want to proclaim publicly. My subconscious has involved me in all these things so that I should have no time to work on the history of diseases manuscript which bores me, and I must admit that it has been very successful. I have also lost a lot of time, as a matter of fact the whole Xmas vacation, with a perianal abcess [sic] which had to be excised. Lucy sells houses. The children grow. For Xmas they got a piano, and now learn to play on it, which is very painful for the innocent bystander.

The aunt who had brought me up, and kept house for my parents for forty-seven years, had a stroke in November and died last week. She was 74, and for her it was a delivery from horrible sufferings, but for my parents it is a catastrophe. My mother (blind) had to be brought to a home. My father is broken. This brings unfortunately an element of great uncertainty into our summer plans, organizational, financial and otherwise. But we hope for the best.

Again thanks for the "Bulletin", and very, very best wishes for the future.

Yours ever cordially,
Erwin

P. S. Please give our best regards to Emmy who wrote us so kindly during your sickness.

"Bulletin" see S. to A. of 5 February 1955. Humboldt paper (Ackerknecht 1955b). "Association" for the History of Medicine.

Sigerist to Ackerknecht, Pura, 24 May 1955

Dear Erwin,

When shall we have the pleasure of your visit? I hope the death of your aunt doesn't affect your plans. This is a real catastrophy [sic] for your parents. Can't your sister take care of them?

Now you must be glad that the Detroit meeting is over. I am sure it was a success as you had your finger in it, but I haven't heard echoes from it.

The content of your letter of 17th February interested me a great deal. How busy you must be. Thank the Lord the academic year is over. I can imagine how trying it must be to have the children practice the piano. I am anxious to see your paper on Humboldt.

My health is improving from day to day and all I have left over is a certain stiffness in my hand and leg, and also symptoms of a motor aphasia, in that I cannot find certain words, but I can dictate, though hesitatingly and I have resumed my work. I do not find it easy, however, as you know I am accustomed to write in longhand which I cannot do at the moment, so that I have to dictate. I resumed my work on the Autobiography and on the History, wrote a paper on Como and the Plinii, finished the Heath Clarc Lectures on the History of Hygiene and wrote a few book reviews. That's all for the time being. When and if you come you will find me in new quarters. Since I should not climb many stairs, I have my study downstairs, where the living room was and we had a bathroom built, so that I have the entire groundfloor at my disposal, and the garden, [...] to go to Milano to see the exhibition of Etruscan art.

With kind regards,
I am,
yours very cordially,
[Henry]

The style of this letter differs from that prior to S.'s stroke. S. dictated to his English secretary, Phyllis Arnold, who joined him in 1954. *Como and the Plinii* (Sigerist 1955b), *History of Hygiene* (Sigerist 1956a). [...]: last line of the first page illegible.

ACKERKNECHT to SIGERIST, Madison, 31 May 1955

Dear Henry:

Thanks ever so much for your letter of May 24th. I was absolutely delighted to see that your health has so greatly improved, and that you are able to work. I hope you don't overdo it. I am looking eagerly forward to embrace you in your new quarters. Our plans have indeed been badly shaken by the death of my aunt, and by a consecutive severe disease of my father. (Diagnosed as allergy. I think it was scarlet fever. He was delirious and ran very high temperatures. There was of course also a strong psychosomatic element.) But I will come and see you, be it only for a few days. In view of the health of my father plans are still fluid, but at present I hope he will stay with us the second half of July in Paris (we have an apartment – but my address is as usual: Musée de l'Homme, Palais de Chaillot, Paris 16e); then at the end of July my father and Lucy and the children will go to Ludwigsburg, while I rush down for a few days to Pura, and also for Zurich where I want to see my uncle, who is not getting any younger either. I will then soon have to go back to Ludwigsburg, as Lucy wants to go on to Berlin and Spain and I cannot leave my father alone with the children. I will then stay a few days in Ludwigsburg, trying also to make a little money by radio speeches, and then return with the children to Paris. This is the present situation, but God knows how it will work out.

The Detroit meeting was neither particularly good nor particularly bad. The program was overloaded, as Whittaker wanted to show […] museums to the people, and I wanted to give them papers, and had to give them plenty in order to duplicate the unavoidable horrible amateur papers which are offered, by qualified invited papers. We had quite a few of the latter variety: Temkin, Rosen, Genevieve (who has developed admirably). The banquet speaker, the chairman of surgery in Michigan, Coller was refreshing in his heresies, showing the surgeons that their progress is actually a gift of the scientists and they are not Santa Claus themselves. One of the main troubles with the Association is that we go more and more to places where there is no strong local group. This is mostly due to the absence of leadership. Those who could provide it (like Temkin who has experience, and a clear idea as to what the Association should do) do not want to, and perhaps are not wanted by the Association to do so. Those who are asked to give leadership, or who want to give it for not altogether altruistic reasons, have either not the experience, or not the abilities. As you certainly heard Ilza Veith was elected secretary-treasurer, and as you have perhaps not heard, had herself immediately voted a salary for secretarial help, which had never been done before. It kind of reminded me of her beginnings. I am sure glad the Detroit business is over. I just returned from the dedication of the new building of the Armed Forces Institute of Pathology in Washington (speech by the President and all the trimmings) to which I am a consultant for one of their appendices, the Medical Museum. It is the first atomic bomb proof public building erected in Washington, looks like a pyramid. But everybody talked about peace, let's hope for the best. As most of those attending were pathologists, I felt at first a little lonely, but was gratified to see that my name was usually familiar to them on account of the Virchow. The damned Humboldt paper is still not yet in my hands, although I have already received the bill for the reprints. Quite accidentally a few weeks ago a new book on Humboldt appeared in English by a certain Helmut De Terra, so called Swiss nobility, but actually a geologist from Munich. Although the man is in many ways an adventurer, the book is, within the limit it has set itself, (a popular biography), not bad at all. Except for the fact that the author has been bitten by the psychoanalytic bug, and [...] makes Humboldt a full-pfledged [sic] homosexual, which he was not, but explains his protection of young men, as the aspirations of a "super-mother", which seems, to say the least, a little far fetched.

Since Detroit I have also finished the index of my text book, which was horrible, and we had the invasion of 250 medical librarians, mostly female, which was no less horrible, but we had also the visit of Lloyd Stephenson [sic] which was nice. We sail June 15th. I have still to write four more German popular papers. I am so commercial this time as I have to pay the whole thing out of my own pocket this time. It's all a horrible rat race, but thank God, it will soon be over.

Very, very best wishes
   Yours ever cordially,
    Erwin

Kindest regards to Emmy

"My uncle": Eberhard Ackerknecht (1883–1968) professor of veterinary anatomy in Zurich. Alfred H. Whittaker, medical historian in Detroit. Frederick A. Coller (1887–1964). Ilza Veith (born 1915) S.'s doctoral student, professor of medical history in Chicago and then San Francisco. Alexander von Humboldt see A. to S. of 23 November 1954. (De Terra 1955). "My textbook" (Ackerknecht 1955a). Stevenson see S. to A. of 3 November 1949. "To pay the whole thing": probably his European trip of 1955.

SIGERIST to ACKERKNECHT, Pura, 20 June 1955
(Original in French)

My dear friend,
   Welcome to you all in this City of Lights. I am looking forward to have you here, but Emmy is disappointed she won't see Lucy and the children. I know your uncle in Zurich, give him my regards.

It goes without saying that you sleep in our house and that you stay as long as possible. I am looking forward to the news that can be exchanged by word of mouth only.

With my very best regards to you
[Henry]

City of Lights: Paris.

ACKERKNECHT to SIGERIST, Paris, 27 June 1955 (Original in French)

My dear teacher and friend,

Thank you so much for your good note of 20 June which I found here. I shall come around 2 August, providing you with the details before departing. Excuse this ugly stationary, but that's all I have in my office presently.

We have been here for a week, but there is still confusion. I have too much to do at the same time (work, take care of the children, see friends, absorb cultural events). Thus, all is done in an imperfect way which gets me nervous. But there will be an end of it.

Best wishes and see you soon
Yours as ever
Erwin

ACKERKNECHT to SIGERIST, Paris, 26 July 1955 (Original in French)

My dear Henry,

We'll all leave Paris on the 1st of August – we can't leave earlier. I shall be in London on August 2 and arrive in Zurich on August 3. I will get in touch with Emmy who wrote Lucy she might be in Zurich on August 3. So I shall see you in Pura on August 4! Unfortunately, I must leave for Stuttgart on the evening of August 6 because of the children.

416

Thus, it won't be for long. Nevertheless, we will be together for a couple of days.

I am very impatient to see you. Best wishes and see you very soon

Yours as ever

Erwin

ACKERKNECHT to SIGERIST, Ludwigsburg, Germany, 8 August 1955 (Original in German)

Dear friends,

After my happy arrival let me thank you so much for your hospitality and the wonderful hours spent in Pura.

My return was good for Ellen for she has a bad cold, and I succeed better than my father in telling her to put on warm things and not to go swimming. The weather here is horrible. I also hope my ulcer will receed under diet and rest.

Excuse my having forgotten to give your maid some money for her holidays. Please give her the enclosed.

Again, many thanks, best regards and wishes, good luck, bonne chance, bon plaisir

Yours

Erwin

P. S. The children were much pleased to receive the chocolate and kerchiffs. They will write you.

SIGERIST to ACKERKNECHT, Pura, 17 August 1955 (Original in French)

My dear Erwin,

Your visit has been an immense joy, and I thank you for having come. I deeply regret that you suffered from your ulcer while with us, and I hope you have recovered in the meantime.

I also thank you for thinking of our maid, but it wouldn't have been necessary. I wish you a good stay and send you my regards

[Henry]

ACKERKNECHT to SIGERIST, Paris, 19 August 1955 (Postcard)

Dear Friends:

I arrived here yesterday with the children. We seem to get along quite well with Sylvia's cooking. Ellen wrote Emmy a letter in Ludwigsburg – but forgot it there. Thus more later.

Very best regards and wishes

    yours ever

        Erwin, Sylvia, Ellen

ACKERKNECHT to SIGERIST, Madison, 20 September 1955

Dear Henry:

This is just to announce to you that we have safely returned three days ago. The mountain of letter [sic] I found on my desk is depressing, the climate as beastly as ever, and the transition to the small town a little difficult, but it will all come out with the wash. I hope and trust that they did send you my little textbook which just came out. I hope you will not be too much disappointed. It is very difficult to do something really good in this framework, and in addition they edited it to death. I very much hope you are doing well. You are probably right now in Zurich for that language treatment.

Very best wishes for its success.

    Kindest regards to you both

        Yours ever,

            Erwin

Textbook: (Ackerknecht 1955a).

Dear Erwin,

Here are the photos. I notice to my horror that I did not have a chance to make one of you alone.

Thanks for your note announcing me the safe return of the family to the wilderness of America.

I just spent a very pleasant month in Zurich, where I engaged full time in rehabilitation exercises. I had speech lessons with a very able speech trainer, with good results. I also consulted a neurologist, had my eyes examined and showed my nose to a rhinologist, who confirmed that my chronic condition was allergic. I also greatly enjoyed the theatres, where I saw Operas and Plays, a charming performance of Giraudoux' "Intermezzo", a typical Giraudoux play that is between dream and reality.

Needless to repeat that I greatly enjoyed the days you spent with us.

With best wishes,

I am,

Yours ever,

[Henry]

SIGERIST to ACKERKNECHT, Pura, 13 October 1955

Dear Erwin,

I forgot to tell you in my last letter that Temkin asked me to review your book for the Bulletin. The book has not arrived yet, but I am expecting it any day now, and you are sure to get a benevolent review in the Bulletin. I will write it as soon as I have read the book.

With kindest regards,

I am,

Yours ever,

[Henry]

"Your book": (Ackerknecht 1955a). "Bulletin" of the History of Medicine.

Dear Henry:

Thanks ever so much for your letters of October 6th and 13th, and the fine photographs. I was very glad to hear that you spent a good month in Zuerich, and equally happy to hear that you are going to review my book for the Bulletin. I only hope this job will not be too boring for you. In such a very elementary short textbook on the level of the American medical student, one can not be profound or brilliant.

I hope you will not mind too much if I am bothering you today with something else. When I had left you in August and had some time to think over the whole situation, I felt that beside the financial problem, the most important thing was to find a scholarly person to help you to finish volume two as soon and as well as possible. I feel that even a competent secretary would probably not be sufficient to do such a job. The archeologist might, but also might not be sufficient. I thought that the person should preferably be a good classical scholar, and that he or she should be English, because he or she would thus be cheaper than an American, more likely to have the required background, and able to write herself occasionally passages when necessary or desired, which, for instance, a German could not do.

I therefore contacted Walter Pagel who is a good personal friend, extremely helpful and efficient and familiar with the British scene. Walter informed himself a little bit, and feels that such a person could be found. In particularly [sic] he feels that it would be worthwhile to approach Dr. Lotte Labowsky whether she would be willing to do this job or not. Dr. Labowsky was for years in charge of the Plato Latinus and lecturer at Sommerville [sic], Oxford. She seems to have some experience in this kind of cooperation.

The main problem is, of course, whether you want yourself to engage yourself [sic] in this direction. And even then many problems remain to be solved. How is the collaborator to be financed? In a way it might be good if the money could be chanelled through Yale, because this would reflect some academic glory on the incumbant, who would most probably be an academic person. One should also know beforehand how long the help would be needed, at what date, and many other similar questions. Needless to say that I am giving the name of Dr. Labowsky here confidentially, as, of course, she has not yet been approached on the project. Please let me know whether this project agrees with you. If so, why don't you contact directly Walter, which would save a lot of unnecessary writing around. If not, just let us forget about it with, I hope, no hard feelings on both sides.

I apologize for being rather short today, but at present I am rather a travelling salesman than anything else. I have just returned from lectures and committee meetings in Chicago, Detroit, Boston and New York and am leaving tomorrow for the same. I am rather frustrated at the moment but hope to get rid of this later in the year, and start doing something more sensible. I very much hope that your health continues being good.

Kindest regards and best wishes
    Yours ever,
      Erwin

Textbook: (Ackerknecht 1955a). "Scholarly person to help you to finish volume two": see comments of S. to A. of 23 June 1954. Walter Pagel see A. to S. of 28 February 1950. Lotte M. Labowsky (born 1905). Somerville, a college at Oxford.

ACKERKNECHT to SIGERIST, Madison, 16 November 1955

Dear Henry:

This is just to thank you for your fine reprints. Congratulations that you are on the publishing front again. This is certainly a great joy and satisfaction for all your friends.

Kindest regards and best wishes
    Yours ever,
      Erwin

SIGERIST to ACKERKNECHT, Pura, 1 December 1955

Dear Erwin,

I wish to thank you for your good letter of October 28, 1955, for which I am awfully grateful, as it shows me that you take a lively interest in my work. I shall certainly be glad to contact Pagel directly, but not before I have tried out the archeologist. She is an extremely nice person to

421

have in the house, Dr. Victorine von Gonzenbach, godchild of Emmy. So I want to give her a chance to show in what fashion she can help me best.

Just now I am writing the lecture I gave in Oxford on the Latin Medical Literature of the early Middle Ages in order to find the way back into philology. The lecture will be published by the English branch of the Oxford Press and then I shall tackle volume 2 and finish it in onestroke [sic].

I had a letter from the American branch of the Oxford Press saying that they will reprint volume 1 as it stands. I had suggested them this procedure as I would not have time to make a new edition. I read [the] corrected German translation and brought it up to date, while I had no control over the Italian translation.

To make a long story short: I shall contact Pagel directly when the time comes, as I have appointed Victorine only until April 1 and as we have to wait and see how our finances will be by then.

I wish to thank you for 4 reprints. I liked the one on George Foster [sic] and Alexander von Humboldt best. Dr. Meek may not have been a great medical historian, but at any rate I was glad to see the excellent photograph of you. How nice that you have "Doktoranden". The thesis on Rasori I liked very much also, but the one on Hospital Diets is quite good too.

Let me thank you once more for your letter and for the spirit it reveals. I am reading your History of Medicine, I like it very much.

> With kind regards I am
> > Yours very cordially
> > > [Henry]

Pagel see A. to S. of 28 February 1950. Victorine von Gonzenbach (born 1921) Swiss archeologist, lecturer in Zurich. Latin Medical Literature (Sigerist 1958). Volume 2 of S.'s *History* was still incomplete at his death in 1957: it was published as a torso (Sigerist 1961). *Georg Forster, Alexander von Humboldt* (Ackernecht 1955b). Walter J. Meek (Ackernecht 1954). Doktoranden: doctoral students. Rasori see A. to S. of 13 May 1954.

ACKERKNECHT to SIGERIST, Madison, 7 December 1955

Dear Henry:

Thanks ever so much for your letter of December 1st. I am quite relieved that you did not take amiss my letter of October 28th, and took it for what it was and is, that is, a sincere attempt to be helpful in a somewhat complicated situation. Let us hope that Dr. von G. can give you all the necessary help, and that it becomes unnecessary for you to get into contact with Walter Pagel. I have also had a few ideas concerning foundations, but I have always forwarded them directly to John Fulton, as this seemed to be the most practical thing and time saving, to have this problem concentrated for the time being in his hands. I still hope and trust that something will come out of his efforts.

The best of luck for the Oxford lectures, and Volume II. It is quite gratifying that Volume I will now be reprinted. I just reread Volume I for the third time, and I must confess that I like it better every time I read it. There is a wealth of material and ideas which one is not able to assimilate all at a first reading. As I am convinced that Volume II is just as good, if not better, I hope so very much that it will be possible to bring it out, and that this tremendous effort of yours should not be lost. I am glad you liked the reprints. I had the satisfaction that the author of the Rasori thesis, Dr. Rossi, got a Fullbright [sic] fellowship on the basis of it, and with the help of Middleton was released from the army, which had already drafted him, to go for one year to Italy and continue work on Italian medical history.

I hope you have meanwhile received my little Gall. My new dean was so enthusiastic about it, that he decided to have it translated into English, and printed. We will this way start a little series "Wisconsin Studies in Medical History". Quite apart from the fact that I like, of course, to have the Gall in English, I am very glad that my dean shows so much interest in my Department, a thing of which I was not sure at all, and for which I had not too much hope, as deans go in this country. His interest means unfortunately also a lot more administrative work, but this is better than the contrary.

I am looking forward very much to your review of my short history. I am so glad you like it. But please tell me also, at least in private, what you do not like in it. Because unavoidably there will be the unsatisfactory passages in an attempt to cover so much ground.

I have just returned from a lecture in Bloomington, Indiana. Compared to that dump, Madison is a metropolis. But in exchange they have it somewhat warmer, while we enjoy now here the usual sub-zero Fahrenheit temperatures and plenty of snow. I am sorry for poor Leo Kanner who will be here as a guest professor in the second half of the winter. I try frantically to do something better than these futile lectures, projects, etc. but have not been very successful so far. Hoping very very much that you are doing well, I am

With my kindest regards and best wishes

Yours ever,

Erwin

"Dr. von G.": Victorine von Gonzenbach, see S. to A. of 1 December 1955. Pagel see A. to S. of 28 February 1950. Fulton see S. to A. of 26 February 1945. Oxford lecture (Sigerist 1958). Volume I of S.'s *History* was reprinted in 1967 only. Rasori see A. to S. of 13 May 1954. (Rossi 1954). Middleton see A. to S. of 7 October 1946. Franz Joseph Gall see A. to S. of 2 October 1947 and (Ackerknecht/Vallois 1956). New dean: Bowers, see A. to S. of 17 February 1955. S.'s review (Sigerist 1956b). Leo Kanner see A. to S. of 5 August 1941.

ACKERKNECHT to SIGERIST, Madison, 21 February 1956

Dear Henry:

I have not heard from you for some time. But I want you to know that I am thinking very often and very cordially of you. I have heard via Lucy and Emmie that you had unfortunately a very upsetting time with some tempetuous [sic] philanthropic friends (I tried to talk sense to them, but I am far away, and letters do not impress people very much) and with Erika. I very much hope that these trials are now over without having damaged too much your health.

I have myself a very unsatisfactory winter. I got myself into too much lecturing and committee work. I have just returned from my twelfth trip since we came back in september [sic]. I was in New York the day before yesterday, and saw the Rosens who send their most cordial regards. He is writing a short book on the history of preventive medicine, which should be finished in March. I have also a lot of work with my course this year, as I have to give an entirely different course, now that the old one appeared in the form of the short history. With all this neither my health nor my research are in very good shape. The only good time was the Xmas vacation, when I wrote a short paper on medical education in 19th century France which gave me a few new ideas. I also enjoyed greatly reading some translations of Hindu medicine, and several books like the one by Filliozat.

424

I can see now why you were so fascinated by Hindu medicine, and I only hope that your results might be published in not too far a future.

Kanner is now here, and giving two excellent lectures every week. I hope the European cold has spared you.

Kindest regards and best wishes

Yours ever,

Erwin

"Tempestuous friends": S. does not touch this subject in his next letter. Erica, S.'s elder daughter. Rosen see S. to A. of 27 March 1945 and (Rosen 1958). "Short paper" (Ackerknecht 1957). Jean Filliozat (1906–1982) French physician and author. Kanner see A. to S. of 5 August 1941. Europe was hit by a cold wave during February 1956.

SIGERIST to ACKERKNECHT, Pura, 28 March 1956

My dear Erwin,

I wish to thank you for your letters of 7th December 1955 and 21th [sic] February 1956 and I did not want to answer them before I could add my book review of your <u>Short History</u>. Here it is at last. The reason why I am so late is that I had a set back of my illness which invalidated me for about five weeks. You may have heard from Temkin that I wrote him five weeks ago that I had it on my "this weeks [sic] program". Well in that very week I suffered the set back from which I am still not fully recovered.

I hope you like the review. I tried to be fair to the book. I read it a long time ago and failed to make notes of some mistakes which you will have corrected long ago. For instance on p. 79 the School of Salerno flourished in the 12th century. And again on p. 96 Paracelsus was supposed to graduate from the university not of Padua but of Ferrara. On the illustration facing p. 136 the name should be not Koelliker but Kölliker; this is a mere printing error. On p. 73 Aetius should be written Aitius otherwise the Americans will pronounce it Aitius. These are just a little obvious errors. I will read the book once more critically since you asked me to point out mistakes.

And now let me thank you most cordially for your Gall which I read with the keenest interest. And I was delighted to hear that your dean has suggested an English translation.

I am sorry for you that you have to give so many lectures. You have my full sympathy as it was my lot for years to have to run around giving lectures. That I achieved something besides giving lectures is a pure miracle or rather it was due to my stubborn energy.

This is all for today. I am anxious for you to see the book review and I shall write soon again.

In sincere friendship I am
    Yours very cordially
      [Henry]

S.'s review of A.'s short textbook (Sigerist 1956b) contains the sentence "I can well imagine that it is going to be a most popular student's textbook". This is indeed what happened, and this for decades since the book was revised and enlarged in many editions. Albert von Koelliker (1817–1905) Swiss anatomist. Gall: (Ackerknecht / Vallois 1956).

ACKERKNECHT to SIGERIST, Madison, 3 April 1956

My dear Henry:

First and above all let me send our most cordial wishes for your 65th birthday. We are so fortunate that we can celebrate it with you, and hope for many happy returns. We hope you will spend pleasantly this day when so many people all over the world will remember you, and we wish you for the years to come all that you could wish yourself.

This congratulatory letter which was planned long ago coincides with my thanks for your letter of March 28th, and the review of my short history, which just arrived. You were certainly very generous and said a lot of nice things about something which in the nature of things is not very exciting. I was horrified by the Ferrara-Paracelsus and the 10th century Salerno school. I was somewhat consoled, finding that in my original manuscript the things were correct. One of the four editors who wiped their red pencil and their shoes on my manuscript, must have slipped these pearls in. But there they stand now and I had overlooked them. There must be more of this. And I would indeed appreciate it very much, if you could draw my attention to it so that at least in future editions these things are eliminated.

We were very sad to hear you had health troubles again, but hope fervently that these things have straightened out by now. I am leading the

426

same rotten life I wrote you about in my last letter, flying next week to Los Angeles, the week thereafter to Durham, North Carolina. I am hoping now for the summer to do some more serious work. I am glad you liked the Gall. I have a lot of work with the translation, as my translator is not too good, and there are indeed very difficult technicalities. There is now a fair chance that my Virchow will come out in German (with Enke, Stuttgart). I hope I will have less trouble there with the translation.

A week ago I heard about the death of Milt. I did not know him, but he seems to have been a fine scholar and it is sad that he had to go so early. On the other hand this puts, of course, the question of his succession. And I must confess that I am very much interested in it, and would be very grateful to you if you could say a good word for me in this situation, unless, of course, you do have a more competent candidate in mind.

Again our very, very best wishes and our kindest regards to the family
Yours very cordially,
Erwin

S.'s 65th birthday was on 7 April 1956. His review of A.'s textbook (Sigerist 1956b). "Ferrara-Paracelsus and 10th century Salerno school" see S. to A. of 28 March 1956. Gall (Ackerknecht/Vallois 1956). Bernhard Milt see S. to A. of 19 January 1951, professor and director of Switzerland's first department of the history of medicine at the University of Zurich, founded in 1951 with the active help of S. Sigerist-Milt correspondence see (Bickel 2008).

SIGERIST to ACKERKNECHT, Pura ?, 9 April 1956, (Telegram)

THANKS FOR LETTER. AM HAPPY TO RECOMMEND YOU TO ZURICH UNIVERSITY PRIMO ET UNICO LOCO. PLEASE SEND CURRICULUM VITAE AND LIST OF PUBLICATIONS.
SIGERIST

ACKERKNECHT to SIGERIST, Madison, 12 April 1956

Dear Henry:
When I came back last night from Los Angeles I found your telegram. A thousand thanks. This is the best thing that has happened to me in a long

time. With your help I should really be able to make it, and this would solve so many of my problems. Among other things I feel that for my work it would be very important if I would come into a more stimulating atmosphere. It would be wonderful if we could again live close together. You will understand that we are extremely excited, and eagerly waiting for all kinds of news. A lot of things would have to be settled before our departure. As a matter of fact I am so full of this project that I went through Seattle, San Francisco, and Los Angeles in a rather detached mood. Chairs, by the way, might come up in not too far a future in Los Angeles, where an anatomist called Magoun is very active, and in San Francisco, where Saunders is now dean. In San Francisco I stayed with Otto Guttentag, who has three very nice children, and a very nice wife, and, of course, we talked a lot about you and he sends his very best regards.

I hasten to close this letter today in order to get the material to you as soon as possible. I am sending two vitae, leaving it to you which you judge to be more appropriate for the occasion.

Thanks again.

Kindest regards and very best wishes

Yours ever,

Erwin

Usually sceptical and pessimistic, A. shows in this letter an optimism which is not realistic in view of the fact that new professors are chosen by the faculty and appointed by the government, so that S.'s influence is very limited. Horace W. Magoun (1907–1991) neuroscientist at UCLA. Guttentag see A. to S. of 12 November 1945.

SIGERIST to ACKERKNECHT, Pura, 14 April 1956

My dear friend,

I sent yesterday a letter to professor Fischer of which I am sending you a carbon. I hope you like my letter. It is fortunate that Fischer, the professor of pharmacology and editor of Gesnerus and member of our Pura circle is Rector of the University, because he has medical history very much at heart. I also sent him an incomplete list of your publications and promised him a complete one as soon as I get it from you. These publications are in my hands and I am ready to submit them to the Faculty if so required. Bad luck has it that your monograph on Malaria in the Upper

Mississippi Valley is just at the bookbinder's to be bound with other Supplements. Do send it to me, your own copy, but by air parcel. I shall return it as soon as I get my own copy back from the bindry.

Your chief competitor for the job is Heinrich Buess and it may well be that a Swiss citizen will be preferred to a "Chaibe Schwab". Your chances are that Buess has a job at the Ciba where he is factory doctor. But who knows what the Faculty wishes to do.

Milt's chair is ein "etatmässiges Extraordinariat für Geschichte der Medizin und der Biologie", that means that you are not obliged to give many lectures. Die Pflichtstundenzahl ist geringer. His stipend was 20 000 Sfr.– but you could get more, first of all an "Ordinariat ad personam" and a larger stipend, if you ask for it. Of course travelling expenses for you and the family and the furniture and the books will be paid by the authorities of the Canton of Zurich.

The Institute consists of the very rich collections of Dr. Wehrli and books from the Zentralbibliothek and objects from the Schweizerisches Landesmuseum. It is located in the tower of the university building, but a separate building is being considered.

Library facilities are ideal in Zurich in that the Zentralbibliothek is particularly rich in old medical books.

I am holding my fingers crossed and sincerely hope that you will get an invitation to join the Faculty of Zurich. Count on me, I shall be doing everything I can to bring you over. I fully appreciate the fact that you are sick and tired of America. I could stand the country only for 15 years. The same length of time that you could stand.

With warm regards I am
    Cordially Yours
      [Henry]

Hans Fischer (1892–1976). Gesnerus, Swiss Journal of the History of Medicine and of Science. *Malaria* … (Ackerknecht 1945). Buess see S. to A. of 3 November 1949; he was also lecturer at the University of Basel. "Chaibe Schwab" Swiss slang for "damned German". Ciba, one of the Basel chemical companies, later part of Novartis. "Milt's chair is" a regular associate professorship for the history of medicine and biology. "Die Pflichtstundenzahl ist geringer": A lesser amount of compulsory teaching hours. "Ordinariat": Full professorship. Wehrli see S. to A. of 19 January 1951. "Zentralbibliothek" Central Library (of Zurich). "Schweizerisches Landesmuseum": Swiss National Museum. S., who loved America, had become ambivalent. A. after criticizing America, would love it again.

SIGERIST to ACKERKNECHT, Pura, 18 April 1956

Dear Erwin,

I am sending by the same mail to Prof. Fischer your Curriculum vitae (the long one), a complete list of your publications and a list of the theses that were written under your guidance in your department. And you will find enclosed a copy of a letter of april [sic] 15 from the rector of the university of Zurich.

Your chances are the very best. Buess is out and Erna Lesky will not accept the chair as her husband is full professor of classices [sic] at the university of Vienna. Artelt could not accept the position either as his wife is professor of medical history at the university of Mainz. So that I am happy to say that your chances are the very best.

I am sorry I got some wrong dates in my letter which I wrote to Fischer but this will be easily corrected as I am sending your Curriculum vitae. I also added your memberships and awards to the Curriculum vitae.

I rejoice more than I can tell at the idea to have you in the same country. Zurich is very close to Pura, only four hours by train.

Emmy and I hold our fingers crossed and send you our warm regards.

Yours ever

[Henry]

Hans Fischer and Heinrich Buess see S. to A. of 14 April 1956 and 3 November 1949, respectively; see also the Sigerist/Fischer correspondence (Bickel 2008). Erna Lesky (1911–1986) Austrian medical historian. Artelt see S. to A. of 14 May 1946, his wife Edith Heischkel see A. to S. of 10 November 1949.

ACKERKNECHT to SIGERIST, Madison, 24 April 1956

Dear Henry:

Thanks ever so much for your letter of April 14th which I received just before leaving for the Association Meeting at Durham on April 18th and which, together with the wonderful letter you wrote to Professor Fischer, was a great encouragement to me. I mailed my malaria monograph immediately by air parcel, and hope it reached you safely. Please do not return it for the time being, as I hope to receive it back from your own hands, when we have successfully finished this whole operation.

Upon my return I found your equally heartening letter of April 18th, together with the carbon of Fischer's letter of April 15th. You have thus received the different lists safely. Buess seems out, which is very important! As far as Erna Lesky is concerned, not only is she tied down to Vienna through her husband, but I do not think that her status (I just recommended her for habilitation) and publications put her quite into the same class as me, in spite of all her qualities. The same holds good for Steudel, or whatever other German might come up, except Artelt. And Artelt will probably be sufficiently tied down in Frankfort through his wife's job. And even him, may it be said with all due immodesty (petit quand je me juge, grand quand je me compare) I would not recognize as my superior. I have some idea concerning the collections, and the library facilities in Zurich, which, quite apart from the general atmosphere and your proximity, make the thing so attractive. I am now waiting for a letter from Fischer. I will of course have to try to get in the way of status and salary something close to my present position. I know they can't match it, and this is really not the essential issue. I also will have to make them understand that a decision would have to be reached either before August 1st, or January 1st, as I cannot resign in the middle of the semester, and semesters start here, unlike in Europe, in the beginning of September, and the beginning of February. The earlier I can leave, of course, the better. I want to accomplish something in Z. The earlier I start, the better my chances.

There is not much to report about Durham. It was the usual social whirl. There were three good papers, one by an historian, Duffy from New Orleans (an Englishman), one by George Moro [sic], a young Italian psychiatrist who happens to be at Chapel Hill, and one by Saul Jarcho, who is really a fine fellow. The rest of the papers be better not mentioned.

We very much hope your health is bearable. I feel ashamed that I had to put this extra burden on you. But I am happy to see that you too are longing for a reunion. Thanks again for all you have done, and let's hope for the best.

Kindest regards and best wishes
    Yours ever,
        Erwin

Fischer, Buess, Lesky see S. to A. of 14 April 1956, 3 November 1949, and 18 April 1956, respectively. Habilitation: Degree in Germany and some other countries permitting to start an academic career. Johannes Steudel (1901–1973) German medical historian. Artelt see S. to A. of 14 May 1946. "Petit quand je me juge …": Small in judging myself, big in comparing myself. John Duffy (1915–1996) medical historian at Tulane University. George Mora (1923–2006) psychiatrist and medical historian. Saul Jarcho see A. to S. of 3 June 1948.

SIGERIST to ACKERKNECHT, Pura, 30 April 1956

Dear Erwin,

I am sending you enclosed a copy of a letter of Fischer and of a letter that I wrote to the Dean of the Medical Faculty in Zurich.

I do not know what Fischer wrote to you but I suppose, if I juge [sic] from his letter, that it is the bare minimum that you could expect in Zurich. Your position is very strong, in that Zurich has no other choice but you. Hence you must not accept the position, unless they are willing to offer a chair similar in status and salary to the position, that you are holding at the university of Wisconsin.

Yesterday I had a phone call from Zurich from Prof. Fanconi, the paediatrician there, who asked me about you, not knowing that I had written to the rector and to the dean. He heard that you were recommended by Schultz. So you are recommended from two sides.

I cannot find my copy of your Virchow book. My library is in chaotic conditions since I moved down to my present study. I am pretty sure that it is in Zurich. But in order to play safe, may I ask you to send it by air parcel. I must have lent out my copy, but I cannot remember to whom.

So much for to-day. I shall keep you informed about further moves.

Your ever

[Henry]

Dean of the Zurich Faculty of Medicine was Paul Henri Rossier (1899–1976) professor of internal medicine. Guido Fanconi (1892–1979). Schultz see A. to S. of 16 May 1946, formerly at Johns Hopkins, was professor of anthropology in Zurich.

Dear Henry:

Thanks ever so much for your letter of April 30th with the enclosed copy of letter of Fischer and your good letter to Dean Rossier. I have meanwhile received my letter from Fischer. I omitted sending you a copy. Please forgive me. I am doing it herewith. I did send you already my answer to Fischer. I hope I found the right tone with him. On the one hand I must insist that they give me somewhat more in the way of salary and status than is indicated in the letter, on the other hand I would not like the thing to go wrong on this issue. As a whole Fischer seems pretty much committed to my candidature, and I am therefore rather optimistic. It is awfully decent that Adolf Schultz has intervened for me. That will certainly help too. A copy of the Virchow goes to you by air mail today.

Nothing new to report from here. The spring is even more abominable than usual. Still occasional ice and snow. And hardly a leaf daring to put its nose out. What a climate! And the intellectual is congenial. I am really looking forward to the time when I will not have to listen to grown-up so called intellectuals talking all the time about ball games. I just re-read for my course your "American Medicine". It is still the only readable history of American medicine. Although from the vantage point of 1956 one would probably look differently at several things. Their progress and regress during the last twenty years has been equally marked. I also endulged [sic] in the melancholic passtime [sic] to read your old reports of the Leipzig Institute (I am sifting my reprints. I will leave a good deal of them here. I read the reports because I try to get an idea of the European level, which, I hope at least, will be higher than the one I am used to in teaching here.) Those were good times.

Thanks again for your kind and energetic help.

Very best wishes, especially for your health, and very best regards to you both

Yours ever,

Erwin

Dean Rossier see S. to A. of 30 April 1956. Schultz see A. to S. of 16 May 1946. *American Medicine* (Sigerist 1934).

SIGERIST to ACKERKNECHT, Pura, 14 May 1956

My dear Erwin,

Thanks ever so much for your letter of the 4th May and for your book on Virchow which arrived safely. Your letter to Fischer of 26th April was a masterpiece, dignified and just in the right tone.

You must be patient as faculty affairs are very slow. The whole apparatus is very clumsy. I will do my best to accelerate the business, but I am not very hopeful that I shall be able to accelerate it. In the meantime I will inquire how much Schultz gets as a salary.

My book American Medicine is just over 23 years old, and I look at the American Medicine now with different eyes. But the historical part I don't disavow.

With kind regards and best wishes to you all, I am

Yours very cordially,
[Henry]

Schultz see A. to S. of 16 May 1946. *American Medicine* (Sigerist 1934).

ACKERKNECHT to SIGERIST, Madison, 22 May 1956

My dear Henry:

Thanks ever so much for your letter of May14th. I am glad that you found my letter to Fischer appropriate. I felt a little insecure, as I have lost the habit of maneuvering in Germanic academic circles with their special lingo and formalities. And, alas, slowness. It is awfully good of you that you try to speed them up. We in turn will try to be as patient as possible. Only this is not purely a psychological problem. If they want me to be there in october [sic], so many things have to be settled here. This is not like taking a train from Frankfurt to Zurich. Shipping space is harder to get than ever, and I had to make reservations for August 22nd, just gambling on the issue, because otherwise I might not get any. Also I will have to resign on August 1st, if I do not want to look much like a heel (They will hate my guts anyhow for leaving the paradise), etc. etc.

Have you seen the essay on Egyptian medicine by Lefebvre? I just reviewed it. I criticised that he ignores your contribution. Otherwise it is not a bad book. Especially his attempt to untangle of what diseases and what medicaments the Egyptians actually talked. And he is rather well equipped to do this. Jonkheere [sic] would have probably done a better book, but he preferred to carp and to throw out tidbits. Well, anyhow, he is dead. The series of biographies edited by K. Kolle "Grosse Nerven Aerzte" [sic] contains some good pieces, although it is somewhat frightening to see how inhuman most of the great men just in this field were. But that is perhaps why they went into it or stayed in it. On the other hand what workers! – I also read the new Diepgen textbook, a task I had always shied away from so far. But if and when I go to Zurich, it is a book I have to count with. It is as pedestrian, as I expected. (As the late Sarton said so nicely about Galen – and he could have said the same about himself – "A man whose knowledge is larger than his intelligence becomes a pedant.") He even has some juicy mistakes. A thing I would not mention as this is almost unavoidable in a book of that scope, if he had not been always so severe with other sinners. He has not departed from his old habit of using other people's ideas and material but nobly ignoring their names. Except his own […] you seem to have studied nothing but American medicine. And Temkin seems not to exist at all. – Artelt is different when it comes to publishing. But on the professional level he continues the great tradition. He has always claimed the greatest friendship for me, and had sworn to announce me immediately any European opening. I have still not yet heard from him concerning Zurich, though I received a most cordial postcard from some meeting. Well, this sure does not break my heart. But such things still slightly surprise me. Such "life crises" as I am going through one now have the advantage of showing you where you stand with people and who your real friends are.

I very much hope your health is bearable. And I hope so much we will spend a few good days together in September. Right now I am incredibly tired but classes are over next week, thank God, and I will retire to the hospital for a few days for some proctological repair, and hope to sleep there extensively.

Thanks again for your efforts.

    Kindest regards and best wishes to you both
      Yours ever,
      Erwin

(Lefebvre 1956). Jonckheere see S. to A. of 23 February 1948. (Kolle 1956). Diepgen see A. to S. of 2 May 1945 and (Diepgen 1949). Sarton see A. to S. of 23 March 1945.

Dear Henry:

I enclose a little sketch which I did for some kind of handbook edited by my friend Fritz Ernst, the medievalist in Heidelberg. I would be very grateful to you if occasionally you could tell me what in your opinion should be added, omitted or changed. I have tried to be fair, except for the two New York illusionists Iagory and Grego, but this is extremely difficult in an object in which one is so much involved oneself.

Have you by the way seen Iago's latest pronouncement on Romantic medicine? In spite of the fact that this time we are at least spared the statement that the new Vienna school and Wunderlich were Romantics, I still feel that his admiration is proportionate to his unfamiliarity with these problematic materials. And I feel that only familiarity can preserve medical historians from a danger which menaces them all. All medical historians are probably in some way dissatisfied with present day medicine, and have a tendency to pick a period of the past where they feel their aspirations were better realized. Unless they are very cautious, they tend to mythologize that particular period. Another recent case in point is I. Snappers [sic] work on Boerhaave. I feel myself this temptation very keenly when dealing with the Paris School. As Galdston is mythologising German Romantic medicine, he must of course ignore serious recent work on the period like that by Rosen or Temkin.

Kindest regards and best wishes

    Yours ever,

    Erwin

"Sketch" see also S. to A. of 1 June 1956. Fritz Ernst (born 1905). "Iago" Galdston and Wunderlich see A. to S. of 2 August 1944 and 6 February 1954, respectively. Snapper on Boerhaave possibly in (Snapper 1956).

My dear Erwin,

I just called up my friend Professor Schinz, who is the Radiologist of the University of Zurich, in order to find out how far your affair had progressed. To my great disappointment I heard that they had only one faculty meeting so far. The next meeting of the Faculty is to be held on June 6th, where the business of the successor to Professor Milt is being brought up for the first time. Schinz has promised to keep me informed of what happens. I was afraid that something might have gone wrong, as I was not invited yet to submit your publications to the Committee, but the Committee has not been appointed yet.

I warned you that faculty affairs are a slow method, and I do not think that you will get an offer from the authorities by August 1st, hence you must reconcile yourself to the idea of probably spending another winter in Wisconsin. I hope my prognosis is wrong, and that a miracle happens that the business will be accelerated, and that we shall meet in September as we hoped for.

I haven't seen the essay on Egyptian Medicine by Lefebre [sic], and it was news to me that Jonckheere had died. I met him for the first time two years ago at the Rome Congress, where he made a very bad impression on me. He had the face of a criminal, but he was a solid worker in the field of Egyptian medicine, and I respected him and admired him.

About Kolle's book "Grosse Nerven Aerzte", I feel that the book should not be arranged alphabetically which does not make much sense, but chronologically. I also criticize that there is no index to the book, not even an index of names. Diepgen sent me his third volume. It is pedestrian as you very appropriately said, and makes frightfully dull reading.

I am sorry to hear that you need some proctological repair, and I wish you that the operation will be successful.

Be sure to hear from me as soon as I have news from Zürich, and I sincerely hope that my prognosis was all too pessimistic.

With warm wishes to you and the whole family, I am,

Yours ever,

[Henry]

Schinz see S. to A. of 18 July 1946. (Lefebvre 1956). Jonckheere see S. to A. of 23 February 1948. (Kolle 1956). Diepgen see A. to S. of 2 May 1945 and (Diepgen 1949); his 3rd volume is actually volume II,2.

SIGERIST to ACKERKNECHT, Pura, 1 June 1956

Dear Erwin,

I just received a letter from the dean of the University of Zurich of which I enclose a copy and naturally I hastened to send him your publications, which went off today in two huge parcels.

I also enclose two passages of a letter from Adolph Schultz, which are selfexplanatory. Schultz is a great pessimist, who accepted the call to the University of Zürich merely because he would have had to retire at 65 in Baltimore, and the age-limit is 70 at Zürich. His American wife is terribly unhappy in Zürich, and this of course depresses him.

Many thanks for your beautiful sketch of Medical History in America. I greatly appreciated the words you devoted to me and my part which I was able to play in this development. You sized me up correctly and intelligently and I have no suggestions for changes of any kind. You handled Iago and Gregory very tactfully.

With all good wishes
    I am yours ever
       [Henry]

Schultz see A. to S. of 16 May 1946. "Sketch" see A. to S. of 25 May 1956. "Iago" Galdston see 2 August 1944. "Gregory", probably Zilboorg, see A. to S. 5 August 1941.

ACKERKNECHT to SIGERIST, Madison, 5 June 1956

My dear Henry:

Thanks ever so much for your letter of May 29th. It was very good of you to ring up Professor Schinz, who together with Loeffler, seems to be quite a power in the faculty. The information is somewhat disappointing, they are really incredibly slow, and this does not help much our practical problems here. But regretable [sic] as this may be, the main thing is that the final results will be positive. We are very grateful to you that you gave us your prognosis. One has to face realities. Let us still hope that the miracle happens, and we meet in september [sic].

As to Jonckheere's facial expression, I fully agree with you. He seems to have had a miserable death. At the time they did not know whether it was an adrenal tumor, or endocarditis. The Kolle is undoubtedly poorly organized. But some of the essays are really interesting. Nothing important has happened here since my last letter. We are in the midst of exams, a particularly boring occupation.

Kindest regards and best wishes to you both, especially for your health

Yours ever,

Erwin

Schinz see S. to A. of 18 July 1946. Karl Wilhelm Loeffler (1887–1972) professor of internal medicine in Zurich. Jonckheere see S. to A. of 27 February 1948. (Kolle 1956).

Ackerknecht to Sigerist, Madison, 7 June 1956

My dear Henry:

Thanks ever so much for your letter of June 1st. It just arrived, when I had written to you. I am very glad to see from the letter of the Dean of the University of Zuerich that they are at least starting to approach the problem. Well, let us hope for the best.

I am also grateful for the passages from the letter of Adolph Schultz. We know now what his "real" salary is. It would be, of course, good to know what his nominal salary is, in order to know what to ask, in order to get such a real salary. He does not say either whether this actual salary is after taxes or not. If it would be after taxes, it would still be less than here, but it would not be too bad. If it is not after taxes, it is indeed considerably less than we get here. But I do not think that it is so much less than what Schultz got at Hopkins. It is a pity that Schultz got into this unhappy situation in Zuerich through his wife. He is otherwise such an agreeable and competent man.

I am very glad you liked my little sketch on medical history in America, and had no changes to suggest. I really tried to be as objective as possible, but in such non-scientific situations I feel always insecure as to the degree of objectivity I might be able to achieve. It is not easy to be objective for me, even when it comes to the past, as nature has built me with strong likes and dislikes.

I am sending you under separate cover a little book by Barzun on Berlioz and his Century. Sylvia gave it to me for my 50th birthday (alas it happened – and the children nickname me since "half-century") and I liked it very much, especially as Barzun is one of the few people in this country who can write. And as I feel rather at home in Paris in 1830. But as on the other hand I do no longer keep books most of the time, and as I feel you might like it too, I take the liberty of passing it on to you. If you have it already or if it does not agree with you, please just pass it on.

Today is that famous faculty meeting in Zuerich and I hope the results will be satisfactory. Thanks again for all you have done in this direction.

Kindest regards and best wishes to you both from all of us

Yours ever,

Erwin

Schultz see A. to S. of 16 May 1946. (Barzun 1956). Hector Berlioz (1803–1869) French composer. Sylvia: A.'s daughter.

SIGERIST to ACKERKNECHT, Pura ?, 8 June 1956 (telegram)

MIRACLES DO HAPPEN. FACULTY JUST RECOMMENDED YOU TO AUTHORITIES UNICO LOCO. ARE OVERJOYED.

SIGERISTS

ACKERKNECHT to SIGERIST, Madison, 9 June 1956 (Original in French)

My dear Henry,

Your telegram has just arrived and made us so joyful! It's wonderful to think that in a few months we will breathe European air. And we will talk together, but not about baseball, I swear! It is also good to see how much you are respected in Zurich.

Lucie who had become most pessimistic is now completely transformed. Despite my inborn pessimism I had never given up hope. Nevertheless, my joy is immense, and so is my gratitude. I just write you this note; it is Saturday, I have no secretary, and I don't want to bother you with my hieroglyphs. But I want to add my thanks for your reprints which arrived

440

yesterday and which I will comment later-on. What a pity that the latest number of "Time" shows Barzun as a dull philistine. Yet he made beautiful things. – How strange that for over 30 years the 30th of June was always a day of important events for me. Enough chatter. Once more all my thanks, best wishes and à bientôt! In friendship

Yours

Erwin

Barzun see A. to S. of 7 June 1956.

Sigerist to Ackerknecht, Pura, 9 June 1956

Dear Erwin,

I receiver [sic] yesterday the enclosed letter from Prof. Schinz which is selfexplanatory. Needless to say that we are overjoyed at the good news. You have in the meantime received our cable; the next step is for the Dean to write to the authorities and you will receive a letter from the Regierungsrat offering the chair to you. It has never happened that the Regierungsrat did not follow a recommendation of the Medical Faculty. How long this will take nobody can tell and I am keeping my fingers crossed that you will get the call soon.

Best wishes

Yours ever

[Henry]

Schinz see S. to A. of 18 July 1946. Regierungsrat: executive council (of the Canton of Zurich). In previous letters both S. and A. complained about the slow handling of their affair. However, in view of the many problems a large faculty has to deal with, it handled this one in rather short time.

Ackerknecht to Sigerist, Madison, 15 June 1956

Dear Henry:

Thanks ever so much for your good letter of June 9th, with the letter of Schinz which confirms your cable of June 9th to which I immediately answered. I hope and almost trust that I will have enough "durchschlags-kraft" for Schinz. Now we have to wait for the Regierungsrat, and to pray that all will still work out in time. As to the Regierungsrat there is still one important question: can I still try to bargain with them, when their finan-cial offer is too measly, or is it an either-or proposition? The thing disgusts me, but I know too well that what I do not get now I will not get for the next ten years. I kind of hope that your answer will arrive before the letter of the Regierungsrat.

I still have to thank you for your reprint "Thoughts on the Physicians [sic] Writing and Reading". It is very charming and should be very help-ful. I was surprised to hear that you are still frightened in entering the lecture hall. You certainly do not sound it. I am also physically completely exhausted after a lecture. My technique of writing papers is very similar to yours. Only that I start out with a rather complete outline of the thing. Your advice to read novels from a stylistic point of view I took already in Baltimore, and it has proved to be very helpful. I like poetry very much, but I have never tried to start the day with a poem. This sounds like a very good idea, and I will try. I feel that you are absolutely right in your re-marks of classics versus new books. It was not pedantic at all, and very good that you got these things on paper.

After a practically unexisting spring we are now suffering from one of these lovely heat waves. I am nevertheless working on a French paper. One of my students who left gave me a wonderful Kurt Weill record. I must play it to you when we come to Pura. Thanks again.

Kindest regards and best wishes to you both

Yours ever,

Erwin

P.S. Many thanks also for the newspaper clipping with the Zürich "tarif". E.

Schinz see S. to A. of 18 July 1946. "Durchschlagskraft": penetrating power; Schinz in his letter to S. expressed his hope that A. will have more of it than his predecessor. Regierungsrat see S. to A. of 9 June 1956. *Thoughts on …* (Sigerist 1955c). Kurt Weill (born 1900) German composer.

SIGERIST to ACKERKNECHT, Pura, 18 June 1956

My dear Erwin,

I got your letters of 7th and 9th June and I hasten to answer them. In the meantime I suppose you have received the clipping which I sent you from the Neue Zuericher [sic] Zeitung that contains the salary scales of the full Professors at the University of Zuerich. To these you have to add Frs. 1,500 to which you are entitled as Director of an Institute. Taxes are not deducted from the salary. What is deducted is a pension fund, old age unsurance [sic], contribution to the University Sanitorium [sic], and similar minor items. Remember that the education of the children costs very little in Switzerland. Gymnasium and University are practically free, or cost only a nominal charge.

I am looking forward to receiving the book of Barzun on Berlioz and his century, as the period interests me very much.

By the way René Sand once told me that Jonckheere was married twice. From the first wife he was divorced for mental and physical cruelty, and on the second he operated, and the woman died under his operating knife.

So much for today. I suppose you haven't yet heard from the authorities in Zuerich. I just had a letter from the Dean, asking me if he could keep your publications for the time being.

With best wishes, I am,

    Yours ever,
      [Henry]

Neue Zürcher Zeitung, a Zurich newspaper. Gymnasium: the German-type high school. Barzun on Berlioz see A. to S. of 7 June 1956. René Sand and Jonckheere see S. to A. of 18 July 1946 and 23 February 1948, respectively.

SIGERIST to ACKERKNECHT, Pura, 20 June 1956

Dear Erwin,

I just received your letter of June 15 and I hasten to answer it. Not that I am afraid that the letter from the Regierungsrat will anticipate my letter. You must be prepared to wait for a long time for this letter to arrive.

Well, if the offer of the Regierungsrat is too measly I would advise you to bargain. Do it carefully so as not to break off bridges. As soon as you get the offer do cable me the sum offered to you and I will advise you by cable what to do.

This is all what I can tell you for the moment.

With very best wishes I am

Yours ever

[Henry]

Regierungsrat see S. to A. of 9 June 1956.

ACKERKNECHT to SIGERIST, Madison, 24. June 1956

My dear Henry,

Thanks ever so much for your letter of June 18th. Excuse me for only acknowledging it today. I just came back from the Hospital. I was there for 5 days for a haemorrhoidectomy. I am still supposed to stay in bed for a week. And I feel like it too. I would never have suspected this minor surgery to be so painful and exhausting. I will write more as soon as I feel better. Then, I hope, there will be perhaps also some news from Zürich! (Yes, I received meanwhile the clipping with the "tarif" from the Neue Zürcher.)

Very best regards

Yours ever

Erwin

"Neue Zürcher" Zeitung, see S. to A. of 18 June 1956.

ACKERKNECHT to SIGERIST, Madison, 2 July 1956 (Telegram)

JUST RECEIVED TELEGRAM FISCHER. GOVERNMENT ACCEPTED FACULTY PROPOSITION AND EMPOWERED FACULTY TO ASK ME FOR CONDITIONS. WOULD IT BE POSSIBLE TO ASK FULL PROFESSORSHIP AD PERSONAM PLUS MAXIMUM SALARY FULL PROFESSOR 28,500 PLUS INSTITUTE DIRECTOR SALARY PLUS MOVING AND PASSAGE EXPENSES.

CORDIALLY ERWIN +

444

My dear Henry:

Yesterday I received a telegram from Fischer (see enclosed copy) – it had dragged for 25 hours in our wonderful Western Union Bureau here – and immediately sent you another telegram (see copy) following your kind offer of June 20th, to consult you by telegram on the matter. I hope and trust the telegram has reached you – Pura is probably more efficient than Madison – and I have even your answer before this letter arrives in Pura. We were of course all very delighted and excited about the Fischer telegram; we had just my friend Gourevitch from Chicago as week-end visitor, and embraced each other. It is a great blessing that Fischer transacts by telegram. This way we can hope to get the thing settled before the vacation starts in Zuerich, and before it is too late here. It better goes this way, because we have paid the boat tickets, have sold the house, and have to leave it anyway in August, and have sold quite a lot of expendable furniture, books, etc. It would be disastrous if we would still have to go back into an apartment before leaving here. We are of course terribly excited and happy about the whole thing.

It is now a week since I am out of the hospital, but I still feel rather low, and have still to devote a lot of time to taking care of my sixty stiches. I have not been able to work too much, but have done some reading: The latest novel by Francoise [sic] Sagan – the girl has definitely talent – and a thick book by the new sociology professor at the Sorbonne Raymond Aron on Vichy, which is unconvincing. Following your advice, I have also read classics, and I am glad about it: Chateaubriand's Mémoirs d'Outre-Tombe and les Confessions de Rousseau. The latter contains even more psychopathology than I remembered, but is quite fascinating.

Let us hope that everything goes on well. Thanks again for your very kind help. I still keep the thing secret, as it would be very disagreeable if my dean hears about it, before I hand in my official resignation, which I cannot do before a final settlement with Zuerich. We very much hope your health is satisfactory. Here it is beastly hot.

Kindest regards and very best wishes to you both

Yours ever,

Erwin

Fischer see S. to A. of 14 April 1956. Gourevitch see A. to S. of 26 May 1950. (Sagan 1955). (Aron 1954). Vichy: The French régime in the unoccupied zone of France 1940–1943. (Chateaubriand 1848). (Rousseau 1798).

SIGERIST to ACKERKNECHT, Pura, 3 July 1956 (Telegram)

CONFERRED WITH FISCHER AND SCHINZ, EVERYTHING O. K., AWAIT MY AND FISCHER'S LETTER.

HENRY

SIGERIST to ACKERKNECHT, Pura, 4 July 1956

Dear Erwin,

I am sorry to learn that your operation was so unpleasant and that you were knocked out for two whole weeks. I sincerely hope that you feel better by now.

In the meantime the book Berlioz and his century arrived, and I wish to thank you for it most warmly. I have also received Lefebvre "Essay sur la Médecine Egyptienne" and what I read I found very good. I am just reviewing the two volumes of Hermann Grapow's "Grundriss der Medizin der alten Aegypter["]. This is an ambitious project that will cover the whole field of Egyptian medicine in at least five volumes. It will contain new translations of all existing medical papyri.

Now to your affair. I wish to confirm my yesterday's telegram which said that I conferred with Fischer and Schinz, in reply to your telegram of the 1st July which I read to both men and asked for their candid opinions. The result of these conultations was the following: –

1) Do ask for a full professorship ad personam.
2) A full professorship ad personam carries a salary of an extraordinary professor. This is somewhat complicated as the full professor is expected to lecture at least ten hours a week, and the extraordinary professor is supposed to lecture only six hours a week. Since you could not get students for ten hours a week, you are entitled to a salary of an extraordinary professor, although you are nominally full professor. Fisher [sic] thought that you could get an additional few thousand francs from a special fund. I would advise you to ask for Frs. 25,000 without insisting on this sum. Don't forget that the purchasing power of the dollar is about 2–3 Frs.
3) You are fully entitled to 1,500 Frs. as Director of an Institute.
4) Fisher [sic] thought that you could not get more than 50 % of your moving and passage expenses. That is what Schultz got.

Fisher [sic] promised me to take the matter up with the authorities without delay. He is anxious that you should come for the winter semestre [sic], but I told him that your dead line was July 31st, so that it is going to be a race against time. It is unfortunate that Vaterlaus who is Regierungs-Rat in charge of education, is a Social Democrat who doesn't believe that Medical History is a necessary subject. Well that is all for today. I am keeping my fingers crossed, and I wish you would find your way clear to come.

With best wishes, I am,
>Yours ever,
>>[Henry]

Berlioz see A. to S. of 7 June 1956. (Lefebvre 1956). (Grapow 1954). Fischer and Schinz see S. to A. of 14 April 1956 and 18 July 1946, respectively. "Extraordinary professor" = associate professor. Ernst Vaterlaus (1891–1976). Information corrected in S. to A. of 20 July 1956.

ACKERKNECHT to SIGERIST, Madison, 10 July 1956

My dear Henry:

Thanks ever so much for your letter of July 4th which arrived yesterday. Basing myself on your suggestion I telegraphed Fischer: "Erlaube mir vorzuschlagen ordentliche Professur ad personam Gehalt Francs 25,000 plus Gehalt Institutsdirektor plus haelfte Umzugs- und Ueberfahrtskosten[.] Ackerknecht". This morning I received a letter from Fischer where he indirectly suggests me better conditions, as you see from the telegram which I just sent him and which is only a repetition of what he suggests. "Bitte gestriges Telegramm annullieren[.] Erlaube mir nunmehr vorzuschlagen ordinarius ad personam[,] Gesamtbesoldung ca. Francs 30,000 dreiviertel Umzugskosten und Ueberfahrt mit Familie[.] Einkauf durch Regierung in Pensionskasse[.] Brauche für Kommen Wintersemester endgueltigen Anstellungsbescheid 31. Juli wenn möglich früher[.] Ackerknecht"[.] This mixup is annoying, and I know it is my fault. I should have, following your instructions, waited for Fischer's letter. But I did not anticipate his letter to differ from yours; and we are of course terribly under pressure with time. There are only five weeks left till we should leave Madison, and six weeks till the boat leaves in New York. I also have to hand in my resignation by

447

July 31st as you fortunately told Fischer again. We are also embarassed through the legends which we have to tell even our friends why to sell the house, books, etc. etc. Thus please forgive me, and let us not take the thing too tragically. I have of course to try to get the best possible material conditions, but this is not the essential point, and as you see I am perfectly willing to make sacrifices, if it is necessary. It is a pity that we did not know earlier that the Regierungsrat is a social-democrat, as we could have worked on him via several friends in Germany who are now social democratic leaders there. Well, it is too late, and I trust things will work out anyhow. Excuse me for being so short and confused today. But you understand our situation. I have now to shoot off a letter to Fischer to explain to him the mixup. If things work out all right we would leave here on August 14th, in New York on August 22, arrive in Paris on August 28th, stay there a week, go then to Zuerich for about a week to watch our things arrive, and for a short orientation. Then we will have to go and see our parents for a few days and then we will come for a few days to Pura, which therefore would be around September 20th. Then it goes back to Zuerich and work can start.

Thanks again and again for your help and kindness.

Very cordial wishes from all of us to all of you

Yours ever

Erwin

First telegram: Propose full professorship ad personam. Salary 25.000 Swiss Francs plus addition for head of department plus 50 % of moving and passage expenses. Ackerknecht.

Second telegram: Please disregard yesterday's telegram. Now propose full professorship ad personam. Total salary Swiss Francs ca. 30,000 plus 75 % of moving and passage expenses. Retirement pay deposit payed by government. For winter term start need confirmation of employment by 31 July, if possible earlier. Ackerknecht.

SIGERIST to ACKERKNECHT, Pura, 20 July 1956

My dear Erwin,

Time is getting short, and I hope that you got the official invitation to join the Zürich Faculty by now.

It is for me to apologize that I misinformed you, but both Fischer and Schinz were unanimous in thinking that you might not get more than

Frs. 25,000 and half your travelling expenses. However, Fischer hinted that some additional money might come out of a special fund, this is why I wrote you to wait for Fischer's letter.

I misunderstood Fischer when he said that the Socialdemocrat Meierhans was in charge of Education. Actually Meierhans is only on the Board of Education. In charge of Education is a man who has the handsome name of Vaterlaus, and it is from him that you will receive the official invitation. He is, if I remember correctly, a member of the Liberal party.

Fischer told me last week on the telephone that all your wishes were granted and accepted by the authorities, and so I trust that nothing will interfere. I fully realize how awkard [sic] the situation must be for you.

On the 21st September we hope to go to Italy for three weeks vacation. We have an American invasion just now. Temkin and family were here yesterday and the day before. Temkin was fully informed, and asked whether you had received the call yet. I had great pleasure in seeing him and talking to him after these many years. The next Baltimorean to be expected will be Horsley Gantt.

I still keep my fingers crossed, and I hope that nothing will interfere.

    With warm regards, I am,
        Yours ever,
            [Henry]

Vaterlaus see S. to A. of 4 July 1956; the literal meaning of the "handsome" name is father's louse. Gantt see S. to A. of 18 September 1948.

ACKERKNECHT to SIGERIST, Madison, 20 July 1956

My dear Henry:

I have not written you since July 10th, because we anxiously waited every day for the final news from Switzerland, but nothing was heard of from Zuerich since July 11th. Thus I had better bring you up to date on the whole situation. On July 10th I reported to you on my second telegram to Fischer. On July 11th I received the following telegramme from Fischer:

"Regierung mit Ihren Bedingungen ordentliche Professur ad Personam Gehalt fr fuenfundzwanzigtausend plus Gehalt Direktor plus mindestens haelfte Umzugs und Ueberfahrtskosten einverstanden[.] Bitte telegraphisch genaues Geburtsdatum Ihrer Frau[.] Gratuliere zur Wahl[.] Fischer Rektor".

I cabled back the same day the following:

["]Prof. Fischer, Rektor, Universität, Zuerich, Switzerland Frau Lucy geboren 27 July 1913[.] Wenn mein zweites Telegramm zu spät für Aenderung von Bedingungen[,] annehme heutige Regierungsbedingungen[.] Herzlichen Dank für Ihre Bemühungen[.] Ackerknecht["]

Now we hoped we would get a final statement as an answer to this telegramme. But as said above nothing has happened so far. I have therefore decided to send Fischer the enclosed letter, if I have no news till tomorrow morning, as there is really not much time left. It is of course possible that I have misunderstood Fischer, and that he regards his telegramme of July 11th as the final notification. But even if I am stuck with my lower offer of July 9th, I still feel I should have a final notification, preferably from the government. Well, we still have ten days to wait and hope, and I very much hope that by now not everybody is raving mad at me. It is a tour de force (and without your help it would have been entirely impossible) to transact such a thing over such distances in such a short and limited period, and difficulties are almost unavoidable. Meanwhile the house gets emptier every day (there are a lot of things which are not worth while taking over, like an old piano, children's furniture, etc.) and we get jitterier [sic] every day although we try hard not to do so. As a matter of fact I am reading voraciously, as I sleep little, mostly material on Paris 1800–1850, which I bought for the library here and French novels (I tried to read German novels, but I can't take them) but everything has a slightly unreal character. We also try to do as much packing as possible (you know what amount of packing and sifting is involved in such a move). We very much hope your health is OK. Please forgive all the trouble I am creating for you. It should now soon be over, and we can enjoy in peace the sweet [?] fruits of these bitter flowers.

Kindest regards and very best wishes to you both

    Yours ever

       Erwin

Telegram Fischer to A.: Government agrees with your conditions full professorship ad personam, salary Swiss francs 25,000 plus addition for head of department plus at least 50 % moving and passage expenses. Please cable date of birth of your spouse. Congratulations for election. Fischer, Rector.

Telegram A. to Fischer: Wife Lucy born 27 July 1913. If my second telegram too late for change of conditions, will accept today's conditions of government. Thanks for your effort. Ackerknecht.

Rector = president of a university.

Ackerknecht to Sigerist, Madison, 24 July 1956

My dear Henry:

The girl comes only day after tomorrow. Thus I better write you long-hand. Thanks ever so much for your letter of July 20th. It was a great relief to have at least some news from Switzerland. No, the final word of that dear Vaterlaus (why didn't his dad buy him an h for the l?) has still not yet arrived! Well, there is one more week to go, – and to wait. Perhaps my "Notschrei" to Fischer (of July 21) which you have seen meanwhile, has some effect. – Let us forget about the financial mixup. It is not essential. And it was all my fault anyhow.

It is good that you write in time about your vacation plans. We will then come to Pura, before we go to Ludwigsburg. (around Sept. 12?)

Yes, I told Temkin in Durham that I hoped to get the invitation. (The only one I did tell.) With him one is safe. He will never tell anybody out of sheer fear of getting mixed up in something. – Also because I want to remain on good terms with him. And through the queer logic of paranoid thought the same man, who would rather die than tell me such a thing, would never forgive me for not having told him. Well, one has to take him how he is. With all his queerness [sic] (which by the way has considerably improved) he has still more brains than anybody else here.

Otherwise we go on waiting, packing, selling, reading etc. Sunday I saw Urdang. I must now start "confessing" to at least a few. To my surprise (he always pretended to be so assimilated) and relief he was enthusiastic and even a little envious. The poor fellow is in bad shape. Bodily his Parkinson progresses slowly, but inexorably. Intellectually he is also steadily going down. Told me as great news who Celsus was, what he wrote etc. But he is firmly decided to have a big celebration for his 75th birthday next year.

Very best wishes and warm regards to you both from all of us

Yours ever

Erwin

"Girl" = secretary. Vaterlaus see S. to A. of 4 and 20 July 1956 (Vaterhaus would mean father's house). Notschrei = cry of distress. Urdang and Celsus see A. to S. of 23 March 1945 and 14 June 1949, respectively.

Ackerknecht to Sigerist, Madison, 25 July 1956

My dear Henry:

I had just mailed a letter to you, when I received the following telegram from Fischer:

Berufung durch Regierung vorläufig abgelehnt. Kommt für Wintersemester nicht mehr in Frage. Brief folgt.

This is in strange contrast to his last telegram, but it is at least clear. We can now try to sell the tickets, move into an appartment [sic] and unpack. I am glad that I was so discrete [sic] about the whole thing here. I will, of course, write you immediately, when I have the letter and see clearer in this strange matter of which Fischer is certainly innocent. If I were not so attracted by Zürich, if that were just some US university, there need be no letter, I would have a Goethe quotation handy as an epilogue to the whole matter. Still they would make a mistake in Z. to conclude from my patience that they can take me for granted.

Ce qui sera difficile ce sera de se retablir [sic] dans une situation que déjà je n'aimais pas avant l'espoir de pouvoir en sortir. Je devrais aller à un congrès, aller en vacances, voir des gens. Je n'ai envie de rien de pareil.

Mon cher vieux, j'espère que tu ne seras pas trop décu, et surtout que ta santé ne s'en ressente pas! D'abord on peut toujours espérer [?]. Et même si toute cette affaire s'effondre [sic], tu m'en as donné au cours d'elle de telles gages d'amitié qu'elle me sera toujours un souvenir plustôt précieux qu'amer.

Très, très amicalment

Toujours ton Erwin

Telegram Fischer to A.: Call declined by government for the time being. Begin winter term no longer possible. Letter follows.

Summary of the two final paragraphs: It will be difficult to find the way back in this situation. I ought to go to a congress, go vacationing, see people, but I'm not in the mood for these things. I hope you won't feel too bad and this affair did not affect your health. Even if the whole thing should evaporate, you have given me such a proof of friendship that the memory of it will be precious rather than bitter.

Ackerknecht to Sigerist, Madison, 31 July 1956

My dear Henry:

I should have had more sense and waited in crying on your shoulder concerning Fischer's telegram. But I did it. And I hasten now to send you 1) a copy of Vaterlaus' product, 2) a carbon of Fischer's letter to me, 3) a carbon of my letter to Fischer, 4) a carbon of my letter to Rossier. There is not much to say about the whole sad story, and not too much to hope, although of course as long as Fischer wants to fight for it, I will be glad to participate.

The government just seems not to want me, feeling that I am "spoilt" and too expensive, and I even doubt whether they want anybody, and were not secretly glad to get rid of that "luxury" through the death of Milt. Otherwise I cannot see why they made me look financially even more exacting than I was. My ulcer has, of course, very vigorously reacted to the message from Zurich and I therefore close. I just had a letter from Temkin who seems to have enjoyed his visit with you tremendously.

Kindest regards and best wishes to you both

Yours ever,

Erwin

P. S. The young man in the P. S. to Fricker is Hans Ris, Hanja Ris' husband. He hesitates. Your telegram just arrived, thousand thanks! yours ever

Erwin

Vaterlaus and Rossier see S. to A. of 4 July and 30 April 1956, respectively. The four letters mentioned explain the complex situation and at the same time support A.'s conclusions in this letter. Hans and Hanja Ris-Wislicka see A. to S. of 28 February 1950. Hans Ris (1914–2004) was a cell biologist

Sigerist to Ackerknecht, Pura, 7 August 1956

My dear Erwin,

I have no adequate words to express my disappointment about the failure of your affair, and I wish to thank you for having sent me copies of the various letters pertinent to it. Apparently you were too expensive for the Regierungsrat, and they were afraid that you might come with other postulates once you saw the Zurich Institute. But I am still hopefull [sic] that the Regierungsrat will reconsider its decision, since you are the only possible candidate. Buess is firmly rooted at the Ciba, where he gets, so I hear, a handsome salary, and otherwise there is nobody around that the faculty can recommend.

I must say that I am somewhat disappointed in Fischer, who congratulated you too early. I fully approve of your letters to him and the Dean. The only objection I have is that you stated a date. Faculties don't like to be rushed. Things must, at the present point, be developed slowly. The only risk you run, is that you may be called for the winter semester 1957–58, that is one year from now. Since this winter semester begins only on the 23rd of October, you cannot expect action to be taken immediately. So be patient.

My love to you and your family.

Yours ever

[Henry]

Regierungsrat, Buess, and Ciba see S. to A. of 9 June 1956, 3 November 1949, and 14 April 1956, respectively.

ACKERKNECHT to SIGERIST, Madison, 14 August 1956

My dear Henry:

Thanks ever so much for your lines of August 7th. Tomorrow we will move and our new address will be 2930 Arbor Drive. It will be quite a change from the rather large house to a small apartment, and unfortunately I will be no longer able to walk to my office as I did during the last nine years. The week thereafter we will go for a few days to Chicago to visit friends.

My stomach is not very good. I had even to give up smoking, and am living on an abominable diet. I have also spent a few days in bed with the ulcer. Otherwise I am working, but my heart is not in it. It is now three weeks that we received that particular "Gruss aus Zuerich," and I find it still somewhat hard to overcome my disappointment, and humiliation.

On the basis of the material provided by Fischer I have thought over the thing again, and I have come to the conclusion that on the part of the director of education (or whoever is behind him) there was never any intention to refill the chair of Milt. When the faculty did not respond favorably to his desire not to refill the chair, he went through the motions of accepting me, accepting even my conditions, but was firmly decided to eventually have me turned down by the Regierungsrat. The way he presented my problem to the Regierungsrat is further evidence of this hypothesis. The financial demands which I actually made were but a pretext for refusal. I would almost bet that when the faculty now will nominate a cheap young man, he will follow the same procedure, that is, accepting him, but have him eventually turned down by the Regierungsrat for lack of experience or some such thing. In my opinion the chair at Zuerich will not be refilled, unless Fischer and the faculty are very strong.

You are absolutely right that I should not have given them a date. It makes me look too eager. As a matter of fact I should never have done so. Well, it won't happen again. We can, on the other hand, of course, not live to the end of our days in a provisorium [sic] in view of a job in Zuerich which probably will never work out. I think if they have not made up their minds by next spring, they never will, and we can without further consultations buy ourselves again a house, burry [sic] our dream of living in Europe or even in the more civilized parts of the U.S., but have a look at them during our vacations. Excuse me for not being more cheerful. You sure deserved more amusing letters from me after all you did for me.

Kindest regards and best wishes to both of you from all of us

Yours ever,

Erwin

"Gruss aus Zuerich": Greetings from Zurich. Milt and Regierungsrat see S. to A. of 19 January 1951 and 9 June 1956, respectively. Provisorium: temporary place. A. often had pessimistic spells like the one in this letter.

SIGERIST to ACKERKNECHT, Pura, 22 August 1956

My dear Erwin,

I thank you for your letter of August 14th and am sorry to learn that your health is not very good and that you had to give up smoking, which I guess is a great sacrifice for you. You must not feel disappointed and particularly not feel humiliated. These are just little incidents which happen in academic life. I am still hopeful that you will be invited to join the faculty in Zürich, although it may take some time. The faculty has really no other candidate but you, and you must not forget that the History of Medicine ranks in Switzerland as a minor subject.

I don't agree with you in your guess that the Government doesn't wish to fill Milt's chair. There is, after all, the huge Wehrli Collection, and the Institute that forces the people to appoint a professor, and I repeat, you are the only serious candidate. Just let things develope [sic]. The faculty, I am sure, is behind you, and we will support your candidacy to the limit. So cheer up and don't let yourself be depressed.

With warm regards to you and your family, I am,
    Yours ever,
      [Henry]

P. S. I am sending you under separate cover a copy of my Heath Clark Lectures which just came out. The first three lectures are new, the last two contain rehash of my former publications.

Milt see S. to A. of 19 January 1951. Heath Clark Lectures (Sigerist 1956a).

Ackerknecht to Sigerist, Madison, 13 September 1956

Dear Henry:

Excuse me for not having answered earlier your very good letter of August 22nd. I was waiting for the Heath Clark Lectures with my answer and I was also physically and morally too depressed to write much. I was very touched by your attempts to cheer me up, but felt unable to share your optimism (also that of Rossier and Fischer expressed in short letters). But it seems I was wrong, as you see from the enclosed. Things actually look rather promising after this letter of Vaterlaus. The Faculty must really have put the screws on the old boy. Of course, I try not to get excited again. And am now better prepared than before July for some last minute difficulties or even failures, as we have worked out some plans which should make the coming years more agreeable, even if we have to stay in Madison.

You are probably now on your vacation in Italy, and we hope that you have an agreeable time. Our vacation was restricted to three days in Chicago, and three days in Door County, a peninsula in Lake Michigan, "famous for its natural beauty", and actually quite pretty. Now the teaching starts again. In spite of all I have succeeded this summer to go over 200 books (Paris Medical Publications, 1800–1850, which I bought for the library here in 1951 in Paris) in view of the book I intend to write "Paris Medicine 1800 to 1850", and have also done some preparatory work for a course in the history of psychiatry for our psychiatric residents which I am starting next week. I am so glad that this time I am able to give you some good news.

Kindest regards and best wishes to you both from all of us

Yours ever cordially,

Erwin

P.S. The Heath Clark Lectures just arrived. A thousand thanks. I read them immediately. A fine book. I liked the Galen and Cornaro best. Somebody should really devote a life-time to Galen. But I guess everybody is scared. Quantitatively he is worse than Virchow, not to speak of his other characteristics. I am glad you defend the Renaissance concept. One can argue about the details, but the wholesale denial that something decisive and rapid happened around 1500 is bunk. (We have an old Dean here, Gellery, who has written a long book on the subject)[.] I have always felt that the dramatic changes in medical illustration, which you once published, were a very convincing argument. Thanks again.

E.

Heath Clark Lectures, Rossier, and Vaterlaus see S. to A. of 22 August, 30 April, and 4 July 1956, respectively. Psychiatry (Ackerknecht 1959). Galen see A. to S. of 22 May 1956. Luigi Alviso Cornaro (1467–1565) Italian humanist and author. Virchow see S. to A. of 27 April 1932.

SIGERIST to ACKERKNECHT, Pura, 18 September 1956

My dear Erwin,

I cannot tell you how happy I am about this sudden turn of events that came much sooner than I had anticipated. I knew that the faculty stood solidly behind you, but I was not anticipating results so soon. Emmy shares my delight. Now it is important that you don't get excited again, so that you may not be disappointed if anything goes wrong, but I am most optimistic as to the end result.

I am delighted that you started Wisconsin Studies in Medical History, and am also delighted that No. I was the translation of your French book. I cannot tell you how grateful I am to you for placing me in the centre of your paper. I read it several times, which is not the expression of vainty [sic] on my part, but merely an expression of my delight over the article.

Day after tomorrow we are going to Zürich for two weeks, and after that for one week to my sister in Basel. I would have preferred Italy, but I am in need of some medical examination, and I long for a change of environment. We hope to go every second evening to the theatre.

Just now Genevieve Miller is typing her paper in the next room that she will deliver in Madrid. We had an endless number of visitors from the United States. The O'Malleys, the MacKinneys, Ilza Veith and her husband, but also old friends and former Leipzig students came to see me, among others Norpoth, whom you will remember as my most brilliant student, who had taken a Ph.D. in medieval philosophy before he studied medicine, then, Deta Meyer who is now Dr. Kunstler, who has an opthalmic practice in Canada and whose husband is a chest surgeon, and Irene Zygoures, who is married to an orthopaedic surgeon, Dr. Lange. Herbert Plügge and his wife are yet to come. He is now full Professor in Heidelberg and in charge of the University Polyclinic [sic].

I am glad that you liked my Heath Clark Lectures. Did you ever get my recollections of my Leipzig period?

With warm greetings, I am,

    Yours ever

     [Henry]

French book: (Ackerknecht/Vallois 1956). "Your paper" (Ackerknecht 1956). Loren MacKinney, professor of medical history at University of North Carolina. Heath Clark Lecture see S. to A. of 22 August 1956. Recollections on Leipzig (Sigerist 1956c).

    Names mentioned earlier:

Lang	S. to A. of 18 December 1945
Norpoth	S. to A. of 14 February 1947
O'Malley	S. to A. of 10 July 1952
Plügge	S. to A. of 18 July 1946
Veith, Ilza	A. to S. of 31 May 1955
Zygoures	S. to A. of 18 December 1945

My dear Henry:

Thanks ever so much for your letter of September 18th (and the post-card drawing my attention to the review in the Scientific Monthly). It was a great pleasure to share the good news with you, and on the other hand this time I remain quiet. We were quite saddened that your news is not so good, and you have to go to Zurich instead of Italy, for health reasons. Let's hope that you can report very soon about good results of your x-rays, and that you have nevertheless a good time in Zurich and Basle. In spite of the diagnostic proceedures [sic] ahead of you, which I know all too well, and the memory of which I do not cherish.

I am glad that all the reprints reached you all right, and that you liked them. It seems almost impossible that I did not acknowledge your Leipzig recollections, as I liked them so very much, and as beyond their intrinsic value they are also a good sign that you have not given up work on the auto-biography. But they might have arrived just in that terrible "Vaterlaus period." I have just read "Libre Histoire de la Médecine Francaise [sic] by Pierre Mauriac. It is, of, course, better than similar short stuff on French medical history. As an outsider (Catholic, conservative) Mauriac has al-ways been more perceptive and has had more ideas on the subject than his countrymen. As evidenced by his work on Claude Bernard. But as a whole I am disappointed. There are less new ideas, and more provincialism, than I had anticipated. In my search for somebody who knows what he is writ-ing about when writing on the History of Psychiatry, I have eventually come across a German, Joachim Bodamer – I found his article in the bibliography of Diepgens [sic] last volume – who fullfills [sic] that re-quirement. Not without the German tinge of mysticism. But that seems unavoidable. Of your innumerable visitors I remember Norpoth, Zygoures, and Pluegge very well. As a matter of fact I knew Norpoth already before Leipzig. Hanja Ris, by the way, just told me that they [?] had turned down the Zurich call. Well, everybody must know what is good for him.

Kindest regards and very, very best wishes from all of us to you both

Yours ever cordially,

Erwin

The mentioned postcard is missing. Leipzig recollections (Sigerist 1956c). (Mauriac 1956). History of Psychiatry probably (Bodamer 1956).

Names mentioned earlier:
Bernard   A. to S. of 21 August 1952
Diepgen   A. to S. of 2 May 1945
Norpoth   S. to A. of 14 February 1947
Plügge   S. to A. of 18 July 1946
Ris   A. to S. of 31 July 1956
Zygoures   S. to A. of 18 February 1945

SIGERIST to ACKERKNECHT, Pura ?, ca. 29 September 1956 (Telegram)

HEARTIEST CONGRATULATIONS. ALL IS WELL THAT ENDS WELL.
   SIGERISTS

ACKERKNECHT to SIGERIST, Madison, 30 September 1956

My dear Henry:
   This is just my last exchange of letters with Vaterlaus. Things seem to progress in a satisfactory way. Otherwise nothing new. – We hope so very much that the result of your examination in Zürich will be satisfactory.
   Very cordially
      Yours ever
         Erwin

SIGERIST to ACKERKNECHT, Pura, 16 October 1956

Dear Erwin,
   I was very pleased to receive your letters of 25th and 30th September, from which I assume that your call to Zürich is almost sure to come. You would not be invited to submit to a medical examination if the Government of Zürich had not made up its mind. I expect that you will receive the official documents in the next few days. I heard from Emmy that you have received congratulatory telegrams from Fischer and your chief competitor Buess.

460

I just spent two weeks in Zürich and one week at my sister's in Bâle, and had quite a good time although I had to submit to several quite unpleasant medical examinations. However, we enjoyed the theatres, particularly the super [?] performance of Torquato Tasso.

I am truly looking forward to your coming to Zürich. I feel rather isolated here although I have many visitors. John Fulton came with his wife to see me. Genevieve Miller spent ten days here between the International Congress of the History of Science and the International Congress of the History of Medicine. I also had the visit of the MacKinneys, of O'Mally, of Anna Tjomsland and many others, but still feel isolated and am really looking forward to your coming to Zürich.

With best wishes, I am,
    Yours ever,
      [Henry]

* Schinz found that I have several diverticula of the colon descendens and he also found a suspicious shadow in the rectum whereupon he advised me to have a rectoscopy performed. The biopsy revealed that I had a mere stenosis of the rectum – thank God not carcinoma – The diagnosis therefor [sic] is diverticulosis coli and stenosis recti which explains the bloody stools. Hemorroids [sic] were not found and the condition does not require surgery. I am much relieved.

Bâle: French spelling of Basel/Basle. *Torquato Tasso*: Drama by Goethe. Anna Tjomsland (born 1880) anesthetist and medical historian.
    Names mentioned earlier:
Buess   S. to A. of 3 November 1949
Fulton   S. to A. of 26 February 1945
MacKinney S. to A. of 18 September 1956
O'Malley S. to A. of 10 July 1952
Schinz   S. to A. of 18 July 1946

ACKERKNECHT to SIGERIST, Madison, 21 October 1956 (Telegram)

JUST RECEIVED CONFIRMATION AND RESIGNED HERE SEE YOU FEBRUARY THOUSAND THANKS LOVE FROM ALL TO YOU BOTH. ERWIN

Ackerknecht to Sigerist, Madison, 22 October 1956

My dear Henry:

Thanks ever so much for your letter of October 16th., and your telegram of the 21st. I still have no official confirmation from the Zurich government, but with congratulation telegrams from you, Rossier, and Buess (sic) and a U. P. release telling in newspapers and over the radio that the government has elected me, there should be no longer any doubt. We are, of course, extremely happy, and I want to thank you once more from the bottom of my heart for all the help and friendship you have given me. I know, without you, I would never have made it. We are looking forward very much to our common life in Switzerland. I am also very glad that this long period of waiting is over, especially as it grew rather embarassing during the last weeks, when my dean almost daily promised me something new, if I would only stay here. He dragged even the President into my office who conjured me not to leave them. But my decision was made long ago. We will leave here on February 1st, and hope to show up in Pura at the end of February.

I cannot tell you how relieved we are to hear that you had no malignancy and did not require surgery. Rectal surgery, even for non-malignant conditions is no fun.

We are rather busy. I have now to revise the German translation of the Virchow, which is finished. I hope to be able to dictate a short history of psychiatry in German before we leave. I do this with great reticense [sic], but I have invested so much time in the subject that I might just as well write about it. There is also objectively a need for the book. But fundamentally I dislike the subject, as no real progress has been achieved. It is an eternal carousel from Soranus to Bleuler. Bringing the book out in German I also will not enjoy the unanimously good reviews I had for my books in English, as my "positivist" approach will be as distasteful to many Germans, as their false profundity is to me. Never mind, the Virchow will have established me. And a little fight for a good cause has its advantages too.

We have an extremely beautiful fall, warm and sunny. As you were the first to tell me that fall is the only good season in the US, you know how beautiful fall can be here. We try to get of it as much as is possible with our multiple occupations. There are also quite a few amusing French speaking people around the campus this fall. Unlike you, we never have many visitors here. But we had one which rather impressed me. It was an old co-student from Berlin 30 years ago who meanwhile has become a famous British newspaperman with the old Scotch name of Richard Loewenthal. As he is a very brilliant man, it was very refreshing. And it was rather strange to see, and also to hear from him concerning others what life has done to our generation.

I cannot close without reporting the tremendous educational advance which we have made in this university. Every second toilet door in the men's toilet (of course not in the women's toilets) has been removed, in order to prevent the exchange of morse signals between homosexuals. His [sic] is not yet quite as good as the new Tuft dormitory where the whole place is wired, but a decisive progress. What a bunch of morons. And I have lived here for 15 years, ten of them in the Midwest.

Nous vous embrassons tous très joieusement et à bientôt

Toujours ton
Erwin

Buess see S. to A. of 3 November 1949. History of psychiatry (Ackerknecht 1959). Soranos of Ephesos (ca. 100 A.D.) Greek author of texts on gynaecology and psychiatry. Eugen Bleuler (1857–1939) Swiss psychiatrist. Richard Loewenthal (born 1908?).

ACKERKNECHT to SIGERIST, Madison, 27 November 1956

My dear Henry:

I have not heard from you for some time, but I hope that it is no sign of any health trouble of yours. The Zurich appointment seems now to have happened so long ago, as meanwhile all these tragic world events have occurred. Some people think we are fools to go to Europe now. I don't. The Zurich story remained a comedy of errors up to the very last. The first I heard about it was through a United Press release. Then I had to wrestle a confirmative telegram out of them in order to finish the ambiguous situation here. The official letter came by ordinary mail only on November 5th! The appointment brought me an avalanche of letters. The local reactions oscillate between hostility and frank envy. You know all that. I was not consulted concerning my succession and had to open a little war with my dean who feels personally offended, and seems not very much inclined to refill my job. He would probably prefer to create a new chair, which would bring more news releases, than just to refill an old one. It would be a pity, as I think I have built up a pretty nice plant here in the course of ten years.

Even without all that I would be busy enough to do my ordinary duties and to prepare for our departure. The revision of the German translation of Virchow is done, and I hope you will not mind that I have dedicated it to you. I have also done five chapters of my little book on the history of psychiatry and hope to finish it before leaving. The visit of a very nice German psychiatrist, Konrad Ernst (brother of the medievalist in Heidelberg Fritz Ernst) enticed me to read eventually "Genie, Irrsinn und Ruhm" by W. Langeteichbaum [sic]. Not bad, but too long (gruendlich). Otherwise here the usual damned ice and snow. I long to leave it and I wish I were two months older.

Kindest regards and very best wishes to you both
    Yours ever,
      Erwin

"Tragic world events": The crushing of the Hungarian revolution by Soviet Russia and the Suez Crisis. History of psychiatry (Ackerknecht 1959). Konrad Ernst (1903–1997). Fritz Ernst see A. to S. of 25 May 1956. (Lange-Eichbaum 1935). Gruendlich = thorough.

SIGERIST to ACKERKNECHT, Pura, 30 November 1956

My dear Erwin,

I do not remember if I thanked you for your latest reprints "Medical Art as a Psychological Safety-Valve" etc. If I did not, I want to do it now with my apologies. However[,] I am sure that I did not acknowledge the receit of your telegram and of your good letter of 22 October.

Enclosed find some clippings that may interest you. I am anxious to see you as soon as you think it possible, because I have some instructions to give you on matters of etiquette that Edolf Schulz [sic] did not know about so that he remained completely isolated. It is too complicated to write you about it. When are you sailing exactly? I can imagine that you are very busy not only dictating your "short History of Psychiatry" but in winding up business.

464

Every spring the Swiss medical historians meet in Pura for a two days conference. Next year as Easter is being late I have the intention of calling the conference March 30 and 31. It will give me an ideal chance to introduce you and I want you to give a paper. Papers are usually half an hour and the discussion takes half an hour. Each participant has a full hours [sic] time to deliver his paper and have it discussed. Think it over. Any subject that you choose will do.

What courses will you give at the university? It is essential that you get into the program of next semester. I do not know what the deadline is for announcing the courses.

So much for to-day. I shall write you soon again. With cordial greetings I am

Ever yours,
    [Henry]

PS: The postman just brings your letter which I am going to answer in a few days

Medical Art … (Ackerknecht 1955c). Adolf Schultz see A. to S. of 16 May 1946; on etiquette and isolation see S. to A. of 1 June 1956. History of psychiatry (Ackerknecht 1959).

ACKERKNECHT to SIGERIST, Madison, 6 December 1956

My dear Henry:

Thanks ever so much for your letter of November 30th, and the interesting newspaper clippings. We are sailing on February 9th on the "United States". There was no earlier boat. We are arriving in Paris on the 14th, which leaves us only two weeks for Paris, Ludwigsburg, and possibly Pura, as I have promised to be in Zurich on March 1st. But I will try to show up as early as possible in Pura, not only on account of the important instructions in "behavior". It is true, it is very important not to start on the wrong foot in this respect.

I am looking forward very much to come to the Pura conference. I would have liked to start out with a paper which has some local flavor (on Schoenlein or Griesinger or Labert [?], or Louis' Swiss pupils), but

I am afraid there will not be enough time for that between March 1st and March 30th. Thus it might be best that I either talk about "Medicine and Science in 19th Century Europe" (deals mostly with educational reasons for the supremacy first of French then of German medicine in the century), but I should perhaps save that for my "Antrittsvorlesung" about which I also will have to talk with you. Another possibility, and perhaps the best one, would be that I give one of the chapters of my book. For this purpose I am sending you a short synopsis. Anyone will do as far as I am concerned. Personally I like the Pinel one best. But I would really prefer to leave it to you to pick the subject.

Fischer sent me a form for announcing lectures for the summer semester. And after some back and forth I have decided to announce: Geschichte der Medizin von den Anfaengen bis zur Gegenwart (2 Stunden), Geschichte der Krankheiten (1 Stunde), Seminar (2 Stunden, Klassiker der Psychiatrie). I am indeed terribly busy. I have now eight chapters. But they are getting more and more difficult. And in addition to everything else I have a lot of speaking engagements by groups who want to hear me once more, and which I cannot always turn down.

Kindest regards and very best wishes to you both

Yours ever,

Erwin

Schoenlein and Griesinger see A. to S. of 4 April 1947 and 13 May 1954, respectively. "Labert", probably Hermann Lebert (1813–1878) French pathologist of German origin, pupil of Schoenlein. Pierre Charles Alexandre Louis (1787–1872) French clinician and epidemiologist. Antrittsvorlesung: Inaugural lecture. "My book" (Ackerknecht 1959). Pinel see A. to S. of 23 March 1945. A.'s Zurich lectures announced:
    History of medicine from the origins to the present (2 hours)
    History of diseases (1 hour)
    Seminar: Classics of psychiatry (2 hours).

Sigerist to Ackerknecht, Pura, 7 January 1957

My dear Erwin,

Last Saturday I sent out the invitations to the Pura Conference. To our Pura cercle [sic] belong the following gentlemen:

Charles LICHTENTHAELER, who is a specialist on Hippocrates, wrote a book "La médecine hippocratique" that was published 1948 in Lausanne. He is quite a nice fellow although I cannot follow his theories on Hippocratic Medicine. He lives in Leysin.

Raymond de SAUSSURE you know of course. He is our specialist on the History of Psychiatry.

Edgar GOLDSCHMID is professor emeritus of the university of Lausanne. You are of course familiar with his books dealing with the History of Pathological Illustrations. Right now he is collecting materials for a book about anatomical wax preparations.

Of the Basle group you know BUESS of course. He has an assistant Nikolaus MANI and a former student of his a Dr. KOELBING. To the Basle group belongs also Dr. KARCHER who is very old and well known for his book on Platter.

From Zurich we may expect Dr. SALZMANN who is a specialist on local medical history of the Ticino. Dr. FUETER who is our link to the History of Science. He is a Ph. D. who graduated with a thesis dealing with the History of Mathematics. Professor FISCHER also belongs to our group.

From Bern we invited Professor HINTZSCHE who is the anatomist of the university and is very interested in Haller, wrote the History of the Inselspital and lately became interested in Chinese anatomy. He was recently in the States where he found a lot of material on this subject.

I invited also Dr. WALKER of Yale who happens to be in this country living with his wife and two children in Gstaad.

I strongly advise you to save "Medicine and Science in 19th century Europe" for your Antrittsvorlesung and to give us a paper on either Pinel or Griesinger at the Pura Conference. Dead line for the announcement of the papers is March first and the Pura Conference will take place, as you know, on March 30 and 31.

The lectures you give in the summer semester could not be better. Your seminary will attract the psychiatrists and those students interested in psychiatry.

I can imagine that you must be swamped with work, but you will have a rest on the ship. Enclosed find a clipping of the series "Heilkunde in drei Jahrtausenden" that I forgot to send you.

With warm regards I am,
    Very cordially yours
        [Henry]

(Lichtenthaeler 1948). Leysin and Gstaad, resorts in Switzerland. Inselspital, the University Hospital in Bern. Antrittsvorlesung see A. to S. of 6 December 1956. *Heilkunde in drei Jahrtausenden* not identified.

New names (Swiss scientists):
Fueter, Eduard (1908–1970) historian of science
Haller, Albrecht von (1708–1777) physiologist and poet
Hintzsche, Erich (1900–1975) anatomist and medical historian. See correspondence with S. (Bickel 2008)
Lichtenthaeler, Charles (1915–1993) medical historian in Lausanne and Hamburg
Karcher, Johannes (1872–1958) physician and medical historian
Koelbing, Huldrych M. (1923–2007) medical historian
Mani, Nikolaus (1920–2001) medical historian in Madison and Bonn
Platter, Felix (1536–1614) physician and anatomist
Salzmann, Charles, dermatologist and medical historian
Walker, not identified

Names mentioned earlier:
Buess   S. to A. of 3 November 1949
Fischer   S. to A. of 14 April 1956
Goldschmid S. to A. of 14 August 1952
Griesinger   A. to S. of 13 May 1954
Pinel   A. to S. of 23 March 1945
Saussure   A. to S. of 23 March 1945

ACKERKNECHT to SIGERIST, Madison, 15 January 1957

My dear Henry:

Thanks ever so much for your letter of January 7th, and the list of the participants of the Pura conference. As Saussure is coming, and as he has written quite adequately on Pinel, and a speech on Pinel would probably bore him, I prefer then to talk about Griesinger (something like Die Psychiatrie von Wilhelm Griesinger). We are now in the middle of the most terrible departure troubles. Since January 1st I have already undergone two banquets and a lot of private farewell parties. And there is still more to come. This will continue in New York. I will really need the rest on the ship badly. I hope I will still be whole by that time. But I have at least finished the manuscript of the little book (about 130 pages). Excuse me for not writing more today. But from your own experience you know how I feel. Anyhow we will soon be able to talk over everything orally.

Looking forward very much to that blessed moment, I am with my kindest regards and best wishes to you both

Yours ever,

Erwin

Saussure and Pinel A. to S. of 23 March 1945. Griesinger see A. to S. of 13 May 1954. "Little book" (Ackerknecht 1959).

ACKERKNECHT to SIGERIST, Paris, 15 February 1957 (Original in French)

My dear friend,

This is just to announce that we have finally arrived in our old Europe yesterday – in pretty bad shape, to be sure, after six painful days on an agitated sea. Nevertheless, we are very happy. A week from now we shall be at Ludwigsburg, in two weeks in Zurich, and the second weekend in March I hope to hug you in Pura. I've seen Nora and her family in New York. They all were fine, and she sends you all her love. Everything else by word of mouth. Excuse me for not writing more today, but my head is still turning.

With best wishes

In friendship yours ever

Erwin

S.'s daughter Nora see S. to A. of 12 February 1946.

SIGERIST to ACKERKNECHT, Pura ?, mid February 1957 (Telegram) (Original in French)

WELCOME TO YOU ALL IN OUR OLD EUROPE HENRY ET EMMY SIGERIST

ACKERKNECHT to SIGERIST, Zurich, 2 March 1957
(Original in French)

My dear friend,

We have arrived yesterday, at last! Emmy has received us very nicely, the apartment is fine, the department a mess. We'll talk about that. Yet I have time enough to rearrange things. I will see you on March 8 or 9. Paris was fine (thanks a lot for your good telegram), Germany was tiring but, after all, my duty. By the way, I have already a contract with Enke (who published my Virchow) for the "Short History of Psychiatry".

Best wishes, friendship, and see you soon
    Yours as ever
      Erwin

My regards to Mrs. Bickel to whom we are very grateful to have let us use her apartment which she so nicely prepared.

The letter-head reads Medizinhistorisches Institut der Universität Zürich. History of psychiatry (Ackerknecht 1959). Marguerite Bickel, S.'s sister, living in Basel, let the A.s have her Zurich apartment as a place to start.

SIGERIST to ACKERKNECHT, Pura ?, early March 1957 ? (Telegram)

LOOKING FORWARD MEETING YOU STATION LUGANO WEDNESDAY 1722 GREETINGS
    SIGERIST

ACKERKNECHT to SIGERIST, Zurich, 11 March 1957
(Original in French)

My dear friend,

As you see, I have well returned, reading "Boulevard" which was so funny that the trip seemed short. Let me thank you and Emmy once more for your unsurpassed hospitality. And special thanks to you for the good counsels which I immediately started to apply. Alas, we don't even have a complete set of the "Zürcher Abhandlungen". But we'll manage. I also immediately wrote to Madison concerning Jarcho as a candidate. I have bought the Swiss "Knigge" etc., etc. My audience with our dear president Vaterlaus was quite satisfactory. He confirmed the existence of the credit of 80,000 Francs, and he promised to deal with the necessary constructions after his return from Japan in mid-April.

I am so happy to have seen that your speech difficulties have so much improved since my last visit and that you are able to continue your work, if at a slower pace. My visit was too short to discuss all that one had wished to discuss, but in the future I shall come frequently.

Best wishes, friendship

Yours as ever

Erwin

"Boulevard", probably a book. "Zürcher medizingeschichtliche Abhandlungen". Jarcho see A. to S. of 3 June 1948. "Schweizer Knigge" (Guggenbühl 1981). Vaterlaus see S. to A. of 4 July 1956.

A.'s hope to frequently return to Pura was not fulfilled: S. died on March 17, about a week after A.'s visit in Pura and this last letter. –

In Zurich A. reorganized the department and its collections, continued his research and publishing and enjoyed his success in teaching. He also married his third wife, Edit Weinberg and retired in 1971, still remaining active and productive despite increasing health problems. He died on November 18 of 1988 in Zurich.

4.3. Literature

Ackerknecht, Erwin H.: *Beiträge zur Geschichte der Medizinalreform von 1848.* Thesis Leipzig 1931. Sudhoffs Arch. Gesch. Med. Naturwiss. 25, 61–183, 1932.

Ackerknecht, Erwin H.: *Paul Bert's Triumph.* Bull. Hist. Med. Suppl. 3, 16–31, 1944.

Ackerknecht, Erwin H.: *Malaria in the Upper Mississippi Valley.* Bull. Hist. Med. Suppl. 4, 1945.

Ackerknecht, Erwin H.: *Incubator and Taboo.* J. Hist. Med. Allied Sci. 1, 144–148, 1946a.

Ackerknecht, Erwin H.: *Primitive Medicine: A Contrast with Modern Practice.* Merck Rep. July 1946b.

Ackerknecht, Erwin H.: *Medieval Medicine.* Merck Rep. October 1946c.

Ackerknecht, Erwin H.: *The Role of Medical History in Medical Education.* Bull. Hist. Med. 21, 135–145, 1947a.

Ackerknecht, Erwin H.: *The Dawn of Modern Medicine.* Merck Rep. January 1947b.

Ackerknecht, Erwin H.: *Hygiene in France 1815–1848.* Bull. Hist. Med. 22, 117–155, 1948a.

Ackerknecht, Erwin H.: *Anticontagionism Between 1821 and 1867. The Fielding H. Garrison Lecture.* Bull. Hist. Med. 22, 562–593, 1948b.

Ackerknecht, Erwin H.: *Cinchona and Malaria in Precolombian South America.* In: S. R. Kagan, ed: "Victor Robinson Memorial Volume". New York 1948c, 23–26.

Ackerknecht, Erwin H.: *Early History of Legal Medicine.* Ciba Symposia 11, 1286–1289; *Legal Medicine in Transition.* – 1290–1298; *Legal Medicine becomes a Modern Science.* – 1299–1304, 1951a.

Ackerknecht, Erwin H.: *The History of the Paris Clinical School 1800–1850.* Yearbook of the American Philosophical Society 1951b, 257–259.

Ackerknecht, Erwin H.: *Villermét and Quetelet.* Bull. Hist. Med. 26, 317–329, 1952a.

Ackerknecht, Erwin H.: *Zur Geschichte der Malaria.* Ciba-Zeitschrift 11, 4810–4817, 1952b, continued 4818–4826, 4827–4831, 4832–4838.

Ackerknecht, Erwin H.: *Rudolf Virchow, Doctor, Statesman, Anthropologist.* Madison 1953a.

Ackerknecht, Erwin H.: *Broussais or a Forgotten Medical Revolution.* Bull. Hist. Med. 27, 320–343, 1953b.

Ackerknecht, Erwin H.: *Dr. Walter J. Meek as a Medical Historian.* In: "Medico-historical Papers by Dr. Meek". Madison 1954, 1–4.

Ackerknecht, Erwin H.: *A Short History of Medicine.* New York 1955a.

Ackerknecht, Erwin H.: *Georg Forster, Alexander von Humboldt and Ethnology.* Isis 46, 83–95, 1955b.

Ackerknecht, Erwin H.: *Medical Art as a Psychological Safety-valve.* Bull. Med. Libr. Ass. 43, 465–471, 1955c.

Ackerknecht, Erwin H.: *Die Medizingeschichte in den Vereinigten Staaten.* Welt als Geschichte 16, 154–157, 1956.

Ackerknecht, Erwin H.: *Medical Education in 19th Century France*. J. of Medical Education 32, 148–152, 1957.

Ackerknecht, Erwin H.: *Short History of Psychiatry*. New York 1959. (German original 1957).

Ackerknecht, Erwin H.: *Geschichte und Geographie der wichtigsten Krankheiten*. Stuttgart 1963.

Ackerknecht to Genevieve Miller of 31 May 1972. Dept. of the History of Medicine, University of Zurich.

Ackerknecht, Erwin H.: *Autobiographical Notes. July 1986*. Typewritten manuscript. Department of the History of Medicine, University of Bern, Switzerland.

Ackerknecht, Erwin H. / Vallois, Henri V.: *Franz Joseph Gall and his Collection*. Wisconsin Studies in Medical History, 1, Madison 1956. (The French original was of 1955).

Allbutt, Thomas Clifford, ed.: *System of Medicine*. New York 1896–1899.

Allen, Raymand B.: *Medical Education and the Changing Order*. New York 1946.

Arcieri, Giovanni P.: *Circulation of the Blood and Andrea Cesalpino of Arezzo*. New York 1945.

Aron, Raymond: *Histoire de Vichy*. Paris 1954.

Artelt, Walter: *Einführung in die Medizinhistorik*. Stuttgart 1949.

Aschoff, Ludwig: *Rudolf Virchow, Wissenschaft und Weltgeltung*. Hamburg 1940.

Aymé, Marcel: *Uranus*. Paris 1951.

Bartels, Max: *Die Medizin der Naturvölker*. Leipzig 1893.

Bartlett, Elisha: *Philosophy of Medicine*. Dordrecht 2005.

Barzun, Jacques: *Teacher in America*. New York, reprinted 1954.

Barzun, Jacques: *Berlioz and his Century*. New York 1956.

Berg-Schorn, Elisabeth: *Henry E. Sigerist (1891–1957)*. Köln 1978.

Berghoff, E.: *Entwicklungsgeschichte des Krankheitsbegriffs*. Vienna 1946.

Bernard, Claude: *Introduction to the Study of Experimental Medicine*. New York 1927.

Bickel, Marcel H.: *Henry E. Sigerist's Annual "Plans of Work" (1932–1955)*. Bull. Hist. Med. 71, 489–498, 1997.

Bickel, Marcel H., ed.: *Henry E. Sigerist. Vier ausgewählte Briefwechsel mit Medizinhistorikern der Schweiz*. Peter Lang Publishing Group, Bern etc. 2008.

Blane, Gilbert: *Elements of Medical Logic*. London 1822.

Bodamer, Joachim: *Seele und Seelenkrankheiten des Menschen von heute*. Hamburg 1956.

Buschan, Georg H. T.: *Ueber Medizinzauber und Heilkunst im Leben der Völker*. Berlin 1941.

Cabanis, Pierre Jean: *Essay on the Certainty of Medicine*. Philadelphia 1823.

Camus, Albert: *La peste*. Paris 1947.

Casanova, Girolamo: *Memoirs*. New York 1930.

Castiglioni, Arturo: *Adventures of the Mind*. New York 1946.

Chamson, André: *La Galère*. Paris 1939.

Charcot, Jean Martin: *Clinical Lectures on Senile and Chronic Diseases*. London 1881.

Chateaubriand, François A. R. de: *Mémoires d'outre-tombe*. Bruxelles 1848–1850.

Chavez, Ignacio: *Mexico en la cultura médica*. Mexico City 1947.

Chertok, Leon / De Saussure, Raymond: *Therapeutic Revolution from Mesmer to Freud*. New York 1979.

Clements: *Primitive Concepts of Disease*. UC Publ. Amer. Archeol. Ethnol. 1932, 216.

Cohen, Bernard I.: *Science, Servant of Man*. Boston 1948.

Constant, Benjamin: *Cécile*. Paris 1951.

Contenau, Georges: *La médecine en Assyrie et Babylonie*. Paris 1938.

Contenau, Georges: *La magie chez les Assyriens et Babyloniens*. Paris 1947.

Cranefield, Paul F.: Studies on the Electrical Characteristics of the Cardiac Injury Potential. Madison, 1951.

Cranefield, Paul F.: *Erwin Ackerknecht, 1906–1988, Some Memories*. J. Hist. Med. Allied Sci. 45, 145–149, 1990.

Crile, George W.: *G. Crile, an Autobiography*. Philadelphia 1947.

Cushing, Harvey: *The Life of Sir William Osler*. London 1940.

Da Cava, A. Francesco: *La Peste di San Carlo visto da un medico*. Milano 1944.

De Terra, Helmut: *Humboldt: The Life and Times of Alexander von Humboldt, 1769–1859*. New York 1955.

Diepgen, Paul: *Geschichte der Medizin*. 3 volumes. Berlin 1949–1955.

Düring, Ingemar: *Aristotle's De partibus animalium*. New York 1943.

Ebstein, Erich H., ed.: *Deutsche Aerzte-Reden aus dem 19. Jahrhundert*. Berlin 1926.

Fee, Elizabeth / Brown, Theodore M.: *Making Medical History. The Life and Times of Henry E. Sigerist*. Baltimore / London, 1997.

Fischer, Anton: *Grundlagen der wissenschaftlichen Erkenntnis*. Wien 1947.

Flexner, Simon / Flexner, James Thomas: *William Henry Welch and the Heroic Age of American Medicine*. New York 1941.

Fodéré, François Emmanuel: *Leçons sur les épidémies et l'hygiène publique*. Paris 1822–1824.

Frankfort, Henri / Frankfort H. A., eds.: *Before Philosophy: The Intellectual Adventure of Ancient Man*. Harmondsworth 1949.

Fulton, John F.: *Harvey Cushing: A Biography*. Springfield, IL, 1946.

Garrison, Fielding H.: *Introduction to the History of Medicine*. Philadelphia 1913.

Garrison, Fielding H.: *Medicine in the Tatler, Spectator, and Guardian*. Bull. N.Y. Acad. Med. 10, 477–503, 1934.

Giraudoux, Jean: *Les cinq tentations de Lafontaine*. Paris 1943.

Glasser Otto: *Dr. W. C. Roentgen*. Springfield, IL, 1945.

Gnudi, Martha T. / Webster, Jerome: *Life and Times of Gaspare Tagliacozzi, Surgeon of Bologna, 1545–1599*. New York 1950.

Grapow, Hermann: *Grundriss der Medizin der alten Aegypter*. Volume I, Berlin 1954.

Guggenbühl, A.: *Guggenbühls Schweizer Knigge*. Zürich 1981.

Guiard, Emile: *Trépanation cranienne chez les néolithiques et chez les primitifs modernes*. Paris 1930.

Guillemin, Henri, ed.: *Journal: 1830–1848, Victor Hugo*. Paris 1954.

Hagelstange, Rudolf: *Venezianisches Credo*. Leipzig 1946.

Hippocrates: *On Ancient Medicine*. Whitefish 2004?

Hirsch, August: *Geschichte der medizinischen Wissenschaften in Deutschland*. München and Leipzig 1893.

Hirschfeld, Ernst: *Romantische Medizin*. Leipzig 1930.

Honig, Pieter / Verdoorn, Frans, eds.: *Science and Scientists in Netherlands Indies*. New York 1945.

Howells, William W.: *The Heathens; Primitive Man and his Religions*. 1948.

Kagan, Solomon R.: *Life and Letters of Fielding H. Garrison*. Boston 1938.

Kagan, Solomon R.: *Fielding H. Garrison; a Biography*. Boston 1948.

Kelly, Howard A./Burrage, Walter L.: *Dictionary of American Medical Biography*. 1928.

Kerillis, Henri: *De Gaulle dictateur: Une grande mystification de l'histoire*. Montreal 1945.

Kisch, Bruno: *Forgotten Leaders in Modern Medicine: Valentin, Gruby, Remak, Auerbach*. Philadelphia 1954.

Koestler, Arthur: *Arrow in the Blue, an Autobiography*. London 1952/54.

Kolle, Kurt, ed.: *Grosse Nervenärzte*. 3 volumes. Vol. 1, Stuttgart 1956.

Koty, John: *Die Behandlung der Alten und Kranken bei den Naturvölkern*. Stuttgart 1934.

Kremers, Edward/Urdang, George: *History of Pharmacy*. Philadelphia 1940.

Kristeller, Paul O.: *The School of Salerno. Its Development and its Contribution to the History of Learning*. Bull. Hist. Med. 17, 138–194, 1945.

Kroeber, Alfred L.: *Three Essays on the Antiquity and Races of Man*. Berkeley 1922.

Kroeber, Alfred L.: *Configurations of Culture Growth*. Berkeley 1969 (1st ed. prior to 1946).

Lain Entralgo, Pedro, ed.: *Historia universal de la medicina*. Barcelona 1972–75.

Lange-Eichbaum, Wilhelm: *Genie, Irrsinn und Ruhm*. 2nd ed., München 1935.

Lefebvre, Gustave: *Essay sur la médecine égyptienne de l'époque pharaonique*. Paris 1956.

Leibbrand, Werner: *Romantische Medizin*. Hamburg 1937.

Levi, Carlo: *Cristo si è fermato a Eboli*. Torino 1945.

Levy-Bruhl, Lucien: *L'Allemagne depuis Leibniz*. Paris 1890.

Lichtenthaeler, Charles: *La médecine hippocratique*. Lausanne 1948.

Lockwood, Dean Putnam: *Ugo Benzi; Medieval Philosopher and Physician, 1376–1439*. Chicago 1951.

Lot, Fernand: *Charles Nicolle, un grand biologiste*. Paris 1946.

Lowie, Robert H.: *Primitive Society*. New York 1919.

MacCurdy, George G.: *Human Skulls from Gazelle Peninsula*. Philadelphia 1914.

Manzoni, Alessandro: *I Promessi Sposi*. Milano 1913.

Marriott, Alice L.: *The Ten Grandmothers*. Oklahoma 1945.

Martin du Gard, Roger: *Les Thibaults*. Paris 1942–43.

Mauriac, Pierre: *Libre histoire de la médecine française*. Paris 1956.

McKenzie, Dan: *The Infancy of Medicine*. London 1927.

Meichsner, Dieter: *Versucht's noch mal mit uns*. Hamburg 1948.

Mettler, Cecilia C.: *History of Medicine*. Philadelphia/Toronto 1947.

Meyer, Hans: *Georg Büchner und seine Zeit*. Wiesbaden 1946.

Miller, Genevieve: *A Bibliography of the Writings of Henry E. Sigerist*. Montreal 1966.

Möllers, Bernhard: *Robert Koch*. Hannover 1950.

Neuburger, Max: *Geschichte der Medizin*. Stuttgart 1906/1911.

N. N.: *Essays in Biology: In Honor of Herbert M. Evans, Written by his Friends*. Berkeley/Los Angeles 1943.

Oesterlen, Friedrich: *Medical Logic*. London 1853.

Olmsted, James M. D.: *François Magendie*. New York 1944.

Olmsted, James M. D.: *Charles-Edouard Brown-Séquard: A Nineteenth Century Neurologist and Endocrinologist*. Baltimore 1946.

Paracelsus: *Four Treatises of Theophrastus von Hohenheim.* Baltimore 1941.

Park, Edwards A.: *Changing Medical Care in our Changing National Life.* The Journal of Pediatrics 31, 599–615, 1947.

Pazzini, Adalberto: *Storia della medicina.* Milano 1949.

Pazzini, Adalberto / Baffoni, A.: *Storia delle malattie.* Roma 1950.

Pearse, Innes H. / Crocker, Lucy H.: *Peckham Experiment: A Study in the Living Structure of Society.* London 1943.

Pickard, Madge E. / Buley, R. Carlyle: *The Midwest Pioneer, his Ills, Cures & Doctors.* Crawfordsville, IN 1945.

Plesch, Johann: *Janos, the Story of a Doctor.* London 1947.

Powell, John H.: *Bring out your Dead.* Philadelphia 1949.

Rebatet, Lucien: *Les Décombres.* Paris 1942.

Richet, Charles: *Le Savant.* Paris 1926.

Ripamonti, Giuseppe: *La Peste di Milano del 1630.* Milano 1945.

Rivera, Diego / Wolfe, Bertram D.: *Portrait of Mexico.* New York 1937.

Rosen, George: *The Specialization in Medicine. With Particular Reference to Ophthalmology.* New York 1944.

Rosen, George: *A History of Preventive Medicine.* New York 1958.

Rosenberg, Charles E.: *Erwin H. Ackerknecht, Social Medicine, and the History of Medicine.* Bull. Hist. Med. 81, 511–532, 2007.

Rossi, Ennio: *Giovanni Rasori (1766–1837) or Italian Medicine in Transition.* Thesis, U. of Wisconsin 1954.

Rousseau, Jean-Jacques: *Confessions.* Paris 1798.

Ruffer, Marc A.: *Studies in the Paleopathology of Egypt.* Chicago 1921.

Sagan, Françoise: *Bonjour tristesse.* Paris 1955.

Salinger, J. D.: *The Catcher in the Rye.* Boston, 1952.

Sarton, George: *Life of Science; Essays in the History of Civilization.* New York 1948.

Sauerbruch, Ferdinand: *Das war mein Leben.* Zürich 1951.

Shryock, Richard H.: *American Medical Research, Past and Present.* New York 1947a.

Shryock, Richard H.: *The Development of Modern Medicine; An Interpretation of the Social And Scientific Factors Involved.* New York 1947b.

Sigerist, Henry E.: *Einführung in die Medizin.* Leipzig 1931.

Sigerist, Henry E.: *Grosse Aerzte.* München 1932.

Sigerist, Henry E.: *American Medicine.* New York 1934.

Sigerist, Henry E.: *The History of Medical Licensure.* J. Am. Med. Ass. 104, 1057–1060, 1935.

Sigerist, Henry E.: *The Historical Aspect of Art and Medicine.* Bull. Hist. Med. 4, 271–297, 1936a.

Sigerist, Henry E.: *The Medical Student and the Social Problems Confronting Medicine Today.* Bull. Hist. Med. 4, 411–422, 1936b.

Sigerist, Henry E.: *An Outline of the Development of the Hospital.* Bull. Hist. Med. 4, 573–581, 1936c.

Sigerist, Henry E.: *Historical Background of Industrial and Occupational Diseases.* Bull. N. Y. Acad. Med. 2nd. series, 12, 597–609, 1936d.

Sigerist, Henry E.: *Socialized Medicine in the Soviet Union.* New York 1937.

Sigerist, Henry E.: *Science and Democracy.* Science and Society 2, 291–299, 1938.

Sigerist, Henry E.: *Kagan's Garrison.* Bull. Hist. Med. 7, 357–362, 1939.

Sigerist, Henry E.: *A Physician's Impression of South Africa.* Bull. Hist. Med. 8, 22–27, 1940.

Sigerist, Henry E.: *Medicine and Human Welfare.* New Haven 1941a.

Sigerist, Henry E.: *Medieval Medicine.* In "University of Pennsylvania Bicentennial Conference: Studies in the History of Science". Philadelphia 1941b.

Sigerist, Henry E.: *Four Treatises of Theophrastus von Hohenheim Called Paracelsus.* Baltimore 1941c.

Sigerist, Henry E.: *Civilization and Disease.* New York 1943.

Sigerist, Henry E.: *Review of Bernard J. Stern, "American Medical Practice in the Perspectives of a Century".* New York 1945. Am. J. Publ. Health 35, 654–655, 1945.

Sigerist, Henry E.: *The University at the Crossroads. Addresses and Essays.* New York 1946a.

Sigerist, Henry E.: *Translation of N. A. Semashko, "Friedrich Erismann, the Dawn of Russian Hygiene and Public Health."* Bull. Hist. Med. 20, 1–9, 1946b.

Sigerist, Henry E.: *Beginning a New Year.* Bull. Hist. Med. 19, 1–8, 1946c.

Sigerist, Henry E.: *A Fifteenth Century Surgeon: Hieronymus Brunschwig and his Work.* New York 1946d.

Sigerist, Henry E.: *Medicine and Health in the Soviet Union.* New York 1947.

Sigerist, Henry E.: *Medical History in the United States, Past, Present, Future; a Valedictory Address.* Bull. Hist. Med. 22, 47–64, 1948.

Sigerist, Henry E.: *Jean Rouelle, un médecin-naturaliste français aux Etats-Unis, au XVIIIe siècle.* Verh. Schweiz. Naturforsch. Ges. p. 210, 1949.

Sigerist, Henry E., ed.: *Letters of Jean de Carro to Alexandre Marcet, 1794–1817.* Baltimore 1950.

Sigerist, Henry E.: *A History of Medicine. Volume I: Primitive and Archaic Medicine.* New York 1951.

Sigerist, Henry E.: *The Autonomy of the History of Medicine and its Place in the University.* Acta med. Scand., Suppl. 266, 109–113, 1952.

Sigerist, Henry E.: *Erinnerungen an Karl Sudhoff.* Sudhoffs Arch. Gesch. Med. 37, 97–103, 1953.

Sigerist, Henry E.: *Preface* to J.J. Izquierdo: "Montaña y los origenes del movimiento social y cientifico de México". México 1955a.

Sigerist, Henry E.: *Como and the Plinii.* Bull. Cleveland med. Libr., New Series, 2: 53–58, 1955b.

Sigerist, Henry E.: *Thoughts on the physician's Writing and Reading.* Int. Rec.Med. 168, 609–615, 1955c.

Sigerist, Henry E.: *Landmarks in the History of Hygiene.* London etc. 1956a.

Sigerist, Henry E.: *Review* of "E. H. Ackerknecht: A Short History of Medicine" (New York 1955). Bull. Hist. Med. 30, 278–279, 1956b.

Sigerist, Henry E.: *Erinnerungen an meine Leipziger Tätigkeit.* Wiss. Z. Karl-Marx-Univ. Leipzig, Math.-Naturw. Reihe 5, 17–21, 1955/1956c.

Sigerist, Henry E.: *The Latin Medical Literature of the Early Middle Ages.* J. Hist. Med. Allied Sci. 13, 127–146, 1958.

Sigerist, Henry E.: *A History of Medicine*. Volume II: *Early Greek, Hindu, and Persian Medicine*. New York 1961.

Sigerist, Henry E. / Miller, Genevieve: *Welcome to the Journal of the History of Medicine and Allied Sciences*. Bull. Hist. Med. 19, 115–117, 1946.

Simmons, Leo W.: *The Role of the Ages in Primitive Society*. Harden, CT 1945.

Simpson, William J.: *Treatise on Plague*. Cambridge 1905.

Singer, Charles / Rabin, C.: *Prelude to Modern Science*. Cambridge 1946.

Singer, Charles / Sigerist, Henry E.: *Essays on the History of Medicine Presented to Karl Sudhoff on the Occasion of his Seventieth Birthday November 26th 1923*. London / Zurich 1924.

Smith, William Gardner: *The Last of the Conquerors*. New York 1948.

Snapper, Isidore: *Meditations on Medicine and Medical Education; Past and Present*. New York 1956.

Stern, Bernard J.: *Society and Medical Progress*. Princeton 1941.

Strömberg, Reinhold: *Griechische Wortstudien*. Göteborg 1944.

Temkin, Owsei: *The Falling Sickness. A History of Epilepsy from the Greeks to the Beginning of Modern Neurology*. Baltimore 1945.

Temkin, Owsei: *In Memoriam: Erwin H. Ackerknecht (1906–1988)*. Bull. Hist. Med. 63, 273–275, 1989.

Valentin, Veit: *Die Geschichte der deutschen Revolution von 1848–1849*. Berlin 1930–1931.

Walser, Hans H.: *Publikationen von Prof. Dr. med. Erwin H. Ackerknecht*. Gesnerus (Swiss J. of the Hist. of Med. and Sci.) 23, 5–12, 1966; 33, 3–7, 1976; 43, 6–10, 1986; 45, 311–312, 1988.

Walser Hans H.: *Zum Hinschied von Erwin H. Ackerknecht*. Gesnerus 45, 309–310, 1988.

Walser, Hans H.: *Zum 10. Todestag von Erwin H. Ackerknecht (1906–1988)*. Gesnerus 55, 176–182, 1998.

Waugh, Evelyn: *The Loved One*. London 1967.

Whitehead, Alfred N.: *Science and the Modern World*. New York 1947.

4.4. Name Index